How to
Sleep Better!

Other books available include:

Motivation, Achievement & Challenges

Understanding & Building Confidence

Managing Stress & Preventing Depression

The Real Benefits of Exercise

Weight Loss & Healthy Eating

Please make a donation if you can

TEXT: BOOK32£5

To: **70070**

Or an online donation via:

www.justgiving.com/healthbooks

www.cymhealth.org

THANK YOU!

How to
Sleep Better!

by

Charlie Wardle

Climb Your Mountain

Copyright © Charlie Wardle 2015

The right of Charlie Wardle to be identified as the author of this work has been asserted in accordance with the Copyright, Designs & Patents Act 1988.

All rights reserved. No part of this book may be reproduced, stored in a retrieval system, or transmitted in any form or by any means, electronic, electrostatic, magnetic tape, mechanical, photocopying, recording or otherwise, without the written permission of the copyright holder.

Published under licence by Brown Dog Books and

The Self Publishing Partnership

7 Green Park Station, Bath BA1 1JB

www.selfpublishingpartnership.co.uk

ISBN book: 978-1-903056-99-8

ISBN e-book: 978-1-78545-000-6

Cover design by Kevin Rylands

Printed and bound by CPI Group (UK) Ltd, Croydon CR0 4YY

Contents

About the author 8

Introduction 9
    Questionnaires 11
    The Sleep Council research overview 13

Part 1 – What Is Sleep and Why Is It Important? 15

- *Definition of sleep* 15
- *What happens to our body while we are sleeping?* 16
- *The different stages of sleep* 17
- *How much sleep do we need?* 19
- *Sleep patterns and body clock* 20
- *General effects and benefits of good sleep* 22
- *General effects and problems of insufficient sleep* 23
- *Sleep debt* 23
- *The best performers get more sleep* 24
- *What is melatonin?* 25
- *Hormones* 26
- *Dreaming* 27
- *Children's sleep* 29

Part 2 – Why Don't We Sleep Enough? 31

- *Temporary or chronic sleep problems* 31
- *Twenty-first-century lifestyle* 32
- *Anxiety* 32
- *Specific worry issue* 33
- *Stress* 34

- Depression 34
- Insomnia 35
- Narcolepsy 37
- Snoring 38
- Sleep apnoea 39
- Nightmares 39
- Sleepwalking and sleep talking 40
- Teeth grinding 41
- Delayed Sleep Phase Disorder 41
- Restless Legs Syndrome 42
- Fibromyalgia 43
- Weight issues 44
- Physical pain and injuries 44
- Bed, mattress, pillows and sheets 45
- Food and drink 45
- Noise 46
- Temperature 46
- Light 47
- Pets 48
- Stimulants 48
- Lack of routine 48
- Jet lag 49
- Not tired 49
- Children 50
- Partner 50
- Shift work 51
- Habit and expectations 51

Part 3 – What Can We Do to Sleep Better? 53

- Invest in better sleep 53
- Stop struggling 54
- Reduce anxiety 55

- Rationalise the worry issue   56
- CBT   56
- Relax and wind down   57
- Specific sleep exercises   58
- Your bedroom   59
- Air quality   60
- Write things down   60
- Write a sleep diary   61
- Sleep-inducing scents   61
- Visualise feeling sleepy   62
- Refocus on something else   62
- Solutions not problems   63
- Consult a doctor   64
- Medication   64
- Herbal remedies   65
- Napping   66
- Bed, mattress, duvets and sheets   67
- Temperature   67
- Light   68
- Exercise and be active   69
- Food and drink   70
- The last hour   71
- Sleep positions   71
- Sounds and white noise   72
- Snooze button   73
- Sleep apps   73
- Traditional sleep monitoring   74

Summary and Moving Forward   75

About the 'Climb Your Mountain' Charity   77

About the author

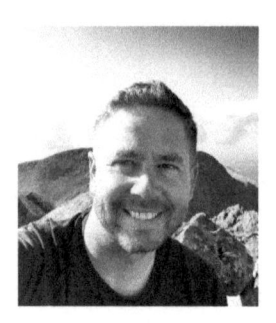

Charlie Wardle founded the Climb Your Mountain (CYM) charity in 2008 with the objective of helping as many people as possible to climb the personal mountain which they may face in their life for whatever reason. CYM provides a wide range of both educational and physical activity opportunities, so that people can help themselves to a healthier and happier life. Previously, Charlie had a successful finance, accounting and marketing career with a number of large blue-chip companies. He is a qualified Chartered Accountant (ACA) and has an MBA from Cranfield School of Management. His passion is health, wellbeing and fitness.

The education and learning side, called CYM Health, offers a range of free health and wellbeing books, courses, workshops, videos, talks and advice which are written, delivered and presented by Charlie. He has spent the last few years researching, reading, thinking, discussing and meeting with hundreds of people in order to build up the knowledge and experience that is then offered to others.

Please read the section at the end of this book to find out more about the Climb Your Mountain (CYM) charity and also please visit the website www.climbyourmountain.org for an online video workshop focusing on this book. Plus make sure you read the other health and wellbeing books in this series.

Introduction

'The best way to see what tomorrow brings is to sleep through the night.'

We spend around 30% of our lives asleep although, as we will see, many people would like that figure to be higher! Sleep is an essential and involuntary process, without which we cannot function effectively. It is as important to our body as eating, drinking and breathing, and is vital for maintaining good mental and physical health. Sleeping helps to repair and restore our brain as well as our body.

During sleep we can process information, consolidate memories, and undergo a number of maintenance processes that help us to function during the daytime. Sleep is crucial to the health of individuals and to the public health of the UK population. We all need to make sure we get the right amount of sleep, and enough good-quality sleep. There is no set amount of sleep that is appropriate for everyone; some people need more sleep than others.

Our ability to sleep is controlled by how sleepy we feel and our sleep pattern. How sleepy we feel relates to our drive to sleep. The sleep pattern relates to the regularity and timing of our sleep habits; if we have got into a pattern of sleeping at set times then we will be able to establish a better routine, and will find it easier to sleep at that time every day. Sleep is a more complex process than many people realise, much of it still a mystery to scientists. During sleep, the body goes through a variety of processes and sleep stages. Good-quality sleep is likely to be the result of spending enough time in all of the stages, including enough deep sleep, which helps us feel refreshed.

Poor sleep over a sustained period leads to a number of problems that are immediately recognisable, including fatigue, sleepiness, poor concentration, lapses in memory, and irritability. Up to one third of the population may suffer from insomnia (lack of sleep, or poor-quality sleep). This can affect mood, energy and concentration levels, our relationships, and our ability to stay awake and function during the day.

Sleep and health are strongly related; poor sleep can increase the risk of having poor health, and poor health can make it harder to sleep. Common mental health problems like anxiety and depression can often underpin sleep problems. Where this is the case, a combination approach to treating the mental health problem and sleep problem in tandem is often the most effective. It is essential for us to better understand the sleep process in order to ensure that we get a regular amount of good-quality sleep.

We can all benefit from improving the quality of our sleep. For many of us, it may simply be a case of making small lifestyle or attitude adjustments in order to help us sleep better. For those with insomnia it is usually necessary to seek more specialist treatment. Sleep medication is commonly used, but may have negative side effects and is not recommended in the long term. Psychological approaches are useful for those with long-term insomnia because they can encourage us to establish good sleep patterns, and to develop a healthy, positive mental outlook about sleep, as well as dealing with worrying thoughts about sleeping.

Introduction

Questionnaires

In preparation for writing this book I sent out a questionnaire to a mixed group of people, male and female, aged from 21 to 67 years old, with a few general questions around sleep. Below are the questions along with a selection of answers which seem reflective of the general population. Take a look and see if any of these answers resonate with yourself.

How do you feel after a good night's sleep?

- *Amazing! I can cope with anything and feel motivated to do as much as I can.*

- *Happier, more energetic, perform better.*

- *Energised & refreshed.*

- *Refreshed, clear mind, better mentally and physically.*

- *Energetic, confident, feeling of just wanting to get out there and do something. More decisive and spontaneous, able to think more quickly and react more appropriately to situations.*

- *Refreshed, bright-eyed, ready to take on new challenges or work hard.*

- *Energised, improved mood, happier, more alert, more confidence in tackling the day ahead and doing more and being more productive.*

How do you feel after a bad night's sleep?

- *It had a negative impact on everything I did. From the moment I got up in the morning, I'd be worrying about whether I would be able to sleep the following night and I was very bad-tempered.*

- *Tired, don't want to do much, not working effectively and efficiently.*

- Tiredness, irritability and a reduced ability to deal with everyday demands.

- Tired, irritable (more so than usual), restless, can't be bothered. Depressed/fed up.

- Grumpy, moody, short temper and attention span. Eyes get puffy, skin looks dull and I look much older which in turn depresses me and has the knock-on effect of a following night's bad sleep because I worry.

- I feel irritable, short-tempered and lack energy.

- Irritable, lethargic, more negative, easier to give up on things, the day becomes much harder.

What are the main reasons for poor sleep?

- Worries, stress, not happy with your life, can't switch off.

- For me, having young children and their lack of sleep can trigger long periods of sleep issues. My middle child didn't sleep through the night until he was 5. Stressful periods of important meetings at work would sometimes mean that I did not sleep at all.

- My husband also snores quite heavily, but I've never been sure if the snoring annoys me or the fact that he's asleep and I'm not does!

- An overactive brain and unnecessary worries about issues.

- Worrying about something, having too much on your mind, being stressed and/or depressed.

- Can't switch off, my mind just thinks of random things i.e. the logic of time and space, how we could possibly logically exist, is sleeping the real world and we live in unconsciousness etc., worry about money, health and work.

- Worrying and thinking about specific issues, being too hot, needing the toilet, knowing I have to get up earlier than usual.

Introduction

Sleep Council research overview

The UK Sleep Council's research reveals that the average Briton goes to bed at 11.15pm and gets just six hours and 35 minutes sleep per night. Men tend to sleep better than women, and high earners sleep best of all, while those on low incomes are most likely to struggle to get the rest they need. While many of us still believe that we need to sleep for eight hours per night, this research indicates that the majority of Britons don't manage to do so: and as many as a third regularly get a worrying less than six hours per night. Although 38% of respondents believe that spending more time in bed – either by going to bed earlier or getting up later – would improve our sleep, more than one in five (21%) think that buying a new bed would have the most positive impact on sleep quality. With this in mind, it's clear that buying a good new bed is a worthwhile investment.

The Sleep Council's research indicates that the average cost of a new bed is £583.05 (or 21p per night over seven years). Given that we spend a third of our lives in bed and that sleep issues are such a common problem, it's staggering that people invest so little in buying a decent bed. Are we really only prepared to pay the equivalent of one fresh egg for our sleep each night? Worryingly, there are several more self-help measures that can help to improve sleep quality, but taking medication (17%) and drinking alcohol (16%) are among the most popular methods that people use to help them drop off. What's more, Britons would rather treat themselves with an over-the-counter remedy (14%) than consult their GP (10%).

It doesn't help that many Britons have poor 'sleep hygiene', particularly with regard to watching television (38%), checking their emails (14%) or using their laptop/tablet (12%) in bed. All of these electrical devices emit bright light which can disrupt the production of the body's natural sleep hormones. What's clear is that one of the best ways to improve sleep is simply to take more exercise. Almost a third of people who exercise daily say that they sleep very well most nights, while those who exercise 5–6 times per week are the least likely to take medication to help them sleep (12%). Exercise also has the added bonus of helping to reduce stress, which is significant given that worry or stress keeps almost half of Britons (47%) awake at night.

So although almost a third of respondents (31%) believe that there is nothing that would improve their sleep, this new research indicates that, in actual fact, we really can help ourselves to sleep better, provided that we are willing to change our habits and make it a top priority to get a good night's sleep.

For more information visit www.sleepcouncil.org.uk

Part 1

What Is Sleep and Why Is It Important?

Definition of sleep

Below are a couple of formal definitions of sleep; however, they don't really go anywhere near describing, detailing and understanding the importance of regular, high-quality, restorative sleep in maintaining good health and vitality for both the human body and mind.

> *'A condition of body and mind which typically recurs for several hours every night, in which the nervous system is inactive, the eyes closed, the postural muscles relaxed and consciousness practically suspended.'*

> *'A natural, regularly recurring condition of rest for the body and mind, during which the eyes are usually closed and there is little or no conscious thought or voluntary movement.'*

Sleep is often seen as time when the body is inactive. In fact, the opposite is true. Sleep is an active, essential and involuntary process, without which we cannot function effectively. Sleep is not a lifestyle choice; just like breathing, eating or drinking, it is a necessity. Sleep is a complex process during which our body undertakes a number of essential activities. It involves low awareness of the outside world, relaxed muscles, and a raised anabolic state that helps us to build and repair our bodies.

Primarily, sleep is for the brain, allowing it to recover and regenerate. During our sleep, the brain can process information, consolidate memory, and enable us to learn and function effectively during daytime. This is why we are encouraged to get a good night's sleep in the run-up to a job interview or exam rather than staying awake all night to prepare. Whilst we sleep, our brain is not only strengthening memories but it is also reorganising them, picking out the emotional details and helping us produce new insights and creative ideas. Sleep affects our ability to use language, sustain attention, understand what we are reading and summarise what we are hearing.

If we compromise on our sleep, we compromise on our performance, our energy, our mood and our interpersonal relationships. Sleep has also been shown to protect the immune system. Animals have evolved to sleep in many different ways. Dolphins can sleep using only one half of their brain at a time. Even hibernating animals have been shown to cease hibernation temporarily, go to sleep (a different, active process), then return to hibernation. Sleep is an inconvenient, time-consuming process, but it is so essential that we have simply evolved to fit it into our lives.

> 'A good laugh and a long sleep are the best cures in the doctor's book.' – Irish Proverb

What happens to our body while we are sleeping?

A good way of looking at what happens when we sleep is that we are charging up our batteries, and without sleep our own batteries lose power and eventually go dead. Sleep is extremely important to both our body and our mind and it is the time the brain directs the body to heal and repair itself, rebuild damaged or worn-out tissues and restore chemical balance.

When you are awake your body burns oxygen and food to provide the energy needed and this is known as a 'catabolic state', where more energy is spent than conserved, thus using up the body's resources. Stimulating hormones such as adrenaline and natural cortisteroids are very active in this state, but as we sleep we move into an anabolic state in which energy conservation, repair and growth take over.

Your immune system becomes active, producing more proteins and natural killer cells to fight off infections and fight disease while your pituitary gland produces human growth hormone. The growth hormone is much more active while we sleep than when we are awake; it promotes growth in children and is essential for maintaining, repairing and renewing muscles, tissues and bones in adults.

The top layer of our skin is made of closely packed dead cells that are shed constantly throughout the day, but during deep sleep the skin's metabolic rate increases and as a result our skin is repaired and improves. So deep sleep can be considered to be 'beauty' sleep and this cannot be compensated for with daytime sleep because the energy needed for tissue repair is not available during daylight, as the body is using this elsewhere.

> **The average Briton goes to bed at 11.15pm and only gets 6 hours 35 minutes of sleep per night.**

The different stages of sleep

Deep sleep is a very refreshing type of sleep, and it is particularly important in helping the brain consolidate what it has learnt during the day. If awakened during these stages, sleepers report feeling groggy and disoriented for several minutes. Eventually, the sleeper will pass into REM (Rapid Eye Movement) sleep. This takes its name from the rapid eye movements that the sleeper displays, usually with their eyes closed, as discovered in 1953 by Nathaniel Kleitman and Eugene Aserinsky.

The frequency of one's rapid eye movements is known as their REM density. During this stage, the brainwaves are similar to those when we are resting, although our breathing rate and blood pressure rise, all our voluntary muscles also become paralysed and our muscle tone becomes relaxed so that we cannot move our limbs. This is a relatively shallow stage of sleep; the average person will have around three to five episodes of REM sleep per night, and the first period is likely to begin about 70–90 minutes after falling asleep. It is during this stage of sleep that we experience dreams. The amount of time spent in the different sleep stages appears to relate to people's mental health. Those who suffer from depression have been shown to have more REM sleep, enter this stage earlier, and have increased REM density. People who suffer from anxiety may spend less time in deep sleep.

Looking at our sleep in more detail, we will typically pass through four stages of non-REM sleep before beginning REM sleep. In total, non-REM sleep accounts for about 75–80% of total sleep in an average adult. This process is cyclical and during a single night we may experience four or five recurring cycles of non-REM and REM sleep each lasting 90–110 minutes. Only recently have scientists begun to understand the process, especially since sleep research has been aided by three measurements:

- Brainwave activity using an electroencephalogram (EEG), which measures electrical activity in the brain.
- Muscle tone through an electromyogram (EMG).
- Movement of the eye via an electro-oculogram (EOG).

Of these three, the EEG is the most important in helping to differentiate between the different sleep stages. While awake, our brain displays a pattern of brainwaves known as beta waves. Beta waves are high in frequency, meaning they occur in quick succession, but they are low in amplitude, meaning they are quite small. Whilst we are awake these waves do not follow a consistent pattern. This makes sense because when we are awake our brain is often doing a number of different tasks, stimulating it in a variety of different ways. When we rest with our eyes closed, our brainwave activity slows down and becomes more synchronised; these brainwaves are known as alpha waves.

Non-REM stage one

The first of the five sleep stages is a form of light sleep, or non-REM stage one. This stage is essentially the bridge between being awake and sleep. Sleepers drift in and out of light sleep and can be awakened easily. During this stage, the person may begin to breathe more slowly and evenly, and the brain produces theta waves, which are smaller and lower in frequency than alpha waves. Muscle activity, measured by the EMG, shows a slowing down of movement and the sleeper may begin to twitch. These twitches are called 'hypnic' jerks and sometimes wake the sleeper, particularly if the jerk is accompanied by the sensation of falling. Since individuals may have some awareness of the world around them, it is in this stage of sleep that some people report out-of-body experiences.

Non-REM stage two and three

Within a few minutes, the sleeper may pass into another form of light sleep known as stage two of non- REM sleep. The sleeper's breathing pattern and heart rate slow down and they become less aware of the outside world. Eye movement stops and sleepers' theta waves become even slower, with the occasional burst of brain activity every minute or so; these bursts of activity are sometimes known as 'sleep spindles'. Stage two non-REM sleep is also characterised by a type of brainwave activity known as a K-complex. A K-complex is a high voltage of EEG activity with a sharp downward spike followed by a slower upward component. This stage accounts for the largest part of human sleep (45–50% of sleep in adults) and is sometimes referred to as true sleep. Like stage one sleep, stage two is also considered relatively 'light' sleep and if sleepers were to be woken up during either of these stages they might deny that they had been asleep at all.

Non-REM stages three and four

Stages three and four are typically grouped together as the last stages of non-REM sleep, also referred to as 'synchronised sleep'. For these stages, sleepers pass from the theta waves of stages one and two to delta waves, the largest and slowest brain waves. There is no real distinction between stage three and four, except typically during stage three, sleep is comprised of fewer than 50% delta waves, and in stage four more than 50% of the waves are delta waves. Thus these stages are often referred to as slow-wave sleep or deep sleep. Sleepers' breathing and heart rate are at their lowest levels, they breathe rhythmically and their muscle activity decreases.

How much sleep do we need?

The general consensus is that on average we need about 8 hours sleep per night and a minimum of 7 hours good-quality sleep for optimum health. However, like with most things, everyone is different and the range of 'how much sleep we need' varies considerably from person to person. Some people are seemingly able to function perfectly well and healthily on less than 6 hours sleep and others seemingly require up to 10 hours per night.

In addition, the quality of sleep is of vital importance and is generally more important than the quantity. Understanding more about your own sleep habits, patterns, quantity and quality will help improve your sleep and therefore your health. You may well be able to live your life on less sleep than is optimal but you will be less productive, less efficient, less effective and will not be performing anywhere near your potential. Do not underestimate the power of good sleep and the health benefits it can bring, as well as the damage poor sleep can do.

The amount of sleep a person needs does depend upon age, though. Newborn babies tend to sleep for an average of 16–18 hours per day, which decreases to about 13–14 hours after one year. Adolescents tend to require more sleep than adults, possibly due to the physiological changes that are happening in the body during this period. As people reach adulthood they tend to sleep 7–8 hours per day. Older adults tend to sleep roughly 6–7 hours per day, but take more frequent naps throughout the day.

Spend some time working out what your level of optimal sleep actually is and see this as an essential 'need' and not a 'hope' or 'desire'. Also, if you sleep with a partner, their optimal sleep levels may differ, which can cause issues. Think about how you feel when you have had a great night's sleep and how long that was for, and put the required effort and focus into endeavouring to achieve this on a regular basis. If you can, then you will definitely see improvements in your overall physical, mental and emotional health.

70% of people in the UK sleep for less than 7 hours per night on average.

Over 40% of people in the UK get less than 6 hours' sleep per night on average.

34% of people in the UK only get between 5 and 6 hours' sleep per night on average.

Sleep patterns and body clock

Equally important as the total amount of sleep is the pattern of sleep. Babies and small children tend to sleep multiple times across each 24-hour period, but as we mature into school years and into adulthood we tend to sleep in one long phase; daytime sleeping decreases and we tend instead to sleep throughout the night. A mechanism called the 'circadian timer' regulates the pattern of our sleep and waking. Most living things have internal circadian rhythms, meaning they are adapted to live in a cycle of day and night. The French geophysicist Jean-Jacques d'Ortous de Mairan was the first to discover circadian rhythms in an experiment with plants in 1729.

Two centuries later, Dr. Nathaniel Kleitman studied the effect of circadian rhythms on human sleep cycles. These rhythms respond primarily to light and darkness. The cycle is actually slightly longer than 24 hours. It is possible to think of a 'master clock' which regulates our circadian rhythms. This clock is made up of a group of nerve cells in our brain called the suprachiasmatic nucleus (SCN). The SCN controls the production of melatonin, which is a hormone that makes us feel sleepy. During sleep, melatonin levels rise sharply. The SCN is located just above our optic nerves, which send signals from the eyes to the brain. Therefore, the SCN receives information about the amount of light in the environment through our eyes. When there is less light, such as during night-time, it tells the brain to create more melatonin

Serotonin is another chemical that affects sleep; it is produced by the brain, with levels of serotonin being highest in the brain when we are awake and active. The brain produces more serotonin when it is lighter outside, which is why most people feel tired at night-time, and why it is a good idea to turn off the lights when we are trying to sleep. Insufficient levels of serotonin are also related to mental health problems such as depression and anxiety.

The immune system also influences serotonin, and therefore influences sleep patterns, which may explain why we need to sleep more if we are feeling ill. As humans are mainly daytime animals, the period during which we choose to sleep is determined naturally by the level of light in the environment, principally due to the setting and rising of the sun. But we can now manipulate light levels through the use of artificial lights, which means that we can continue activities long into the evenings. People who work night shifts may wish to reduce the level of light they are exposed to during the daytime in order to sleep, and can do this through the use of blackout curtains.

The story of the Copiapó mining accident in Chile in 2010 shows the importance of light for circadian rhythms. Miners' sleep–wake cycles were completely disrupted in the absence of sunlight. The National Aeronautics and Space Administration (NASA) consultants advised the miners to segregate their space into working, sleeping and recreation areas. They used the lights on their helmets and the headlights on the mining trucks to create a communal 'light' area. The sleeping area was kept dark, meaning that the miners could regulate the daylight cycle artificially and maintain a regular pattern of sleep. This is an extreme example, but in fact, even moderate changes in lighting can affect our internal circadian timers. Sleep patterns vary greatly; some animals are diurnal and tend to sleep during the night-time, and others are nocturnal and sleep mostly during the daytime.

Within humans, each person's circadian timer is set slightly differently; some people function best in the mornings (larks), others best in the evenings (owls), and many of us are somewhere in between. Some people suffer from what is known as circadian rhythm sleep disorder, which is an extreme end of this spectrum, but is often associated with mental health problems. An extreme 'owl' may have delayed sleep phase syndrome, tending to fall asleep and wake up very late. An extreme 'lark' may have advanced sleep phase syndrome, rising very early in the morning but plagued with sleepiness in the evening. These irregularities can become problems, depending upon what we are trying to do in life, although for some they can prove to be an asset. Similar effects are commonly seen in people whose sleep pattern is disrupted due to external factors, such as working regular night shifts (particularly after working regular day shifts in the weeks beforehand).

Another example is jet lag, which is caused by travel between different time zones. Both shift work sleep disorders and jet lag are very common expressions of circadian rhythm disorders. Humans are not designed to be awake during the night and asleep during the day. People who regularly work night shifts are thought to be at a greater risk of cancer and heart disease. International flight crews are also at elevated risk of cancer, possibly due to repeated disruption of circadian rhythms. Disruption of sleep and circadian rhythms is also documented in people who suffer from bipolar disorder, although it is unclear whether the circadian timer or sleep homeostat is responsible for the underlying sleep disturbances.

General effects and benefits of good sleep

> *'Sleep is the golden chain that ties health and our bodies together.'*
> *– Thomas Dekker*

There are numerous benefits to having good sleep on a regular basis, for our physical, mental and emotional health. Physically good sleep will allow our bodies to grow, repair, rebuild and maintain our cells, tissues, muscles and organs. Our immune systems will function much more effectively in fighting off illness and boosting our defences.

Mentally , good sleep will allow our brains to process and store information, improving our memory and making us more alert and able to concentrate and focus better. Emotionally, our moods will be elevated, we will have more enthusiasm and generally be much more positive in our approach to the day ahead.

As can be seen from the answers in the questionnaire section there are a range of clear and obvious benefits from a good night's sleep and continued good sleep. And if you have built up a period of good sleep then the occasional 'blip' will be much easier to handle and have less damaging effects on your health.

General effects and problems of insufficient sleep

There are many effects and potential effects of insufficient sleep or sleep deprivation. A lack of sleep can have serious effects on the brain's ability to function. With just one bad night's sleep you can feel groggy, grumpy, irritable and forgetful, as well as lethargic; you can struggle with concentration and your attention span shortens considerably, whilst your judgement can also be impaired. Additionally you may eat a worse diet or miss exercise and physical activity opportunities as a result, which further impacts on your health and wellbeing.

With prolonged period of poor sleep the issues will be worse. You will age more rapidly, be more susceptible to colds, flu, infections and other illnesses and be more susceptible to emotional problems like depression and anxiety. Furthermore, your risk of obesity, heart disease, diabetes and other serious conditions is increased and you will be more irritable, have worse judgement, lower concentration, make poor decisions and be more likely to cause an accident for yourself or others.

Driver sleepiness is the cause of around 20% of accidents on long journeys.

Sleep debt

'Sleep debt' is the commonly used term for the difference between how much you should ideally have slept and how much you actually did sleep, and this can then become cumulative over a number of days. So let's say you would ideally have 8 hours' sleep but only manage 6 hours then your sleep debt would be 2 hours. And then let's say this is repeated for the following three days, which would mean your cumulative sleep debt has risen to 8 hours.

If the pattern continues and your sleep debt increases, then the likelihood is that the effects will start to shift from short-term sleep deprivation symptoms to more concerning and dangerous longer-term sleep deprivation symptoms. These will potentially have quite a negative impact on your life in many ways as they affect you physically, mentally and emotionally.

So it is useful to be aware of your sleep debt amounts and really focus on reducing the debt. Think about how you 'owe' your body and mind sleep if you have fallen into debt and how it is possible to manage this debt, stop it increasing and put in plans to reduce it. Many people will be aware that they have sleep debt but perhaps do not realise the extent of it and how dangerous the build-up could potentially become.

Apart from detrimental symptoms like feeling tired, being sluggish, having poor concentration, being grumpy, lacking motivation, eating badly, ageing prematurely and many more, this cumulative sleep debt can cause serious accidents. For example, it is estimated at least 20% of car accidents are due to sleep debt, and many well-known disasters have been attributed to sleep deprivation, such as the Exxon Valdez ecological disaster; it is also thought to have played a major role in the Space Shuttle Challenger disaster. So it is not just your life that can be seriously affected by sleep debt and sleep deprivation.

'The worst thing in the world is to try and sleep and not to.' – F Scott Fitzgerald

The best performers get more sleep

One of the most influential studies of human performance, conducted by Professor K. Anders Ericsson and published in *The Psychological Review* found that elite performers needed 10,000 hours of deliberate practice to reach levels of greatness. It sparked a debate around natural talent versus countless hours of practice, but another element that came out of the study was to a large degree overlooked. His findings suggested that sleep was a further factor that significantly contributed towards success and peak performance. On average the best performers slept for 8 hours 36 minutes whilst the average person slept for only 6 hours 51 minutes.

So if you want to be successful, beat your competition and perform at the best of your abilities there is a strong correlation between this and the amount of sleep you get. There is also much to be said for increased productivity as a result of extra sleep. Rather than staying up late or waking up early so you get more work done, it is more likely that with extra sleep you will be far more productive, more focused and energised. So to get more done, try sleeping more!

What is melatonin?

Melatonin, a hormone produced in the brain's pineal gland, is responsible for the regulation of the body clock in each individual. Interestingly, the release of this hormone is largely controlled by exposure to natural light, or a lack thereof.

Melatonin production is first triggered in the evening, but the hormone continues to be released throughout the hours of darkness that follow (the conventional sleeping period). Levels of melatonin then drop with the breaking daylight and its production is suppressed until the next evening. Due to its dependence on a person being in a dark environment, melatonin is often referred to as the 'hormone of darkness'.

It is precisely this link between darkness and melatonin that informs advice to keep your bedroom dark and free from light-emitting electronics, as research has shown that both melatonin production and deep sleep phases are better maintained in the dark. The introduction of electric light in the nineteenth century is often described as having had a negative influence on sleep. Before we had light bulbs and lamps in our homes, our circadian rhythms were dictated by natural light. People would wake with the first light of day and retire to bed early in the evening as darkness fell.

The invention of artificial light, however, allowed people to make use of the evening after the sun went down. This change to our daily schedules is thought to have brought about changes in our sleep schedule, pushing our bedtime ever later. Electric lighting continues to impact on our sleep, not least because we are now able to work late into the evening and even throughout the night.

Some research has suggested that melatonin supplements taken ahead of bedtime can help speed up the process of falling asleep and even improve sleep quality. There are limitations to this research, however, as it has only been conducted over a short time period. Thus far, this has prevented reliable conclusions being drawn about melatonin as a long-term solution for persistent poor sleep.

Additionally, sleep is influenced by other factors than melatonin production and, as with many other prescription and over-the-counter sleep aids, the benefits of melatonin supplements do not persist once people stop taking them. In the UK and parts of Europe, melatonin is licensed for those over the age of 55 with chronic insomnia, for whom it has shown evidence of sleep improvement.

Melatonin supplements are a relatively recent addition to the sleep aids market, having only gained popularity over the past decade or so. Research has only just begun to scratch the surface of the potential effects of melatonin, both negative and positive. It remains a future challenge, therefore, to answer questions such as when to take melatonin for sleep, or which melatonin dosage is best.

Melatonin is often seen as a 'natural' product when compared to prescription sleeping pills, but this does not mean it escapes associated side effects. So far, reported side effects of melatonin have included dizziness and headaches, but long-term use of melatonin sleep aids has yet to be investigated.

Hormones

A hormone is a chemical released by a cell or gland in one part of the body that subsequently affects cells in another part of the body. In essence, hormones are chemical messengers, travelling in the bloodstream to tissues or organs. They are involved in many different bodily processes, including metabolism, growth and development, reproduction, sexual function and mood.

There is a close link between sleep and hormones. A clear demonstration of this is when women become pregnant. Pregnancy is associated with alterations to reproductive hormones, oestrogen and progesterone, which typically rise throughout pregnancy and peak at term. This increase may initially be associated with elevated sleepiness in the mother, often resulting in an increase in total sleep time and daytime napping. The distribution of sleep stages – deep sleep and REM sleep – may also be altered at this time. Developing physical changes in the latter stages of pregnancy (third trimester) have also been proposed as disturbing sleep in the majority of women. Similarly, during the menopause, sleep disturbance and insomnia symptoms are very common, and have been linked to decreased levels of oestrogen and associated hot flushes.

Specific sleep stages may also be related to certain hormonal releases. For example, it has been well documented that during deep sleep there is an increase in the release of human growth hormone, which stimulates cell reproduction and regeneration. Interestingly, a recent study by Lampl and Johnson (2011) found that infant growth spurts were associated with increased and more consolidated sleep, and the mechanism thought to explain this relates to increased deep (slow-wave) sleep and the associated increase in growth hormone.

Finally, sleep loss and sleep disturbance have also been shown to impact negatively on hormonal balance. For example, the appetite-suppressing hormone, leptin, has been found to be decreased after several nights of sleep restriction. Similarly, the appetite-stimulating hormone, ghrelin, has been found to be increased after sleep restriction. Alterations to these two hormones due to sleep loss may, therefore, encourage people to seek out extra calories!

Dreaming

Dreams have been a subject of awe and inspiration for thousands of years, appearing in the oldest works of literature, such as the *Epic of Gilgamesh* (c.2200 B.C.), as well as in recent Hollywood blockbusters such as *Inception* and *Shutter Island* (2010). Some people are better at remembering dreams than others and many people believe that dreams are a gateway to understanding our feelings, thoughts, behaviours, motives and values.

The theoretical link between dreaming and eye movements during sleep was made as far back as 1868, and the explicit connection between REM sleep and dreaming was made almost a century later. It is possible that our eyes move because we are following the images of the dream in our sleep. Since we all experience REM sleep, we all have the potential to experience dreams. Still, the purpose and function of dreams remains unclear.

There are many theories on the meaning of dreams. Some scientists believe they serve no real purpose, while others believe they are integral to our mental, emotional and physical wellbeing. The most well-known theory comes from the Austrian neurologist Sigmund Freud, who founded the school of psychoanalytic thought. According to Freud, dreams are subconscious wishes. He believed that the images, thoughts and emotions experienced in a dream were attempts by our unconscious to resolve a conflict in waking life, and that the process of dreaming allowed for an interaction between the unconscious and the conscious.

One theory is that the part of the brain involved in emotions, sensations and memories becomes more active during REM sleep, so the brain may attempt to make sense of this internal activity and the result is a dream. Dreams may therefore be the result of signals generated within our brains. Another theory suggests that dreams may help humans to maintain sleep by keeping the mind occupied, so that we don't wake up. It suggests that dreams may entertain the brain so that other areas can rest and recover, and without this kind of diversion the brain would keep telling us to wake up.

However, these are merely theories, and the exact reasons why we dream are still uncertain. What we do know is that dreams are associated with an abundance of a chemical called dopamine in the brain. Dopamine is a neurotransmitter (a chemical that transmits signals within the brain) that helps to direct our attention to important things in our environment. Both dreams and hallucinations involve deregulation of dopamine production.

It is thought that dreaming may be similar to some of the symptoms of schizophrenia, since they appear to have similar neurochemical backgrounds. Dreaming and REM sleep are also strongly related to major depression, and people who suffer from this illness often display more frequent rapid eye movements than normal – literally, people with depression dream more. It actually appears as though getting too much REM sleep can increase our vulnerability to depression.

Interestingly, many antidepressants aim to limit REM sleep. One night of sleep deprivation, particularly the deprivation of REM sleep, may relieve depressive symptoms in the short term. However, this cannot be recommended as a treatment for depression since individuals become susceptible to symptoms again once they have repaid their sleep debt. More importantly, the negative consequences of sleep deprivation can be far more damaging. A possible side effect of many antidepressants is an increase in vivid dreams and also nightmares.

'The future belongs to those who believe in the beauty of their dreams.'
– Eleanor Roosevelt

Children's sleep

Many children will also suffer from poor sleep, which can have many negative consequences and affect both the body and the mind. Good sleep is even more important for children in some ways as their bodies are developing and growing and sleep plays an essential role in this. Poor sleep can cause issues that mean potential growth and development will be compromised in all areas of the body, including muscles, bones and organs including the brain.

Sleep patterns are likely to vary considerably at different ages, with younger children more likely to go to bed early and wake up early, while teenagers are more likely to go to bed later and wake later. However, it is important to be aware of your children's sleep and chat to them about any problems, particularly if they are showing any signs or symptoms of poor sleep. Many children will experience anxiety, stress and depression, which can affect sleep or lead to other issues with school or friends.

Most children now have computer games, mobile phones, iPads, computers and other devices that they use in their bedrooms and can significantly impact on their sleep. Be aware of the potential dangers, as reports show that many children are sleeping less, with this type of technology issue being a major cause.

Another factor is lack of exercise and activity, which means that children are not tired enough to sleep well, even though they may feel tired. Compounding this problem is poor diet – and the number of overweight children is rising. Generally if you are overweight you will do less physical activity, feel more tired and continue to consume an unhealthy diet, which can lead to poor-quality sleep, which then continues this negative cycle.

Children who exercise and are more active will generally sleep better, so try to encourage this as well as providing and promoting healthy eating, because this will help to create a positive, healthy, more productive and happier cycle whereby children will sleep better, have more energy, be more productive and do more activity, to then sleep better and so on.

There are other issues that may apply, including having nightmares, being scared of the dark, wetting the bed, sharing a bedroom with siblings and general sleep hygiene.

Encourage your children to be open and talk about any sleep-related problems and make them aware of how important sleep is. Good-quality sleep will help them perform better at school, be more alert, have more energy, eat more healthily, do more physical activity and overall be happier, which of course is much better for the parents and will help them sleep well, too!

Part 2

Why Don't We Sleep Enough?

There are many reasons why so many people do not sleep well and do not get enough sleep for a productive, healthy and happy life. There is also a clear and growing trend that our sleep is getting worse and our average time asleep is reducing. In this section we look at a variety of factors that may contribute to this trend; it is recommended that you consider each of these in terms of your own personal situation and identify those areas that do or may apply to you.

Temporary or chronic sleep problems

There are effectively two different types of sleep problems, which can be described as either temporary or chronic. Temporary sleep problems, as the term suggests, are those that effect people on a temporary basis and for temporary reasons. For example, you may be going through a very difficult period at work with a lot of stress and issues to deal with, which then impacts on your sleep. Other factors such as not eating properly, not exercising, drinking too much coffee etc., may all add to the main problem of overthinking and anxiety related to the work issues. This type of sleep disturbance is essentially a temporary problem with fairly clear reasons; if addressed correctly it can be resolved fairly quickly and should only ever be a temporary problem.

A chronic sleep problem is defined as one which persists for a much longer period of time and could be due to a number of different factors or indeed one 'permanent' issue. There can be a wide range of 'permanent' problems and types of chronic sleep issues, but for the individual it is usually considered an ongoing battle rather than a temporary problem.

27% of people in the UK say they sleep poorly on a regular basis.

Twenty-first-century lifestyle

Particularly as technology continues to evolve we have at our disposal more and more gadgets that we use in our everyday lives. Many of these are beneficial and helpful and can add to our quality of life in terms of communication, information and entertainment. However, there are also downsides, which include the effect this modern twenty-first-century lifestyle has on our sleep.

For example, having access to and using our smartphones or tablets at night-time can be detrimental to our sleep both in terms of the light and its effect on our eyes and melatonin levels and also the fact that our minds don't switch off easily when using these devices. In addition, we can be woken up by texts and calls etc. during the night if they are left on.

Also, throughout the day we are exposed to so much communication stimulation in the way of texts, emails, social media etc. and are constantly having to make decisions, meet deadlines, think about events, respond to questions, etc., that it can be difficult to switch off and properly relax. So much stimulation and our resulting fast-paced lives undoubtedly impact on our sleep, and unless these factors are addressed it is likely to get even worse.

> *'Some people don't sleep because they have insomnia. I can't sleep because I have internet connection!'*

Anxiety

Many people struggle with general anxiety issues that are often a result of their own insecurities and this can lead to several problems, including sleep-related issues. If you are anxious, you tend to worry about many things and overthink a lot of situations, circumstances and events, which can be past, present or future. This general worry and overthinking is usually negative and non-productive, leading to further concerns and increased overthinking. It can become a vicious cycle and one that is hard to break out of.

The more insecure you are, the more likely you are to worry, overthink and suffer with general anxiety, and these insecurities can continue to build, which will only make the situation worse. Such insecurities could be a result of many factors over a long period of time and can often be traced back to childhood or particular events from the past. If they are not understood, worked on and addressed then the problems are likely to remain or get worse, and if this then affects sleep it will in turn potentially lead to further worries and issues.

If you then become worried about not sleeping, anxious that you are not sleeping enough, or go to bed concerned that you will not sleep, then it is likely you will indeed have a poor night's sleep. Then if you are tired as a result you will tend to be in a more negative state of mind, which will only add to the general anxiety.

Millions of people in the UK have anxiety issues of this nature that become part of such a vicious circle and therefore difficult to escape from. You may be unable to switch off the worry button in your head, then chastise yourself for worrying, then think about the effects of not sleeping because of the anxiety. It keeps you awake most nights because you can't switch off and it becomes more of an expectation or a habit, compounding the issue even more.

'Dear Mind, please stop thinking so much at night. I need sleep!'

Specific worry issue

Although millions of people will suffer with general anxiety, the majority of people will not, and therefore this factor isn't of too much concern for them. However, pretty much everybody from time to time will have a specific worry issue. It could be anything, for any reason and at any time. Perhaps it is a work-related issue, a relationship problem, a financial concern or a health worry.

If you go to bed and you have a specific worry issue then it can often be very difficult to remove this, ignore it or think of something more positive. You can find yourself restless, unable to think about anything else and, of course, getting a bad night's sleep. Nearly everyone can relate to this and it can be incredibly frustrating because you know you shouldn't be thinking about it and you know that it will impact on your sleep, yet no matter how hard you try you cannot help but worry about the issue.

It may be for only one night, which hopefully won't be too damaging or cause too many knock-on issues, but sometimes the specific worry issue will go on for days or even weeks. Then there are much more damaging consequential effects. Apart from the direct lack of sleep you may become, for example, grouchier, even more lethargic, short-tempered, your diet may get worse, you may stop exercising or you may become physically ill. None of these will help with your sleep and before you know it the sleep issue has become more of a problem than the initial specific worry issue.

Stress

Stress can take many forms and will affect people in different ways, but similarly to anxiety and specific worry issues, stress will often be a primary factor in poor sleep. Not being able to switch off, thinking about all the responsibilities, pressures, expectations, work demands, family demands, health issues, money worries, etc., which can all cause stress, means that your sleep and quality of sleep will be put at risk.

A build-up of stress can have physical, mental and emotional effects and because it usually builds up over time you may not be as aware of the consequences that result from stress compared with other factors.

> **54% of women and 40% of men say stress and worry keep them awake at night, causing sleep issues.**

Depression

There are several types of depression and a wide range of levels of the illness, but one of the common symptoms of depression in general is poor sleep. Typically if you are depressed then you will have more worries, more anxiety and more stress than would be considered normal, but there are other factors that also can contribute to poor sleep.

And poor sleep can then become part of a vicious negative circle where the more tired you are combined with the less time your body has to re-energise and recover means the depression is likely to worsen and sleep becomes even more of an issue. In addition, the quality of sleep can be affected by depression, so even if you stay in bed longer you may not be sleeping well and often in these periods the thinking time is negative and the worries are compounded. So poor sleep can affect depression and depression can affect sleep.

Many people take antidepressants and some of these can directly affect their sleep. For example, effectively slowing the body and mind down to help with some of the effects of depression can make the body yearn for more sleep. So if you are unsure, discuss with your doctor the potential side effects that could impact on your sleep.

Insomnia

'A sleepless night is as long as a year.' – Chinese proverb

Most of us have experienced a sleepless night, which, although upsetting, is nothing to worry about since the sleep debt can be repaid over the course of the next few nights. The inability to fall or remain asleep over a period of several nights is known as insomnia. People with insomnia have poor-quality sleep, may be unable to get enough sleep, and may wake up for long periods during the night, resulting in fatigue during the daytime.

Insomnia is a psychophysiological disorder, which means that it is a combination of our thoughts, behaviour, emotions and physiology. Insomnia can be acute (lasting less than a month), or it may develop into a chronic, long-term condition. Essentially, insomnia is associated with arousal of our mind and body. Typically people complain of a racing mind and get into a vicious cycle of poor sleep, concerns about poor sleep, and patterns of thoughts and behaviour that are unhelpful. This means that the normal operation of the sleep debt and circadian mechanisms is interrupted. The result of a series of sleepless nights can be serious. Insomnia is by far the most common sleep complaint in the general population.

Sleep quality is of paramount importance to our health. People who have slept poorly are likely to suffer from fatigue, sleepiness during daytime, poor concentration, irritability, memory loss, depression, frustration and a weakened immune system. Fatigue – feeling weary and lacking in energy whilst awake – is the most common problem associated with poor sleep. This is different to sleepiness because it doesn't necessarily increase the likelihood of falling asleep. Signs of sleepiness include yawning, muscle ache and drifting off to sleep. Furthermore, poor sleep can make us less receptive to positive emotions, which in turn can make us feel miserable during the day, and may increase the likelihood of us developing depression.

Evidence from experiments involving rats suggests that in extreme cases sleep deprivation may even be fatal. Indeed, there is an extremely rare genetic disorder called fatal familial insomnia, affecting around 100 people worldwide. This usually begins between the ages of 35 and 60, and leads to death several months later. Poor sleep can also affect the circadian timing mechanism. Keeping an irregular sleep pattern can make insomnia worse. People who suffer from insomnia are likely to feel the effects of sleep deprivation throughout the daytime. It may be tempting to catch up on sleep by 'grazing' at opportune moments across the day, but even though this temporarily recoups a small amount of sleep debt, unfortunately it also disrupts the sleep pattern.

A person with insomnia may get into a habit of sleeping in short shifts throughout the day, which may then make it difficult for them to sleep at bedtime. The problem with napping like this is that the person only sleeps for short periods of time. This means that they are likely to get lots of light sleep without ever passing through all the sleep stages; in particular, they fail to achieve the essential deep sleep necessary for restoration of mind and body, and fail to recover their sleep debt. Sometimes insomnia can be related to physical health problems. Most of us will have experienced an illness that has made it harder to sleep because of physical discomfort or irritation, such as a blocked nose or sore throat.

Our mental state is perhaps even more important in allowing or preventing insomnia from developing from an acute into a chronic problem. This refers particularly to our thoughts and attitudes about sleeping. For example, some of us, after suffering several consecutive sleepless nights, may become anxious that we have not had enough sleep. This type of thought process is likely to lead to thinking about the problems associated with not sleeping. This can lead to anxious thoughts, which can then lead a person to see themselves as failing to sleep well. These thoughts perpetuate a negative cycle, making it even more difficult for the person to sleep. Many of us may recognise this behaviour if we have watched the clock during the night. This is a very common activity for people who suffer from insomnia, where the clock starts to be used as a gauge to monitor sleep performance. This pressure to perform in turn makes it more difficult to sleep.

Sleeping poorly increases the risk of poor mental health, which is often neglected when aiming to improve health and wellbeing. Insomnia is inextricably related to mental health. Many of us will have experienced a sleepless night through worrying about an upcoming event, such as an exam or a job interview. A prolonged period of stress or worry can also seriously affect our ability to sleep. In a sample of roughly 20,000 young adults, lack of sufficient sleep was linked to psychological distress, and a history of insomnia has been shown to increase the risk of developing depression. Unsurprisingly, anxiety and depression are also common causes of chronic insomnia.

People who suffer from depression may experience sleep disturbances which disrupt the process of falling and staying asleep. The sleeper may wake intermittently throughout the night, or wake early in the morning and be unable to sleep again. Furthermore, insomnia is a common complaint in people who suffer from schizophrenia, and some schizophrenia medications can profoundly affect a person's ability to maintain constant sleep. People visiting sleep disorder clinics with the complaint of insomnia often have another underlying mental health problem. This type of insomnia is more difficult to treat since it involves treating the underlying problem as well as the insomnia.

Narcolepsy

Narcolepsy is a chronic, neurological sleep disorder that causes excessive daytime sleepiness and inhibits a person's ability to control their sleep and wake cycles. People with narcolepsy repeatedly become drowsy during the day and can find themselves falling asleep, often in inappropriate places and at inappropriate times, without much ability to control it. These unplanned sleep episodes are often known as sleep attacks and can last for just a few seconds up to several minutes.

The actual cause of narcolepsy is still unknown, but research suggests that it may be due to a deficiency in the brain's production of a chemical called hypocretin. It is generally a lifelong condition that is not curable and of course can have a major impact on a sufferer's life. However, it is important that narcolepsy is not misconstrued as insomnia because of the extreme tiredness, as they are two very different conditions and the treatment and management of each should be considered separately.

Cataplexy is also common in people with narcolepsy, often brought on by emotion such as laughter. Cataplexy is defined by a sudden loss of muscle tone, which can often leave the sufferer paralysed for a short term and can clearly be a significant issue.

Snoring

> *'Laugh and the world laughs with you. Snore and you sleep alone!'*
> – Anthony Burgess

Of all sleep problems, snoring may seem one of the more innocuous. However, it can cause problems for the partners of snorers, whose own sleep quality may be affected. Strictly speaking, snoring is a respiratory problem heightened when a person is sleeping, not a sleep problem in itself. Snoring is very common; approximately 37% of UK adults snore. It is twice as common in males as females, although post-menopausal women are more likely to snore than pre-menopausal women. Partners may find their own sleep disturbed and may need to sleep in separate rooms.

There is a suggestion that after snorers undergo surgery to stop snoring, the sleep quality of their partners improves. The snoring sound is produced through a partial obstruction in the airway, within which the organs that help us to breathe vibrate. The muscles relax at the base of the tongue and the uvula (the small fleshy piece which hangs at the back of the throat). The relaxation of muscle tone can cause the airway (composed of nose, throat, mouth and windpipe) to become partially or completely obstructed. Other possible causes that can restrict airflow can be jaw problems or nasal congestion.

A person's size and body shape can also have an impact on whether they are likely to snore. For instance, people with shorter, wider necks are more inclined to snore because the muscles around their windpipe cannot support the tissue that surrounds it when they sleep. Alcohol also increases snoring, since it relaxes the tissue at the back of the throat, causing it to collapse into the airway and vibrate more easily. There are a number of treatments for snoring, most of which rely on unblocking the breathing passage, such as nasal strips and sprays. Still, if snoring becomes a problem, it is better to seek professional medical advice first.

37% of people in the UK snore, and twice as many men as women.

Sleep apnoea

Snoring during REM sleep is often a sign of obstructive sleep apnoea, a potentially serious respiratory problem. While sleeping, an individual will experience pauses in breathing or shallow breath. Sufferers may stop breathing for up to minutes at a time, potentially starving the brain of oxygen. Normal breathing usually resumes, with the individual often making a loud snort or choking sound, causing the airway to unblock, waking the individual up and disrupting their sleep. Obstructive sleep apnoea occurs in approximately 3–7% of adult men and 2–5% of adult women. It is more common in older people and in those who are overweight.

Both smoking and alcohol also increase the risk of developing it. Sufferers may find themselves waking up sweaty, with a dry mouth and a headache. The frequent waking throughout the night can lead to insomnia, excessive fatigue and sleepiness during the daytime. Undiagnosed obstructive sleep apnoea is associated with increased likelihood of hypertension, cardiovascular disease, stroke, sleepiness during the daytime, and motor vehicle accidents. The most widely used treatment for obstructive sleep apnoea is positive airway pressure. The sleeper wears a special mask over the nose or mouth during sleep, whilst a breathing machine pumps a stream of air into the nose or mouth through the mask.

Nightmares

Many of us will have experienced a nightmare from time to time. This is defined as an intense, frightening dream that wakes the sleeper in the throes of panic. Usually nightmares occur in the early morning and often they are influenced by frightening experiences that have occurred during the day. Recurrent nightmares are said typically to occur as a result of anxiety. People who suffer from post-traumatic stress disorder (PTSD) can experience distressing dreams or nightmares as a consequence of past traumas, and may experience significant interruptions during REM sleep.

Occasionally, we may experience an episode of sleep paralysis; this happens after waking suddenly from REM sleep, which often happens following a nightmare. Our muscles are paralysed during REM sleep, but during an episode of sleep paralysis they remain paralysed for a short period of time after waking. In old English folklore, sleep paralysis was said to be due to supernatural forces sitting or pressing down upon the sleeper's chest.

Sleepwalking and sleep talking

Sleepwalking (somnambulism) and sleep talking (somniloquy) are perhaps more commonly reported sleep issues than you may think. Both activities occur during deep sleep (stages 3 and 4), and are unrelated to dreaming, with people rarely recalling them upon waking. Sleepwalking most commonly occurs in children between the ages of five and twelve years; 15% of children in this age group are said to walk in their sleep at least once. It is much less common in adults, occurring in about 2–5% of the adult population, the majority of whom began sleepwalking when they were children.

Sleepwalking is more likely to occur when people have been sleep-deprived, drinking alcohol, or under stress. Sleep talking occurs in about 4% of adults, though again more frequently in children. This can range from non-verbal utterances to eloquent speeches, which occur several times during a night's sleep. The speech may or may not be comprehensible to listeners. Sleep talking rarely presents a serious problem. In fact, it is much more likely to be problematic for the partner if they are disturbed during the night on a regular basis. Sleepwalking can become a problem when people run the risk of injury, either within the house or if they go outdoors.

Some sleepwalkers conduct activities during their sleep such as cleaning. It can also be associated with bedwetting; it is not uncommon for people to urinate in closets and cupboards during a sleepwalking episode. In extremely rare cases people conduct violent activities. In the UK, a man unknowingly strangled his wife while on a caravan holiday. He thought he was fighting off some assailants whom he believed had broken into their caravan. He was acquitted of all charges on the grounds that he was not conscious and not in control of his actions.

Teeth grinding

Grinding one's teeth is also known as 'bruxism', and is sometimes accompanied by clenching of the jaw. It can occur during the day or at night. During the day, it is often in reaction to certain feelings or events. During sleep, however, bruxism is characterised by automatic teeth grinding and rhythmic jaw muscle contractions. In one study, 8.2% of the general population were estimated to grind their teeth at least twice a week during sleep, and 4.4% were reported to fulfil the criteria for a full diagnosis of bruxism.

It was also found to be more common in those who regularly consume large amounts of caffeine, alcohol and nicotine. Importantly, bruxism can be symptomatic of underlying stress and anxiety; one study found that roughly 70% of sufferers attributed their teeth grinding to these causes.

Delayed Sleep Phase Disorder

Delayed Sleep Phase Disorder (DSPD), sometimes known as phase lag syndrome belongs to a group of sleep disorders known as circadian rhythm sleep disorders, whereby individuals experience a chronic pattern of sleep disturbance due to changes in the circadian timing of their sleep, relative to what their social and physical environments dictate. For example, an individual whose circadian rhythm, or 'body clock', is delayed may find that their ideal time for sleep is 4am with a rise time of 12 noon. This schedule does not match the typical sleep window of most adults; and thus the main problems of those with DSPD relate to attempting to fall asleep (before their body clock is ready to) and attempting to wake up in the morning (before their body clock is ready to). The latter can be a significant problem if the individual has to commence work at 8 or 9am, leaving them with partial sleep deprivation.

Circadian rhythm sleep disorders in general lead to excessive daytime sleepiness as well as periods of insomnia, due to the shift in the natural, circadian timing of an individual's sleep window. DSPD in particular, tends to describe sleep–wake schedules which are delayed by two or more hours from the 'normal' so, for example, an individual found themselves becoming sleepy at 4am and waking naturally at 12 noon. Other than this offset, DSPD does not cause 'abnormal sleep' and tends to follow a reliable pattern over a 7-day period.

People with DSPD are commonly referred to as 'night owls'; however, those with DSPD do not choose their waking hours, generally falling asleep very late at night and waking in the late morning or afternoon. DSPD will often lead to individuals being labelled as having insomnia but, importantly, they have no difficulty falling asleep if allowed to follow their internally set sleep pattern.

Treatment for DSPD includes a variety of lifestyle changes such as improvement in sleep hygiene habits; for example, restricting caffeine intake in the hours before bed, keeping to a regular schedule and only using your bedroom for sleeping. Alternatively, 'bright light therapy' may help to reset the body clock, using controlled exposure to strong light levels shortly after waking, or prescribed melatonin.

Restless Legs Syndrome

Restless Legs Syndrome (RLS), also known as 'Ekbom syndrome', is thought to affect between 5 and 10% of adults. The syndrome is characterised by uncomfortable or painful feelings in the thighs, calves and feet, which result in overwhelming urges to move the legs. These feelings are often experienced as crawling or tickling sensations in the skin or leg muscles and range from the mildest of feelings to the most severe and debilitating sensations. The symptoms of RLS may not be restricted to night-time and, in the most extreme situations, can significantly impact on daily quality of life.

RLS sufferers tend to begin experiencing the 'itching' or 'tickling' sensations in their legs during periods of rest, only finding relief by moving their legs and, whilst some may only experience RLS very rarely, others will report experiencing these symptoms every day.

RLS is most often discussed in relation to sleep as the urge to move the legs often proves to be strongest at rest. The majority (as many as 80%) of individuals with RLS experience several episodes of jerking leg movements during the night, called periodic limb movements (PLMs), which may seriously fragment their sleep, often without them knowing. Compromised sleep quality and sleep continuity ultimately impairs next-day functioning, through increased levels of sleepiness and fatigue.

There is still much debate and disagreement surrounding the causes of RLS, which may be associated with underlying health conditions, including anaemia (iron deficiency),

Parkinson's disease and reduced kidney function. In these cases, RLS would be given as a 'secondary diagnosis'. Alternatively, RLS may present on its own, being given as a 'primary diagnosis'. In these cases however, there is often no obvious cause of RLS and it may be seen to run in the individual's family.

Most research into the causes of restless legs indicates low levels of the neurotransmitter dopamine to be key. Dopamine is important in the control of muscle movements, meaning that low levels of the chemical may play a role in the involuntary leg movements seen in RLS.

RLS may not require treatment if the symptoms experienced are very mild; however, several lifestyle changes may be advised. These include avoidance of caffeine and alcohol and participating regularly in exercise alongside stopping smoking if you do so. In cases of RLS caused by other conditions, people may find that treatment for their primary diagnosis may also improve their RLS. However, in more severe cases of RLS, people may benefit from medication to adjust dopamine levels.

Fibromyalgia

Fibromyalgia is principally characterised by chronic widespread pain, fatigue and heightened response to tactile pressure. This chronic condition results in marked daytime distress and dysfunction. Poor, non-restorative sleep and insomnia are very common in patients with fibromyalgia (in as many as 95% of diagnosed patients), along with impairments in cognition (especially concentration and memory), headaches and depression.

Approximately 2–4% of the population experience fibromyalgia, and the condition is a lot more common in women than men. Although the underlying cause(s) of fibromyalgia is not yet clear, a number of theories exist, and include altered pain processing, changes in levels of specific neurotransmitters, stress reactivity and psychological factors. The many symptoms can to a degree be managed through medication, therapy and diet, though regular consultation with a specialist is recommended.

Weight issues

Your weight and size can have an impact on how well you sleep, for several reasons. Extra weight can cause snoring and sleep apnoea, which can then affect your sleep (and your partner's). With weight gain, your body deposits excess fat wherever it can, including the lining of your throat, so your breathing passages get narrower and narrower, making you more likely to snore.

Additionally, being overweight or obese can lead to more physical pain, like joint, muscle and back pain, which may well disturb sleep patterns. You may also sweat more at night and feel hot, which can affect sleep. Overweight people are more likely to feel tired, and do less physical activity as a result, so although they will feel tired their body has not been active enough to induce proper sleep.

Being overweight may also affect your confidence and self-esteem and contribute towards anxiety and depression, which will then impact on your sleep. You are more likely to have an unhealthy diet that adds to the issues and of course, this cycle can develop in a negative way, whereby poor sleep leads to less activity, unhealthy eating, lowering of mood and then poor sleep again. One of the best ways to improve sleep if you are overweight is to focus on reducing your weight through more exercise and improved healthy eating. The improved sleep will, in turn, help towards increased activity, improved mood and healthier eating.

Physical pain and injuries

It can be very difficult to sleep if you have any form of physical pain or injury and although it may be for only one or two nights for some, it can be for a prolonged period of time for others. It could also be related to an injury even though the pain may not be a factor; for example, you may have broken your leg or arm and be in a cast, which causes you problems sleeping.

While writing this book I was stung by a wasp, and for about three nights in a row I struggled to sleep as a result of the itching and pain from the wasp sting. So it could even be something like that which causes sleep issues and although only temporary it can still be very frustrating and have negative knock-on effects in your life.

Some people, though, will live in constant pain or go weeks on end with a painful injury or physical condition that causes pain and consequently impacts heavily on their sleep and ability to sleep well.

Bed, mattress, pillows and sheets

Make sure you don't underestimate the importance of your bed, mattress and sheets as this can be a major cause of poor sleep. People will have different preferences when it comes to mattress types; whether they prefer a harder or softer mattress, for example. The size of the bed can also make a difference, particularly if it is too small.

The duvet size, the sheets, the blankets, the pillows etc., can all be factors too, whether that is because they are too big or too small, poorly fitting or not clean. Often people will go weeks or months without changing the sheets or duvet covers, and apart from the obvious problems with cleanliness this can also have an effect on your sleep and quality of sleep. Good sleep hygiene is important; it is all about keeping up good habits related to your bed and bedroom in any way that can affect your sleep.

'Goodnight, sleep tight... don't let the bed bugs bite!'

Food and drink

What you eat and drink can have a big effect on your sleep, especially the nearer to bedtime you consume these. Not everyone is the same and different foods and drinks will affect people to varying degrees, but it is likely that your sleep will be affected in some way as a result of your food and drink consumption.

It is quite likely your sleep will be interrupted by needing the toilet during the night if you drink anything close to bedtime. So be sensible with how much fluid(s) you consume as you near bedtime and ensure you go to the toilet just before you go to sleep if you can. Also, as previously mentioned, be aware of any foods and drinks that contain caffeine as this stimulant is likely to impair your ability to get to sleep. Some foods will be much harder for your stomach to digest than others, too. It is not recommended you eat much close to bedtime and certainly not any big meals.

Additionally, good sleep can help you eat better and more healthily as it increases your production of the digestive hormone leptin, which helps prevent you eating too much, and sleep also causes a decrease in the production of the digestive hormone ghrelin, which boosts appetite. So a good night's sleep decreases your hunger and you are less likely to eat the unhealthy foods you may crave when you don't sleep well.

Noise

Sounds that occur during your sleep are quite likely to have an effect on your quality of sleep, as it is only in the very deep sleep that noise has to be at a very high level to wake you up. At other times fairly low noise levels and sounds can be noticed and thus cause issues. Humans have pretty good hearing and our senses are aroused instinctively if we hear unexpected or loud noise, because it could be a threat. Chemicals can be released to make us more alert and aware, which is exactly the opposite of what we want when trying to sleep!

You may live near a busy road, a train station or even an airport runway, which could all cause noise problems. Or perhaps you live in a busy area, have factories nearby or have particularly noisy neighbours. Perhaps within the house there could be squeaky floorboards, swinging doors or noisy pipes. The noise could also be generated by your partner, the kids, pets or housemates.

Some noises will be out of your control and may only cause occasional problems, but if there are frequent or constant noises that disturb your sleep or cause sleeping issues in any way then you should look to see what can be done to improve the situation.

Temperature

The temperature of your room and bed can play an important role in your sleep quality, whether that is being too cold or too hot. All of us will have a preferred temperature for the best-quality sleep and despite all the modern advances in heating, air conditioning, fans, duvet tog sizes, etc., many of us will still struggle at times with being too hot or too cold.

Feeling so cold that you are shivering, or all you can focus on is being too cold, so that you cannot sleep, is not a pleasant experience, although this tends to be less common than feeling too hot. Those summer nights when it is so hot and stuffy, you spend hours trying to sleep with no success and then, like other sleep issues, this starts to have further negative knock-on effects, and the longer it goes on the worse the issues.

Sleeping with a partner can also affect the temperature, and often people will feel too hot when up close to a partner as their body temperature is far higher than is comfortable for sleep. Two different people can have different temperature preferences, so being aware and sensitive to this issue can be important.

Light

The light in the room where you are sleeping can have an effect on many people. Some like to have a light on for various reasons whilst trying to sleep or during the night. Some don't mind the bright light of the morning sun coming through the windows, whilst others cannot sleep at all at with any light coming in and especially not the sometimes very bright natural sunlight.

Personally, I struggle with bright light when trying to sleep, so during the summer months I try my best to black out any natural sunlight coming through the blinds/curtains in my room. This has some benefits, in that I am then not woken up at 4, 5 or 6am depending on the time of year. However, there is a downside in that my natural body clock has more difficulty adjusting and I miss that sometimes very beneficial natural awakening from sunlight, which can seemingly provide natural energy and make you feel more awake in the morning.

Everyone is different and you should try to work out to what extent light influences your quality of sleep and then seek some solutions if needed.

Pets

Nearly all pets will have a different sleep pattern or preferred sleep pattern to their human owners and this can cause issues. Many dog or cat owners, for example, will often talk about how their pet woke them up early by licking their face, barking or meowing at the door or knocking something over! Or it could be an issue at night while trying to get to sleep, or indeed at any point during the night something may happen involving the pet or pets that disturbs your sleep.

All pets are different and of course the health and wellbeing of the pet is paramount, but you must remember that your health is extremely important, too, and getting good sleep is a key factor in your health and wellbeing. So if your pets are causing some issues look at possible solutions or compromises that could help the situation.

Stimulants

I'm sure most people are aware that caffeine is a stimulant and for most people it would not be advisable to have caffeine before trying to sleep. However, many people will not be aware that many drinks and foods contain caffeine. The caffeine can have an effect for several hours after drinking and additionally many other foods, drinks and substances can be stimulants that will also have an adverse effect when you are trying to sleep.

Apart from coffee, other drinks that often contain caffeine include tea, sports drinks and energy drinks. Chocolate and other sweets can often contain caffeine too. Nicotine is also a stimulant, as are other more destructive drugs like cocaine.

Lack of routine

One of the most effective ways of sleeping well is having a constant and predictable routine for sleep and the times you go to bed and wake up. Your internal body clock can be very good at setting itself when you go to bed and wake up at the same time every day and keep to this routine. However, if the times you go to bed and wake up are constantly changing and there is a lack of routine this will very often cause poor sleep.

If in a typical week you wake up one day at 6am then the next day at 8am, then the following day at 6.30am and perhaps a 9.30am on a weekend, coupled with irregular going-to-bed times, then your body clock is compromised and your sleep patterns affected, which will more often than not mean your sleep is affected negatively. Perhaps you have a job with shift patterns where one week you work days and one week you work nights and it can be very difficult to adjust to these differences and by the time you have adjusted it is time for you to change shifts again.

Jet lag

Most people who have travelled either on business or on holiday to different time zones will have had their sleep affected in some way as the body tries to adjust. The wider the time-zone change the more likely you are to experience problems; this is commonly known as jet lag. For example, if you fly to California which is typically 8 hours behind the UK, then you may be expected to wake up at 8am their time, but your body clock would not have adjusted, so it is effectively only midnight!

It can take many days to adjust once in a destination, and again when you return it can take many days to adjust back, so potentially for a long period of time during and after a visit you can be struggling with sleep patterns and sleep quality.

Not tired

Although this book is focused on poor sleep and how to improve your sleep, we have all experienced times when we just don't feel tired! You may want to go to sleep at a certain time or feel you should, but for whatever reason you just don't feel tired and certainly not tired enough to fall asleep.

It could be due to oversleeping the night before or having a sleep during the day or having a very relaxed, low-activity day where you have not used much energy. Sometimes there can be seemingly no logical explanation. You simply don't feel tired, and of course it then becomes very difficult to sleep; often you will end up worrying about the fact you should be sleeping but can't and how this will have an impact on everything else.

Unfortunately there is likely to be a downside at some point if you don't sleep because you are not feeling tired.

Children

Most parents will say that their sleep is affected negatively at times because of their children. Whether that's babies or young infants crying, or illness, or teething, or needing nappy changes, etc., or perhaps from wetting the bed, nightmares, waking up early, wanting attention, needing feeding etc., there are many reasons why children can affect your sleep.

Of course, the child's or children's health and wellbeing should be a priority, but it is a fact that most parents will have their sleep interrupted and quality of sleep reduced because of their children, and it becomes a battle to try and work out how best to cope with the situation and do the best that is possible.

> **'People who say they sleep like a baby usually don't have one!'** – Leo J Burke

Partner

If you share a bed with a partner, you may at times, or indeed very frequently, be affected by them, whether that's due to snoring, moving about, talking, making other noises, getting into bed or getting out of bed at different times, using phones, iPads, other gadgets, being too hot, etc.

In any relationship there is a need to compromise, but quite often the sleep of one partner and sometimes both is adversely affected, which in turn can cause some of the sleep issues mentioned. Some couples will sleep in separate beds or separate rooms to overcome this, or it could be a case of investing in a larger bed or certain sleep aids for one or both that could help, plus, of course, discussing any issues with each other to see if things can be improved.

> **The world's loudest snore was measured at 111.6 decibels... similar to a jet plane!**

Shift work

Many people will do shift work, which is effectively any work that is not the normal daytime 9–5 routine. So it could be someone who works say 6am to 2pm or from 1pm to 9pm as an example. It also includes those people who do night shifts of say 10pm through to 6am and then also those who may work 3–4 days on and 3–4 days off but with longer shifts of say 12 hours at a time. There are many different types of shift work and most will have a detrimental impact on your sleep.

Humans have evolved over nearly two million years such that their natural cycle was to sleep at night-time and work or be active during the day. It's only in very recent times that we have had factories, hospitals, supermarkets, hotels, etc., where this has given rise to a large amount of shift work. Good-quality sleep usually happens when you are in sync with your natural body clock and you have a regular and consistent routine, so going to bed and waking up at the same time every day. Most shift work will not allow that or will compromise this in some way. Additionally if you have a partner who has a different sleep pattern and working hours then the issue is usually made even worse.

If you have no choice but to work shifts then you really need to make the extra effort to work out what you can do to help improve your sleep quality within the constraints of your shift working hours.

Habit and expectations

Many issues that people have relating to their physical, mental and emotional health can continue partly as a result of expectation and it becoming a habit. People can get used to thinking, feeling, behaving, reacting and acting in the same way through habit and their expectation being the same. So when it comes to poor sleep, the problem can also be prolonged or unresolved as a result. If you expect not to be able to sleep, if your mindset is one that is resigned to a bad night's sleep, waking up early, not being able to switch off, having your sleep interrupted, etc., then this will only increase the chances of these detrimental things happening.

Try to get out of that mindset and habit, and start afresh. Aim to have new, fresh, more positive expectations and believe that you will be able to change the habit and improve your sleep. Just because you have struggled in the past doesn't mean that has to continue. Don't let a negative habit or negative expectations remain.

> ***Pythons sleep for around 18 hours a day while giraffes sleep for less than 2 hours!***

Part 3

What Can We Do to Sleep Better?

In this section of the book we look at a wide variety of practical things that could help both the quantity and quality of your sleep. Read through each one and think about how much of a factor it could be and how you could try the suggestions. Some will not be relevant or practical for you but many will be, so read them with an open mind and remember how important sleep is to your life!

Invest in better sleep

Ideally we would be spending nearly one third of our entire lives asleep and we know that sleep is extremely important to our health and happiness. It has such an influence on our lives, for better or worse, so it makes sense that we should invest in better sleep. How much is your health and happiness worth to you? How much of an effect is sleep or lack of good sleep having on your life? How much would you pay if you could guarantee a great night's sleep?

If sleep is a problem then take some time to consider how important it is to you and what effect it has on your life. Then consider what you can do in terms of investing in better sleep, which could be financial investment or time investment or both. As an example, you could buy a new bed or mattress, which could be a lot of money, but actually if it meant a difference to your quality of sleep over many months or indeed years is likely to be money very well spent.

Or take the time out to really understand your sleep issues, whether that's reading, researching, reflecting, thinking, talking to a specialist, etc., then invest that time because it is likely to pay back and be a great investment.

There will always be things you can do that could make a difference to your quality of sleep, and although they may involve a cost or your time, make sure you think clearly about all the benefits that could occur as a result; rather than seeing things as a cost look at them as an investment in your health and happiness.

'Sleep is the best meditation.' – *the Dalai Lama*

Stop struggling

If you have sleep problems, whether long-term or temporary, then it is likely to play on your mind for much of the time. So in addition to all the consequences of poor sleep both physically and mentally there may be other downsides. During the day you may well be thinking about your lack of sleep and be anxious about whether you will sleep that night or be looking back on your previous poor night's sleep. This additional anxiety is counterproductive.

As much as you can, stop struggling! Stop thinking about your sleep problems. Stop focusing on the negative aspects and concerns around the problem. Accept that you can't change anything about the past and worrying about the next night won't help. And if you are lying in bed unable to get to sleep, or you wake up during the night and then can't sleep, try your best not to focus on that. The more you struggle the worse it will be. Accepting the situation and then focusing on what you can do in the way of potential solutions will be more beneficial.

If you find yourself lying in bed unable to sleep, rather than focusing on the fact that you can't sleep try the tactic of accepting it and stop struggling. Try to focus on what might work in a productive way and relax. That is far more likely to work than struggling and getting more wound up by the situation.

'Man should forget his anger before he lies down to sleep.' – *Gandhi*

Reduce anxiety

Anxiety is a very common and debilitating issue for both men and women and can affect people of all ages. There are many direct consequences of anxiety, one of which is having difficulty with sleeping, which of course then has knock-on negative consequences. So how can people reduce their anxiety levels effectively?

If you understand why you feel anxious and what is happening with the brain then you are much more likely to be able to reduce your anxiety. In terms of the brain, it is likely that the middle part called the amygdala is much more active when experiencing anxiety. You may feel insecure, under threat, unsure about what will happen, be jumping to conclusions without all the facts, being irrational, more emotional, oversensitive and more reactive. These are instinctive thoughts and behaviours based upon your survival instincts and are there to protect you in certain situations. However, it is very unlikely that your worries warrant such an extreme survival approach.

Think about the anxiety issues you have. Do you need to be in survival mode in this way? Nobody is going to attack you or kill you and you have almost certainly dealt with the same or similar issues in the past and got through it OK. If your thoughts were rational, less emotional and reactive, more reflective and pragmatic, based upon known facts and put into perspective then it is very likely your anxiety would dramatically reduce.

You can control your thinking and reduce your anxiety by recognising the difference between the rational and irrational thinking, the reflective and the reactive, and the emotional and the balanced. The more you recognise the difference and change your thought processes, the less anxiety you will face, and the more you practise this the easier it becomes. With less anxiety your sleep will definitely improve, which in turn will have many further positive benefits. Better sleep will naturally reduce your anxiety too, so it becomes a very positive and productive cycle. Understand, recognise, reflect, manage and practise, and then keep practising.

'I want to sleep but my brain won't stop talking to itself!'

Rationalise the worry issue

Most worries that people think about and that play on their mind are really not worth worrying about. Additionally, there is probably not much you can do about it anyway, so the worry is unproductive and a waste of time. Now that is easy to say but it is much more difficult to accept and then to change your thinking in practice. However, by rationalising the worry issue it becomes easier to accept and once accepted it is then easier to stop thinking about it.

Rationalising the worry means stepping back from the issue and reflecting on it and then trying to take a neutral, unbiased view. Something that usually works well is imagining it is a good friend with this worry issue and they are asking you for advice. What would you say to them? You are likely to take a more pragmatic, level-headed approach to the problem and will look to show that worrying isn't the answer.

Usually there are two possibilities – one is that there is nothing that you can do about the issue as it is out of your control. The second is that you will do your best to manage, prevent, sort out or deal with the issue when you can. Either way there is no benefit in worrying about it, as all this does is have a negative impact on you physically, mentally and emotionally, including affecting your sleep.

In general, women tend to worry and overthink issues more than men typically do. The rates of anxiety, stress and depression tend to be higher in women and these conditions can cause sleep issues.

> **Men appear to sleep better than women with 30% of them saying they sleep well most nights.**

CBT

Cognitive behaviour therapy (CBT) is a relatively new therapy, but is becoming increasingly popular and effective in helping people with a variety of issues linked to their thoughts, feelings and behaviours and can thus also help with sleep. It is really about finding techniques that work to correct a person's negative way of thinking and to correct self-destructive and damaging behaviour. Issues such as phobias, obsessions, stress, anxiety, depression, eating disorders, substance abuse, addictions and sleeping problems can all be helped with effective CBT. In fact, in recent years, CBT has proved the most effective treatment for insomnia.

A lot of sleep problems are an effect of other issues that CBT can help with, as people change their thinking and behaviour and understand more about their negative habitual thought processes, so that they develop more positive and beneficial behaviours. You can 'unlearn' the negative thoughts and replace them with much more productive, positive thoughts.

CBT courses and workshops are now often available through your doctor and the NHS, plus there are online courses and many books that are accessible. Although it can take time and a lot of practice, the results can be very effective and can go a long way towards improving many aspects of health and wellbeing.

Relax and wind down

Modern life can be very hectic, busy and stressful and many of us will struggle with being able to relax and wind down sufficiently to then be able to sleep once we go to bed, and then sleep well. You cannot expect to be able to be asleep straight away if you are still buzzing, excited, anxious, stressed, etc., and have not relaxed or wound down enough.

So try to ensure as you approach the time you would typically go to sleep that you are doing things that will help you to relax. Try to take your mind off any worries, stresses or issues of the day. Try not to overthink too much or concern yourself with things that you cannot do anything about right now. Perhaps watch some TV or a film, read a book or magazine or have a nice warm bath.

The more relaxed you are then the greater the chances of you sleeping once you go to bed; once in bed either continue to wind down further perhaps by reading or listening to some relaxing music or try to switch off and sleep straight away.

Specific sleep exercises

Relaxation and breathing
Stressful lifestyles, working late, and watching intense television shows or the news are some of the factors that can contribute to the mind racing and being unable to wind down. It's essential to know the importance of being relaxed before bed, and to have the knowledge of effective relaxation techniques to apply in order to experience deep, restful sleep.

Relax your body
This can be done in bed and works by relaxing separate groups of muscles. It is also effective to visualise each set of muscles being relaxed as you go through the exercise:

- *Tense a muscle by contracting and flexing for between seven and ten seconds. Don't strain the muscle.*

- *Visualise the muscle being tensed and feel the build-up of tension.*

- *Release each muscle abruptly, then relax, allowing the body to go limp before going on to the next muscle.*

- *Keep other muscles relaxed whilst working on a particular muscle.*

Breathe
The effects of deep breathing are largely psychological, but it can bring about a very positive physiological response in the body. It can normalise the heart and respiration rate and relax you, taking away some of the stresses and anxiety that you may have.

As well as relaxing you before bed, you can use this breathing exercise whenever anything upsetting happens, and before you react. It can be done anywhere because you don't have to lie on your back.

- *Sit up with your back straight and place the tip of your tongue just behind your upper front teeth, and keep it there throughout the entire exercise.*

- *Practice exhaling with your tongue in this position. It will be easier if you purse your lips.*

- *Now close your mouth and inhale through your nose for four seconds (counting one one thousand, two one thousand etc.).*

- *Hold your breath for seven seconds then exhale through your mouth, taking eight seconds to exhale completely.*

- *Repeat three to four times and try to be accurate with the counting.*

Try to do this regularly, as the more you do the better you will become and the greater the benefits; if you can get into a routine of doing this every evening before bed you should see the positive effects.

Your bedroom

As far as possible and practical you should ensure your bedroom is primarily about sleeping and make it as conducive to sleep as you can. You should associate your bedroom and your bed with as few other distractions as possible. Apart from sleep and sex, the fewer other things you do in bed the better. Having that strong, consistent association between your bed and sleep will allow you to focus on sleep and more likely improve its quality and quantity.

If you have lots of other things going on in your bedroom which are not sleep-related then these potential distractions or associations with non-sleep activities could be detrimental to your sleeping habits. So for example, watching TV, playing computer games, eating food, working, using work-related equipment like a laptop or a phone, plus in-depth conversation with your partner, can all be a bad influence on your sleep.

Air quality

Ensuring that you have plenty of fresh, good-quality air in your bedroom can play an important role in your sleep. A stuffy, poorly oxygenated room is not going to help, so it is a good idea to open doors and windows letting fresh air pass through when possible. There are practical issues like potential noise or the cold that can at times prevent this, but by using your initiative and planning in advance it is possible to ensure clean, fresh air does circulate through your room, aiding your breathing and sleeping.

Also, be aware of potential allergies that could come from pollen, general dust or dust-mites, particularly if you have asthma or hay fever, and if necessary seek advice or do air-quality tests if you think this may be a problem.

Write things down

Sometimes while we are lying in bed unable to sleep it is helpful to write things down on a notepad if certain thoughts pop into our head. Keeping a pen and pad near your bedside can be useful so that if you are worrying or thinking about issues then you can write them down and tell yourself you will come back to them in the morning.

It could be that you have a fantastic idea or thought and in a similar way you are likely to be better off by writing it down and then forgetting about it so you can sleep and come back to it in the morning. Otherwise you may not be able to stop thinking about it, then get excited, release some adrenaline and your sleep will definitely be compromised.

You may wake up with a particular thought, idea or issue and writing it down could help you relax again and go back to sleep. Knowing that you have documented it should mean you don't have to worry about remembering it or focusing on it when it would be better for you to be sleeping. You could try writing a 'worry diary' whereby you jot down your worries and concerns, which may help you to leave them on your notepad and not in your head at bedtime.

Write a sleep diary

If you have the discipline to write a sleep diary for at least two weeks then you are likely to gain a really good insight into your sleep patterns and behaviours that could be very beneficial and informative and thus provide valuable information to help improve your sleep in the long term.

Write down information such as the times you went to bed, how long it took to fall asleep, the time you woke up, the time you got out of bed, whether you awoke during the night and if so for what reasons, how you felt during the day and if you had any daytime naps. Also, try to include other information like the food you ate and eating times, alcohol and caffeine consumption, plus any exercise you did and when. Also, write about your levels of stress, anxiety and relaxation, and any particular worries or issues that have affected you.

If you can do this over a minimum two-week period then you can analyse the information in detail, perhaps with a friend or partner, and see if there are some key elements and factors that stand out. Look for both the good and bad factors and see if there are things that clearly work or do not work and what things have the most effect on you. By doing this and reflecting upon it you may well find some interesting and very helpful insights and conclusions. It is definitely worth a go if sleep is a problem for you.

Sleep-inducing scents

There are certain smells and scents such as lavender, geranium, chamomile and ylang-ylang that can activate the alpha-wave activity in the back of your brain, which can help to relax you and therefore provide a better environment for falling asleep and aid you in sleeping more soundly.

So perhaps try mixing a few drops of these essential oils with some water in a spray bottle and use a little on your pillows and sheets. You could also try having a bowl of pot pourri in your bedroom. Additionally, if you find yourself sleeping away from home in a hotel, friend's or family's house for example, then you could take it with you and use it to help replicate your own normal sleep environment and thus aid your sleep.

Visualise feeling sleepy

You could try visualising stages of going to sleep whilst you are lying in bed trying to sleep. Focus on yourself and visualise how it would look and feel to be very tired, relaxed, yawning, feeling drowsy, switching off and then falling asleep. Focusing on this and really visualising yourself doing it could actually help you fall asleep.

It will hopefully take your mind off other thoughts, will help you wind down, and you can almost trick your body and mind into sleep through this visualisation. It may not always work or it may take practice to make it effective, but it is worth trying as you have nothing to lose and it could make a big difference.

So again, go over in your head how it would look in an ideal situation where you were tired, feeling drowsy, relaxing and drifting off to sleep in your bed and if necessary keep repeating this visualisation technique. The more you practise the better you will become at it and the more effective it will be.

Refocus on something else

You may go to bed with a whole mix of thoughts or perhaps something very specific that is occupying your mind and preventing you from sleeping. Although it is never as easy as it sounds, try to refocus your thoughts on to something else. Make it something relaxing, positive or productive.

A few things I have tried with success over the years include visualising a gym workout, packing for a trip or thinking about a spa day. So with the gym workout I will visualise the gym with the weights and machines and then go through in my head the different exercises and routines and which muscles I will be working and keep going through the wide range. I may start with some bicep curls, then some tricep dips focusing on my arms, then some sit-ups and chest presses, etc. Basically I go through in my head a routine that I am familiar with, until I fall asleep. This is positive, productive, familiar and relaxing and will often work well.

With packing for a trip or holiday, again it is visualising what I need to pack, putting stuff into bags or suitcases, then maybe I will think about the journey by car or taxi or to the airport. Ensure you visualise something that is positive and relaxing. At the spa day example, think about sitting in a Jacuzzi, doing a few lengths of the pool, going for a body massage and sitting in a sauna. If you are familiar with these things that are also positive, productive and relaxing it will be more likely that you can switch off from the more distracting, worrying, anxious thoughts that may prevent you from sleeping. Come up with your own ideas and ways to refocus and find out what works best for you.

Perhaps you could try visualising your favourite place or a tranquil scene such as a lake or a mountain, the sounds of a gentle stream, or a walk in the woods. Retrace your steps on a favourite walk, taking particular notice of the sounds, the scents, the colours, the feel of the earth beneath your feet and the light as it filters through the trees. Observe the wild flowers, or fungi, or the different leaves on the trees above your head. Or just fix in your mind a certain scene – a lake is always great – and note the stillness, the reflections and the sound of absolute silence.

> *'It is a common experience that a problem difficult at night is resolved in the morning after the committee of sleep has worked on it.'* – John Steinbeck

Solutions not problems

If you find yourself worrying or thinking about a particular problem or several problems and you cannot switch off from it then try as much as possible to think about potential solutions rather than the problem itself. If you are not sleeping then you may as well use that time productively and focus on coming up with solutions. You should also find that focusing on solutions is more positive and productive, and will give you more chance of relaxing and feeling less anxious, so is more likely to help with sleep.

So whatever the problems, keep telling yourself to think about solutions instead. For example, it could be work issues that are occupying your mind. An important meeting or presentation coming up, too much work to do, a work colleague causing you problems, a member of your staff who is not performing, etc. Turn your thought process to working out possible solutions like how you will prepare and plan, who you should talk to and how you will approach it, what help is available, then prioritise your time and realise you cannot do everything, set up a meeting with a mentor, etc. The more productive your thoughts the better it will be for you, and the more you practise this the easier it becomes.

Consult a doctor

If you are really struggling with your sleep, particularly if it seems to be a longer-term, ongoing issue, then you should consult your doctor for advice. There may be additional help or suggestions available. The doctor may discuss medication, may provide some helpful literature or ideas or they could refer you to a specialist or a sleep lab for further analysis and assessment.

Poor sleep is a very common problem, yet people are often reluctant to seek professional help. There may not be any miracle cures or quick fixes but there may be some helpful advice and things to take away either to try out, or to consider how they might be beneficial.

Also, it could be that your sleep problems are more a result of a different condition, illness or health problem, which could be identified by discussing them with the doctor. Often there will be specific underlying reasons for your difficulty sleeping and if they are addressed, managed or treated then your sleep may well improve significantly. So don't be afraid to go to your doctor, as you have nothing to lose and potentially a lot to gain.

Medication

The most common and well-known treatment for insomnia is sleep-inducing medication, also known as hypnotics. The most common type of hypnotic is a group of drugs called benzodiazepines, the most well-known being diazepam (Valium) which is used to treat anxiety and acts as a muscle relaxant, and has been around since the early 1960s. Similar drugs like temazepam can be useful for short-term insomnia, but there is little evidence to suggest that they are appropriate for chronic insomnia. They may also cause side effects and possibly a sense of drowsiness during the day.

Another commonly used group of drugs developed more recently are the benzodiazepine receptor agonists; sometimes these are called 'Z drugs' since many of their names begin with the letter 'Z' (zopiclone and zolpidem, for example). There are various other groups of drugs that may potentially be prescribed for insomnia; melatonin receptor agonists aim to promote sleep by increasing the amount of melatonin in the body, orexin antagonists aim to limit the hormone orexin, which is related to being awake, and some antihistamines and (rarely) opioids can be used as sedatives.

Some antidepressants do have a sedative effect, and research has shown that people who were treated using a combination of sleeping medication and antidepressants showed greater improvements in depressive symptoms than people who used antidepressants only. However, the British Association for Psychopharmacology advises against using antidepressants in the treatment of insomnia as there is limited evidence indicating their efficacy in this application. It is difficult to gauge how many prescriptions are written for hypnotics because many of these drugs are prescribed for problems that are not directly sleep-related. And again, the side effects from these drugs may cause debilitation and other common physical problems.

Up to 40% of people with insomnia may self-medicate with hypnotics that are available without a prescription, and many people also drink alcohol to aid sleep. Hypnotics may be effective for short-term acute insomnia, particularly for conditions like jet lag. However, they only act on the biological, neurochemical factors to help us sleep.

Many people develop tolerance to hypnotics and become physically or psychologically dependent, or suffer withdrawal symptoms such as anxiety, depression and nausea. Some types of hypnotic, such as benzodiazepines, can cause 'rebound insomnia', which is often worse than the original insomnia symptoms. Also, hypnotics can have a range of side effects. The National Institute for Health and Clinical Excellence suggests that hypnotics should only be used after other measures have been tried, and then only for short periods of time, such as 2–4 weeks maximum.

> *More than 10 million prescriptions for sleeping tablets are issued each year in England alone.*

Herbal remedies

Many different varieties of natural sleep remedies are available and promoted as sleep aids, with mixed evidence as to their effectiveness. However, some have been shown to work and they are certainly worth exploring as long as you have done some research and are careful. Many chemists and other health shops will sell a range of herbal sleep-aid products but please read the labels and if possible discuss them with a pharmacist for additional advice.

Examples of herbal sleep aids include melatonin, valerian root and chamomile and can come in different formats like tablets or tea bags. Be aware that they can potentially cause some side effects such as headaches and stomach upsets.

However, as with most things, people react and respond differently so it is certainly worth trying a wide variety of remedies to discover for yourself if they work or not. Speak to friends and colleagues to see if they have tried any herbal remedies and what their experiences were.

Napping

There are mixed views on whether napping during the day can be a good thing or not. Obviously for many people it is not possible or practical – your work colleagues and bosses may not appreciate you having a twenty-minute nap under the desk during the afternoon!

If you are sleeping effectively at night then there should be no need to have additional sleep time or naps during the day. Also, having naps could cause sleep problems at night as you may not feel tired enough to sleep when you go to bed, and it can affect your natural sleep cycle, so be aware of these potential issues.

On the other hand, if you do struggle with sleep at night and have the opportunity to fit in a nap during the day it could be beneficial and provide you with some additional energy and motivation. Some people swear by the benefits. However, if the nap is too long (say more than 30 minutes) you are in danger of feeling more drowsy afterwards so if you do nap make it a 'power nap' of around 20 minutes.

Bed, mattress, duvets and sheets

It should go without saying that the right bed for you will make a difference to your sleep quality and quantity. Whether that's the right size, a firm or soft mattress or a special supporting one, it is worth finding out as best you can what is the optimal bed for you and investing in it. Of course, the sheets, blankets and duvet are also important, and again think about investing in these for your long-term health and happiness rather than as just a one-off expense. Change and wash your sheets and covers often and think about your bed and bedding as not only vital for sleep but also for your overall wellbeing.

A great example of the importance of having the right mattress, sheets, duvet, etc., so that you sleep as well as possible is what Team Sky do for their cyclists (Team Sky are the British-based professional cycling team who have had major success with the likes of Sir Bradley Wiggins and Chris Froome winning the Tour de France). They have a general philosophy called 'marginal gains' which is effectively saying that there are literally hundreds of factors that contribute to or affect the performance of the team and if they can improve all of these even by very small 'marginal gains' then the cumulative effect will become significant and make a real difference.

So when it comes to sleep, Team Sky ensure that they take their own pillows, sheets, mattresses and duvets with them throughout the different tours and numerous different hotels. This means the cyclists have consistency each night and are much more likely to sleep well, which is a very important ingredient in helping them perform at their best.

Temperature

I'm sure everyone has experienced at some point that horrible feeling of being so hot at night that you just can't sleep no matter what you do. No duvet, no covers, no sheets, no clothes, windows open, fans on, etc., yet still it is too hot and uncomfortable too sleep. Conversely you may have had those nights where you are so cold that you are curled up and shivering and unable to sleep. The latter example tends to be less common because of heating and decent duvets etc., but the former problem can be much more common as people tend not to have air conditioning at home.

Your body temperature plays a key role in how well you sleep and this changes at different stages of sleep. Typically you need to be cool in order to provide the best environment for sleep and although everyone is slightly different you should consider how you can have the optimum temperature for you.

Apart from opening windows, having fans (stand-up and ceiling), using air conditioning, lighter-tog duvets, fewer blankets, fewer nightclothes on, etc., think about other things you can try that might help. That could include on very hot nights sleeping in a separate bed to your partner so you are both more likely to sleep better, or a cool bath/shower prior to sleep to reduce body temperature could be beneficial.

Light

Light is vitally important to our sleep cycles and can, for many people, play a major role in their sleep – both negatively and positively. In general terms, when you are asleep your surroundings should be dark with no light at all. So ensuring that no artificial lights are on and no natural light can get through from windows or doors is essential.

Many people have experienced a bedroom light being switched on during the night that wakes you up, and then it is often hard to get back to sleep, or a bright ray of sunshine peeks through your curtains and wakes you. Your brain will naturally react by suppressing the release of melatonin and prepare itself to be awake and alert.

So to prevent your brain and body waking up prematurely because of light make sure you do all you can to mitigate the risk, which can include wearing an eye-mask, using blackout blinds, time-sensitive artificial lights, etc. And ensure the light bulbs in your room are not too bright or, even better, are on a dimmer switch.

Conversely though, light can be helpful in ensuring you don't sleep for too long and there is a danger that if all light is cut out and you wake up with your alarm then you will feel groggy Many people like to use artificial wake-up lights that slowly get brighter over many minutes before an alarm is set off. This prepares the brain, signalling that wake-up time is approaching and users will often feel much more alert and awake when they open their eyes.

Part 3 – What Can We Do to Sleep Better?

Exercise and be active

Being more physically active and doing more exercise is very likely to help you sleep better. So apart from all the other fantastic benefits of exercise, the fact it is a proven way to improve your sleep should be a good motivator to do more. There are several direct reasons why exercise helps people to sleep better, as well as several indirect reasons.

The human body is designed to exercise regularly and has evolved on the basis of being very physically active, so it makes sense that the natural cycle includes activity during the day and rest (sleep) at night. This basic concept has served humans well for many hundreds of thousands of years, so if we don't exercise and are not physically active it makes sense that our sleep could be affected. There is that common saying that after a hard day of physical exertion 'you will sleep well tonight'. And this is generally true.

Exercise also helps to keep us healthy generally, both physically and mentally, so examples like keeping our weight down, having stronger lungs, a healthier heart and lower blood pressure, reducing stress and worry, feeling more confident, etc., are all helpful in the pursuit of better sleep.

Be careful not to exercise vigorously too late in the day and close to bedtime as the various positive chemicals and hormones released as a result of exercise will make us more alert and energised for a while and it may be more difficult to wind down ready for sleep. So be sensible in what you do and when you do it but be assured, exercise and physical activity will help you to improve your quality of sleep.

People who exercise five to six times per week are least likely to take medication to help them sleep (12%, compared to a national average of 17%) and visit their GP (5%, compared to an average of 10%), which suggests that this could be the optimal amount of exercise needed to improve sleep. Indeed, those who don't take regular exercise are more likely to sleep badly: 11% of those who exercise less than once every six months sleep very poorly most nights, compared to the 32% of those who exercise daily who say they sleep very well most nights.

'A well-spent day brings happy sleep.' – *Leonardo da Vinci*

Food and drink

There are three substances that are key to understanding how nutrition can affect the brain chemistry that promotes good sleep:

- Tryptophan
- Serotonin
- Melatonin

What is tryptophan? All protein foods are composed of amino acids and tryptophan is one of them. It is the rarest of the amino acids, and is found in foods like turkey, steak, chicken and pumpkin seeds, and to a lesser extent in peanuts, sunflower seeds, beans and milk. Tryptophan is important because when it reaches the brain, it converts to an important chemical called serotonin.

What is serotonin? You may have heard of serotonin because of its connection to drugs such as Prozac, which are known as selective serotonin reuptake inhibitors (SSRIs). Serotonin is actually a chemical that carries messages between brain cells (neurones) and other cells. Decreased serotonin levels can lead to anxiety, depression, and increased cravings for carbohydrate foods. At night-time, serotonin undergoes two metabolic changes to become melatonin, the chemical that induces sleep.

What is melatonin? Melatonin is a hormone that helps to regulate the body's circadian rhythm and promotes restful sleep. It is produced from serotonin in the evening to help us sleep.

Always combine a protein food with a low to medium glycaemic index carbohydrate food to optimise tryptophan levels and boost serotonin.

Avoid buying melatonin supplements from the internet (they are only available on prescription in the UK). Taking them may disrupt your own natural melatonin production and potentially suppress your ability to produce this important hormone, ultimately making sleep problems worse.

The last hour

What you do during the last hour leading up to you going to sleep or trying to go to sleep can play a vital role in your sleep success. Ideally during the last hour you will be relaxing and winding down and effectively preparing for a good night's sleep. Factors such as not eating or drinking, not exercising, not watching anything too stimulating (like a horror film!), not exposing yourself to bright lights, not working or thinking about difficult issues that may play on your mind, and of course going to the toilet, can all help towards better sleep.

Having a constructive bedtime routine can also help, as well as trying to go to bed at the same time each night and avoiding any stimulants such as nicotine and caffeine. Try to switch off phones, computers, electrical devices and anything else that may stimulate the brain or affect your eyes.

Sleep positions

Have you ever thought much about your own sleeping position? Do you have a favourite or one you find yourself getting into naturally? Most people have what they would call their normal sleeping position and the most common is the foetal position, replicating how a baby in the womb tends to position itself.

There are three main sleeping positions with variables of each: side, back and stomach. Sleep specialists recommend sleeping on your side in order to rest more comfortably and decrease the likelihood of interrupted sleep. While there are many variations of sleeping on your side, all of which are beneficial in helping to alleviate insomnia and chronic sleep deprivation, the most comfortable position involves bending the knees slightly upwards towards the chest area. For those with a bad back, consider placing a pillow between your legs to alleviate pressure on your hips and lower back. Sleeping on your side is actually encouraged for those suffering from back or hip pain, and pregnant women, since this position doesn't increase pain in these areas.

If you prefer to sleep on your back, be careful, as it may actually induce lower back pain and even episodes of apnoea which interfere with normal sleep and restfulness. However, if you prefer to sleep on your back, there are a few minor alterations to this position that you can make to help you sleep more soundly. Try placing a soft pillow or rolled-up towel under your knees to facilitate the natural curve of the spine.

If you like sleeping on your stomach, you're in for a bit of bad news, as sleep professionals don't recommend sleeping on your stomach because it causes strain on your lower back and possible neck pain. People who sleep on their stomach report increased restlessness caused by frequent tossing and turning in an effort to get comfortable. If you do sleep on your stomach use an extremely soft pillow or none at all so as not to put your neck at an awkward angle. For those with sleep problems to begin with, it's best not to sleep on your stomach.

Sounds and white noise

It is fairly obvious and accepted that various sounds and noise whilst sleeping can have an impact on your sleep. There can be many examples of unwanted noises, some of which will be unexpected, and it is natural for you to wake up, be startled, be alert or at the least restless as a consequence. So trying to eliminate these unwanted sounds and noise is important in getting a good night's sleep.

However, certain noise and sounds can actually be helpful and aid you in sleeping better. It has been shown through studies that consistent, expected, known sounds can be effective and many people use gadgets and apps that create certain sounds with great success. Try using 'white noise' apps and see if it works for you, as a constant background noise can be remarkably effective at improving sleep. Your body and brain will get used to the noise and having it consistently played during the night wherever you may be sleeping will provide a kind of security and normality that in turn helps reduce anxiety and create a relaxed atmosphere.

Other sounds to help you fall asleep can work, such as ocean waves on a beach, or the type of music you find at holistic therapists to aid relaxation. It is worth a try!

Snooze button

How many of you use the snooze button on your alarm clock or phone? It is so often tempting to press the snooze button once the alarm goes off and think 'just a few more minutes'. Then the alarm goes off again and you think perhaps one more snooze, then again and again!

So many of us use the snooze button and unfortunately it doesn't do us much good. The short, broken, 'snooze sleep' is a very ineffective type of sleep. It is not restorative sleep and will do little to help our body and mind; essentially it is just wasting our time as we could either be getting proper, effective sleep or be up and being more productive.

Take the snooze button challenge, which is to force yourself to get up as soon as the alarm goes off and never use the snooze button again (OK, maybe on a special occasion!). You will find once you are in the habit of waking up as soon as your alarm goes off that you can set it to a later time and you are more likely to get a longer, deeper, more effective sleep.

Sleep apps

As technology continues to advance and access to smartphones rapidly increases, it is likely that very soon our personal devices will have apps that automatically track the steps we take, the calories we burn and the time we spend sleeping.

Modern smartphones include devices called 'accelerometers', which measure movement. These are used, for example, to detect the phone's orientation in order to switch the screen between 'portrait' and 'landscape' modes. Sleep recording apps use this same technology to monitor your movement throughout the night, gathering information about how long you slept and how many times you woke up, based on how much you moved.

Many sleep apps also feature a 'smart alarm'. Most often, these are intended to wake you up within a window of 'lighter' sleep, in order to minimise 'sleep inertia', the period after waking in which you may feel groggy and disorientated as you transition into wakefulness.

It is important to note however, that there are many factors that can affect how you feel on waking, and that the majority of mobile phone sleep apps have little or no clinical evidence to back up any claims.

There is also a wide range of wearable self-tracking devices available, many of which offer sleep tracking. The devices are usually worn on your wrist or attached to clothing, and sync with mobile and/or web-based applications, which allow you to view the data these devices collect.

The majority of wearable devices use accelerometers, similar to those used in mobile phones, to track movement. Some also feature additional technology to track factors such as temperature, heart rate and skin conductance.

Traditional sleep monitoring

Sleep monitoring is usually carried out by experienced technicians, in sleep laboratories or special sleep centres. A number of physiological parameters are assessed in these places to monitor patients' sleep in order to identify and diagnose disorders and look at best treatments.

Electrical activity in the brain is measured by electroencephalography (EEG), which is used to differentiate between wakefulness, sleep, and different stages of sleep. Muscle activity is measured using electromyography (EMG), because muscle tone also differs between wakefulness and sleep.

Lastly, eye movements during sleep are measured using electro-oculography (EOG). This is a very specific measurement that helps to identify Rapid Eye Movement or REM sleep, during which we often dream. This multi-assessment protocol is usually called polysomnography (PSG), and it remains the only clinically reliable sleep-tracking tool. Despite this, the simpler tracking offered by devices and sleep recording apps can still help give people a better understanding of their sleep.

Summary and Moving Forward

I hope the book has provided you with plenty of information and therefore improved knowledge about sleep and the many associated factors, issues and benefits. This should now help you to improve your own sleep and also be in a better position to help friends and family who may struggle.

Sleep is essential for both body and mind, yet despite it being so important, many of us do not sleep well and many of us do not invest the time, effort and money to improve our sleep. We are all different as individuals regarding how much sleep is optimal for us and there are a wide range of causes and effects of bad sleep, so it is vital that you look to understand the reasons and factors, both good and bad, particular to you.

If you do struggle with your sleep on a regular basis then firstly try to stop struggling and thinking negatively about the problem, as this won't help. Recognise and accept there is a problem and then look to understand why and then what you can do about it. There will always be an explanation, though sometimes hard to find, so do your research, be patient and you can solve your sleep problems.

There are so many potential causes for poor sleep, though stress, worry and anxiety are the most common reasons. Try to identify the factor or factors that are relevant to you and your sleep issues. Then focus on addressing and dealing with these. There are also many effects that can be caused by poor sleep, so be aware of the full extent of these.

Ensure you treat your sleep with the respect and attention it deserves. Sleep is so important for your health and happiness for so many reasons that you really must make an effort in getting good-quality sleep on a regular basis. Invest some time and money where necessary. For example, a new bed and mattress may cost several hundred pounds but it will last for years and if it helps you sleep better it is a great investment.

Be aware that technology can be a real hindrance to your sleep, especially using phones, tablets and computers in the bedroom. Checking emails, texts, Facebook and Twitter will affect your sleep both because your mind can't switch off and because the light from the devices will play havoc with your eyes and melatonin levels, thus affecting your ability to sleep.

If your partner struggles with sleep or is a big cause of your issues then try to help and support them in improving their sleep or seek compromises so that you minimise the negative effects. And if you feel it's necessary, seek expert advice by first discussing the issues with your doctor but then by being referred to a specialist sleep lab or sleep disorder centre.

Getting good-quality, regular sleep is wonderful and has such a positive and beneficial impact on your life, and this can apply to you. By understanding more, looking for the causes and working on overcoming these, by taking more time, making more effort and investing more money, you can make a huge difference to the amount and quality of your sleep. It is worth it – so stop struggling, recognise the issues and seek out the answers – because they are there. Best of luck!

'Your future depends on your dreams – so go to sleep.'

About the
'Climb Your Mountain' Charity

The Climb Your Mountain (CYM) charity was set up in 2008 by Charlie Wardle with the aim of helping anyone who felt they had their own personal mountain to climb in life. CYM offers advice, support, information, education, activities and opportunities for people to help themselves improve their health and happiness and effectively climb their own personal mountain.

Everyone will go through difficult times in life which may include work issues, relationship problems, financial pressures, health concerns, low confidence, anxiety, depression, social isolation, bereavement, etc., and Climb Your Mountain (CYM) offers a range of opportunities for people to help them through these difficult times in a number of ways.

CYM Health offers a range of free practical, easy- to-read, informative self-help books, as well as free online video workshops on the same topics for people to view and benefit from. Charlie Wardle also delivers talks, seminars, courses and workshops to the general public and to companies on a range of health and wellbeing topics.

To fund the charity and be able to offer all the free CYM Health services, the CYM Challenges division offers a range of fantastic trips and challenges across the UK and also some overseas trips. Anyone can participate in these great-value trips and challenges and have an amazing experience whilst also helping to support and fund the charity.

To find out more about the charity:

Website www.climbyourmountain.org

Email info@climbyourmountain.org

We rely heavily for funding on people making donations and raising money from taking part in trips and challenges. If you can help by making a donation please go to

www.justgiving.com/climbym

or get in touch and take part in a trip or challenge with us!

You can also TEXT a £5 donation to the charity

TEXT: BOOK32£5

To: 70070

Or an online donation via:

www.justgiving.com/healthbooks

THANK YOU!

NORTH SHIELDS

The Wilkinson's Lemonade Factory Air Raid Disaster

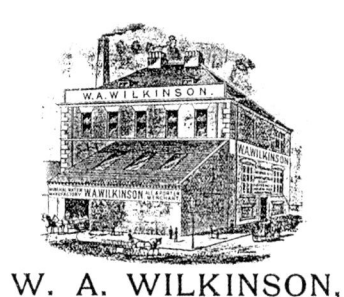

W. A. WILKINSON,
Wholesale and Family
Ale, Porter, Wine, and Spirit Merchant.

PETER BOLGER
2019

© Peter Bolger 2019

All rights reserved. No part of this book may be reproduced in any form by electronic or mechanical means, including information storage and retrieval systems, without permission in writing from the publisher, except by a reviewer who may quote brief passages in a review.

ISBN: 978-1-78972-254-3

For Karen Louise and Alexander Robert
In memory of Bobby, Monica, Gerry and Daniel

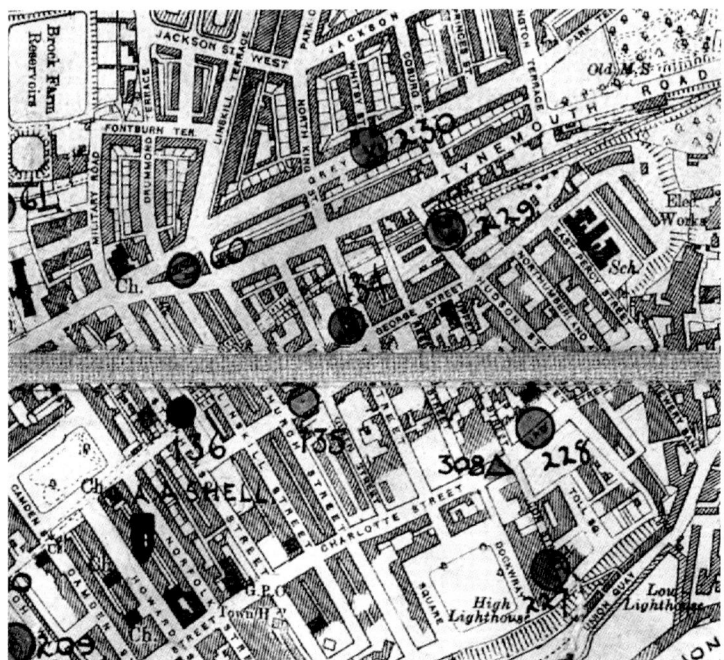

Borough bomb map showing bombs which fell on North Shields. Bomb no 134, in the centre of the image, shows the location of the direct hit on Wilkinson's Factory Shelter.

Contents

1	Introduction	1
2	Questions?	3
	Briefing: By numbers	6
	Briefing: Where was Wilkinson's?	7
	Briefing: The East End	9
3	Air Raid Disaster	12
4	Aftermath	19
	Briefing: Wrong building, right place	33
5	Wilkinson's Heroes	38
6	The Victims A–Z	50
7	Victims by Street	72
8	The Injured	77
	Briefing: Casualties controversy	80
	Briefing: Forgotten victims	81
9	Shelter Stories	82
	Briefing: The worst air raid disaster?	124
10	The Mineral Water King	126
	Briefing: What did the buildings look like?	137
11	Wilkinson's Voices	140
	Briefing: After the raid	160
12	Bombing the Borough	162
	Briefing: Which plane?	184
13	Wilkinson's Shelter: Sodom & Gomorrah	186
	Briefing: In the news again	191
14	Afterword	192
15	Thanks to . . .	194

1 Introduction

My mam wouldn't go to Wilkinson's that night, despite my dad saying we must if there was a raid on. She said it would be too noisy with the accordion player. We lived opposite the factory on King Street. "We'll take our chances here", she said. We hid under a table in the bedroom. Just as well we stayed put. When my dad found us, he cried. I'd never seen a man cry before.

[Jessie Dial – 13 years old in 1941]

This book is the story of one specific, tragic event in the life of a town.

In 1941, a single bomb from a lone enemy plane scored a direct hit on W. A. Wilkinson Ltd's lemonade factory in North Shields. The building and the tons of machinery, glass and chemicals stored on the upper floors, collapsed down into the public air raid shelter located in the basement.

Of the 192 people sheltering inside, 107 were killed. 43 of them were children. Entire families were lost. It was by far, the heaviest single bomb death toll in the North East of England during World War Two. It was also one of the worst air raid disasters anywhere in the country.

This is the story of that night - Saturday 3rd/Sunday 4th May 1941. It is, of course, not just one story. There are hundreds of personal stories and memories from survivors, eye-witnesses, relatives, friends and local residents. There are also tales of outstanding heroism, incredible rescue and lucky escape. Inevitably too, there are shadows cast of official incompetence, and of corners cut. Mistakes were made.

The threat posed by massed bomber attack had not been faced before. Local Authorities were dealing with the unknown. To a degree, they were playing catch-up, trying to ensure civilians were protected, before the bombs dropped for real. It was later than they thought.

Wilkinson's is an amazing story. It is also an unfinished story.

I warmly invite you to get in touch and share your family experiences and memories of the disaster.

The book is a companion to the northshields173.org website. The site explores the disaster fully and updates regularly. Contact details are published there and also on the Facebook page. Just search for "north shields 173".

I hope you find the book interesting and perhaps thought-provoking, as an account of what our townsfolk experienced one Spring night not that long ago. I hope you find it too, a sincere and respectful memorial to those we lost.

Peter Bolger

North Shields 173 was the telephone number for W. A. Wikinson Ltd. I sometimes wonder, in lieu of a time-machine, how fantastic it would be to be able to call that number now.

And then I wonder, just what would I say, when it was answered?

2 Questions?

Whenever I mention Wilkinson's...

I either get a look of incomprehension or sometimes, a wistful smile and a comment along the lines of "my uncle/grandma/cousin was in that shelter".

Some people are well informed about the disaster. However, occasionally, I'll be told the most outlandish tales and re-spins of local myths; of shot down German pilots being marched through Shields after the bombing, of hundreds being killed, of bodies left behind in the debris. And, my favourite...."The site is haunted, you know?"

But most commonly, I get a question, asked with explicit disbelief.

"Why did they put an air raid shelter in Wilkinson's in the first place?"

For people new to this, here's a very quick primer. W. A. Wilkinson Ltd made lemonade and a wide variety of other mineral drinks. Their factory was a converted private residence, already 140 years old in 1941.
A decision was made in 1940 by the Tynemouth Emergency Committee to locate a public air raid shelter for 188 people in the building's basement. Locals (and presumably the Borough Surveyor's team) knew that the factory's heavy machinery, glass and the chemicals used to make the lemonade were all stored on the floors directly above this basement.
W. A. Wilkinson's obviously knew too and perhaps kicked up a fuss about the inherent dangers. Not that they could have prevented the requisitioning of the basement anyway. We shall never know. Whatever, from the outset, despite (again unproven) claims that the factory had reinforced floors, the air raid shelter suffered certain local "unpopularity"

as a potential death trap. It is also true, however, that the shelter was very popular with many local residents.

So, a controversy that's been going on for 75 years. This book attempts to get to the bottom of it. I also ask other questions like: Who used the shelter? What sort of area was it? Why was the shelter so popular? What happened afterwards? How was the rescue conducted after the building collapsed? Was anyone blamed for the decisions taken? Is there a memorial for the victims? Did the business survive? Why was Wilkinson's forgotten? Where did the German bomber come from?

The answers to all of these are in the pages which follow. Maybe you have your own questions and perhaps you will find answers in the information below.

Throughout the book, I refer to "the shelter". More correctly, it was a basement public air raid shelter. Basement shelters obviously inherited the footprint of the host building. From this and from survivor descriptions, often vague and sketchy, we have a picture of how the shelter was organised.

What we don't have are any photos. There simply are none. No doubt, walking around that part of North Shields with a camera in 1941 would get you swiftly locked up.

The shelter is of course, a critical part of the story.

We know that access to the shelter was via an entrance on King Street, down some wooden steps and into the basement which had been divided into 3 distinct "rooms".

There was a family room (Room 1), an entertainments room (Room 2) and at the far end, a smoker's room (Room 3). There is a degree of uncertainty, as people who have described the shelter refer variously to "the front" of the shelter, or "the back", or the "far end". I have made best efforts, with some guesswork to provide an orientation.

These informally designated spaces were not closed off from one another – one could walk through from one end to the other. They were separated

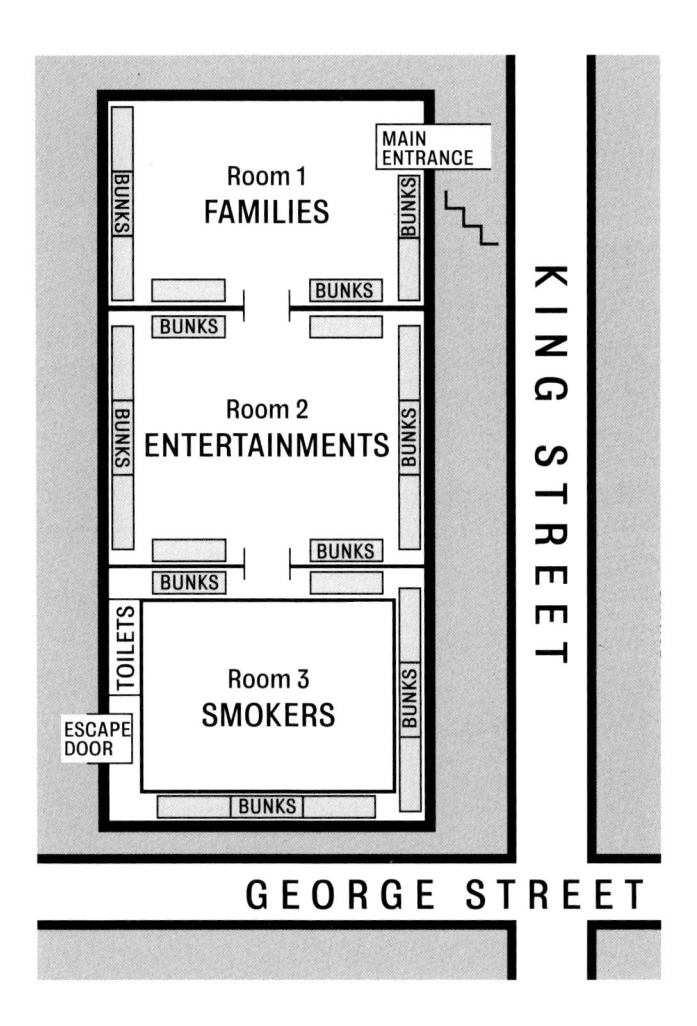

```
                    MAIN
                    ENTRANCE
  BUNKS  Room 1           BUNKS
         FAMILIES
              BUNKS                K
    BUNKS                          I
                                   N
  BUNKS  Room 2           BUNKS    G
         ENTERTAINMENTS
                                   S
              BUNKS                T
    BUNKS                          R
  TOILETS                          E
                                   E
  ESCAPE  Room 3          BUNKS    T
  DOOR    SMOKERS

              BUNKS

              GEORGE STREET
```

by blast walls installed when the basement was commissioned as a shelter. There were plenty of bunk beds for those wanting to sleep away the air raids. Often there would be music and singing – a regular accordion player was fondly remembered – and regulars enjoyed a relaxed and friendly atmosphere.

Let's take a trip back in time together.

It's Saturday night, 3rd May 1941. It's gone past 11pm. The air raid alert sirens have just sounded. What shall we do? Shall we stay at home? Or should we meet our friends, as usual, at Wilkinson's?

What would you do?

Briefing

By numbers

Aircraft involved	1
Number of bombs	4 (1 direct hit)
Estimated number in shelter	192+
Maximum capacity of shelter	188
Total number killed	107
Number who died in the shelter:	100
Number of military personnel killed	4
Number who died in hospital from injuries	7
Number admitted to hospital	36
Number treated at First Aid Centre (Kettlewell School)	16
Number of local streets with victims	21
Number of children under 16 killed	43
Number of males killed	51
Number of females killed	56
Number of victim households	56

Highest family death toll
- 6 members of the CHATER family (Mother, Father and 4 children)
- 6 members of the HALL family (Mother and 5 children)
- 5 members of the KAY family (Mother and 4 children)
- 4 members of the GERMAIN family (Father and 3 children)
- 4 members of the HARMAN family (Mother and 3 children)

Highest household death toll
7 (CURRAN/GLYNN/SMITH families sharing same house)

Youngest victim
Robert Shearer aged 3 months

Oldest victim
Emma Curran aged 80

Gallantry medal recipients: 3

Briefing

Where was Wilkinson's?

Given the distance of time, now over 75 years since the disaster and the partial redevelopment of the immediate area, there is some confusion as to the location of W. A. Wilkinson Ltd.

Waters are muddied for some too, by the fact that Wilkinson's had two sites; a main factory comprising manufacturing/warehouse/shop and offices and, over the road, a large stabling yard for the horses, carts and latterly the delivery lorries. This yard became the main site after the bombing.

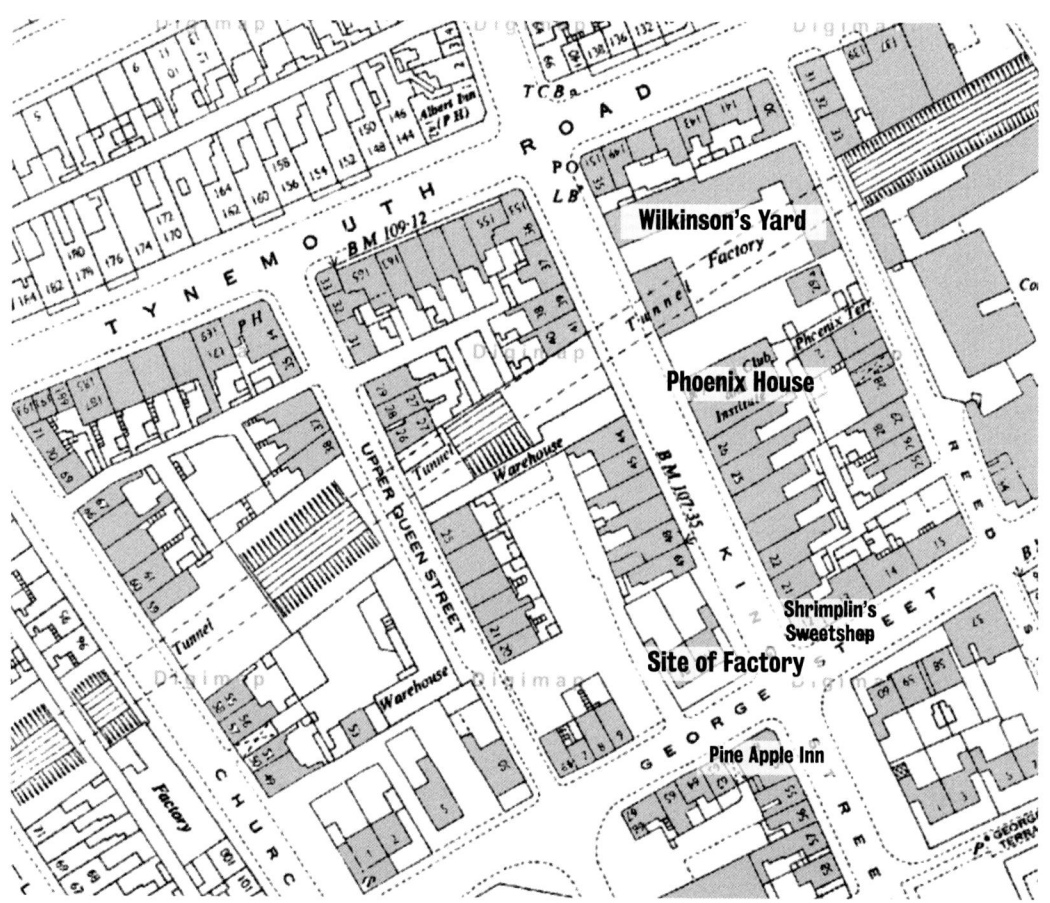

Categorically, Wilkinson's was not on the site of the current King Street Club, nor was it on the site of the East End Youth and Community Club, although this latter building is a mere bottle spin away, abutting the side entrance to the factory.

Walk past this building and stop outside the 2 houses on the corner plot. Wilkinson's was located at the current numbers 10 and 11 George Street.

W. A. Wilkinson Ltd at 51 King Street and 10 George Street

Two council houses were built on the site in 1946. There is a report that the homes were first offered to survivors of the disaster who, unsurprisingly, declined them. By 1978, the *Weekly News* reported that the house at 11 George Street had started subsiding despite having had 65 tons of concrete poured into the foundations. The houses had started to tilt with cracks appearing in the walls. A decision was taken to demolish both houses to prevent any injury to tenants. The houses were rebuilt.

Wilkinson's Yard at 34 King Street

This became a builders' yard – Clifford Leighton's and then Jeffrey Alexander's, after the business closed in the early 1960s. The buildings were demolished in 1983 and the rubble was sold off to form the foundations of the Metrocentre. Images of the yard during demolition can be found in John H Alexander's book, *Memory Lane, North Shields*.

Phoenix House at 27 King Street

Home of W. A. Wilkinson and family. It was sold in 1928, as stipulated in William Arthur's will, and became a CIU Club. Now the site of King Street Club.

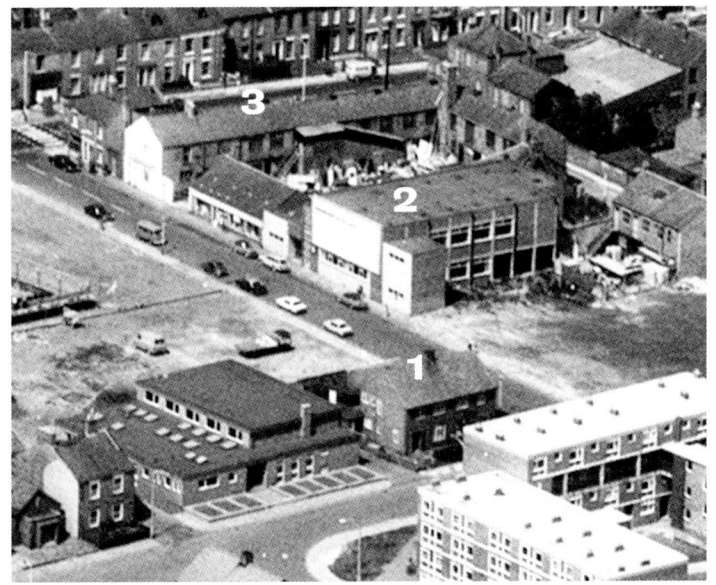

1. The site of Wilkinson's, now with two houses, on the corner of King Street and George Street. 2. King Street Club. 3. Wilkinson's Yard.

Briefing

The East End

North Shields is situated on the north bank of the River Tyne in the North East of England. It is eight miles (13km) north-east of Newcastle upon Tyne. The town is bordered to the north by Whitley Bay, to the east by the village of Tynemouth, to the west by Wallsend and to the south by the River Tyne. North Shields is part of the Metropolitan Borough of North Tyneside.

North Shields was originally a small fishing village restricted to a narrow strip of land alongside the river, hemmed in by a steep bank, with the Bank Top, 70ft (25m) above.

As conditions by the river became overcrowded and insanitary, the Bank Top area began to be developed. In 1763, Thomas Dockwray built his eponymous Square, a development of elegant town houses. He encouraged others to build there and the area became popular with those of status wishing to escape the deprivations of the riverside. Rook's Map of 1827 shows the burgeoning development of the town on a north-south axis to suit patterns of field ownership. Early developments included roperies which, when discontinued, became the long continuous terraces of housing and businesses, extant in 1941, orientated north-south. One of the early buildings was Mathews' Hall, built c1800 with an extensive garden, cottages and large conservatory. It would be taken over later in the century as the manufacturing base of W. A. Wilkinson..

Indicative of the town's growing prosperity, North Shields became part of the County Borough of Tynemouth when it was founded in 1849. The Borough's coat of arms carried the motto "Messis Ab Altis", "Our Harvest is from the Deep", a reference to the bounties enjoyed by its citizens from the sea and the coal beneath the earth.

However, the Bank Top area lost popularity relatively quickly as poor drainage and unreliable water supplies caused expense and inconvenience. Poor drainage would cause the closure of the Dockwray Square trench air raid shelter in 1941 as locals refused to suffer the often-flooded conditions.

A railway line to Tynemouth was built in 1845, cutting across the north end of the Bank Top (and dividing the Mathews' Hall property).

The wealthy moved west to Northumberland Square, which saw a prospering commercial/retail sector develop. The north west including Preston and Chirton found favour, as did eastwards to Tynemouth and the coast, as convivial areas in which to live.

For the poorest of the working poor, and there were many, life still revolved around work based on river/sea and manufacturing activities. Homes in squalid, cramped conditions had sprawled up besides and along the many steep steps leading to the Bank Top. This area of town began to acquire a notorious reputation.

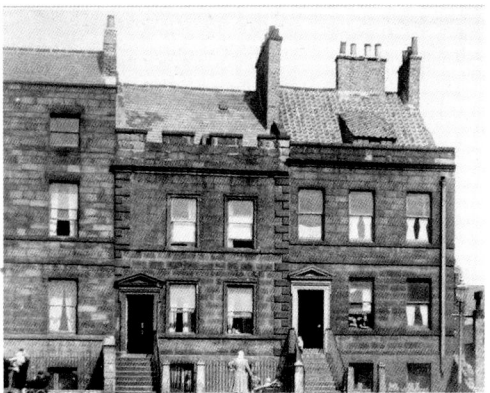

Dockwray Square housing c1949.

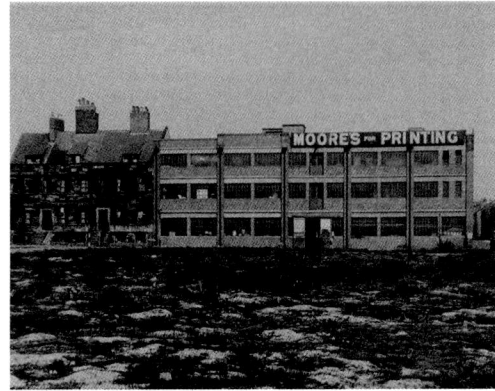

Dockwray Square – housing and industrial use side-by-side c1949.

The comic actor Stan Laurel, of Laurel and Hardy fame, grew up in North Shields and lived at No 8 Dockwray Square between 1897 and 1901. It is said that the steps down to North Shields Fish Quay inspired the famous piano moving scene in "The Music Box". By the 1930s, the same bank sides by those steps were being cleared of the slums and the residents relocated.

Dockwray Square itself had become slum tenements. The homes in the surrounding grid of streets; King Street, George Street, Church Street, were better but there was little or no green public or indeed private space. It was an area of back yards without gardens. This would cause a major headache at the outbreak of war when air raid shelter provision was being planned.

In the late thirties, the area was a grid of tightly packed houses, small businesses, pubs and shops and schools. The majority of the houses, typical of the area, were terraced and often sub-divided into flats and bedsits, with several families often residing at the same address.

In 1940, the Home Office granted permission for Tynemouth Corporation to rent the basement of W. A. Wilkinson Ltd as a public air raid shelter, for the use of those without adequate protection in the event of an air raid. There would be many. No gardens, meant no Anderson shelters. The hastily constructed brick surface shelters, often shoddily built in back yards and in back lanes, failed to attract real public confidence. Wilkinson's was an obvious choice for those in the surrounding streets. Its suitability as an air raid shelter is discussed later.

Wilkinson's shelter then, was very much in a working class, poor part of town.

It served a specific set of streets and specific family and neighbourhood groups, many of whom knew each other. They shared similar homes. The menfolk worked with their hands. In the shelter that night there were; bakers, butchers, carpenters, shipyard painters, stevedores, lorry drivers and cartmen. The women were commonly occupied with "domestic duties", or they worked in shops, or in the fish trade, or in the Tyne Brand canning factory. Some were still domestic servants. Money was always tight. It was a tough area. Decent people with hard lives. A real community.

The East End was also, in wartime, a dangerous place to live and work. The area was a direct target of the Luftwaffe. Enemy maps and aerial photos show marked targets including the nearby railway line and the electricity station on Tanners Bank. There were also myriad riverside targets, especially the Fish Quay and the shipping, merchant and Royal Navy on the river. It was also a convenient place to dump bombs before the long trip over the sea back to base. Other than the disaster at Wilkinson's, the area escaped being flattened. Amazingly.

In 1934 the area was densely populated, housing some 6,214 residents. The War accelerated a population decline already underway. By 1959, some 4,000 of the original residents of the East End had moved away due to slum clearance and other causes. The population then was, 2,243, a reduction of 2/3 from the 1934 figure.

From 1960, Tynemouth Corporation proposed to redevelop the area catering for a total population not exceeding 2000 people. As part of this plan, local public house licensing was carefully monitored and the less frequented, older establishments forced to close.

Poor quality housing replaced poor quality housing. The flats which replaced the demolished terraced houses soon gained a reputation for damp and were associated with anti-social behaviour. However, many of the "flatties" enjoyed a strong sense of community and identity together. The flats were demolished themselves within 25 years, to the relief of many.

The latest round of re-development continues apace as the area becomes once again a desirable place to live. Dockwray Square has been rebuilt with more than a nod to its former elegance. Views of the river are at a premium, as is access to the Fish Quay with its growing restaurant and gastro-pub scene. The old shops and pubs are long gone. The street grid has been altered. Things certainly 'ain't what they used to be'.

For a comprehensive and very readable account of the early history and development of North Shields, Danny Lawrence's *"From Shiels to Shields"* is a must-read.

3 Air Raid Disaster

Saturday 3rd May / Sunday 4th May 1941 (Night 609)

The following is based on survivor and eye-witness accounts.

Night 609. Blackout begins: 21.14 BST, ends: 05.21 DST
Public Alert (Newcastle Warning Dist): 23.12 BST, All-Clear: 04.11 DST

Special Constable Mathew Layzell threw on his police overcoat. It wasn't that cold, but it might turn a bit in the early hours. Closing the front door carefully behind him, he stepped into the street. Deserted. Eerily quiet. And pitch black of course. Not a glint of light. He switched on his service torch – a dim trickle of light barely illuminated the pavement ahead.

Exiting Belford Terrace, he made his way down to the Police Box on the corner at Washington Terrace. Not a soul about.

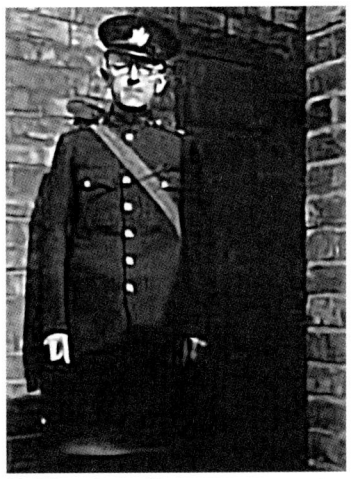

Matthew Layzell.

A faint crackle. Incendiary bombs over in South Shields.

IBs usually meant some heavy bombing coming someone's way.

On cue, the siren began to wail…a plainsong of death, he always thought. The sound cut through him every time.

Ahead, a familiar shape, waiting. Special Inspector Joseph Stuart.

He'd best hurry though. Good friends as they were, the older man liked a prompt start to their beat.

. . . .

Earlier that evening, Mrs Ellen Lee had left the Warden's Post at Kettlewell School, clutching a new notebook and pencil. Mrs Lee was the shelter warden at Wilkinson's, the old pop factory over the road in King Street. Barely keeping up ,were her son, Albert and daughter Hilda. Unlocking the shelter door, Mrs Lee looked behind and said:

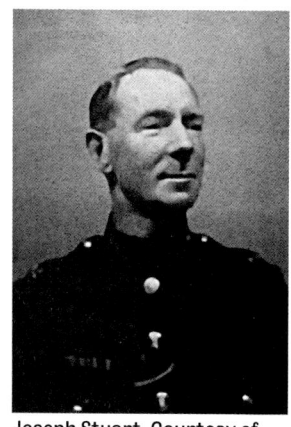

Joseph Stuart. Courtesy of Matthew Layzell.

"Come on now, usual jobs please, bunks and toilet, bunks and toilet…I'll check the emergency flashlights."

She set them to work – a quick check that everything was neat and tidy in Room 1 and then she moved through to Room 3 and unlocked the emergency exit which opened up into George Street. Room 3 was the smoking room. Not for much longer. She was going to have to have a word. She'd already been warned about the smoking from her section boss. Yes, she'd have a word. Not tonight though. Not tonight.

She picked up the notebook, strode up the 3 steps to the entrance and pushed the door open.

People were already milling around waiting to get in. She knew them all of course. They lived in the surrounding streets and were shelter regulars.

"Come on Nellie, lerrus in", someone shouted.

The tally of arrivals grew steadily in the notebook.

. . . .

"Let's get to it then", said Inspector Stuart moving off over the road and down Washington Terrace. They'd do a couple of circuits before returning for a cuppa. Hopefully, despite the alert, it would be an uneventful night.

As usual, they'd be checking the black-out and keeping an eye on any stragglers on their way home. There'd always be a few, especially if there was a dance on at Galaland.

If there was a raid on, they guided folk to the nearest shelter – the trench shelter at the corner of Tynemouth Road at Northumberland Park was the least popular, it was never dry and a few hours in there was like a punishment. Next nearest was East Street and then Wilkinson's on King Street. Constable Layzell had deep misgivings about Wilkinson's. If a bomb hit that old building then there'd be all Hell to pay.

They moved quickly along, past St. Augustin's Church and down to the road junction. All quiet. Some shapes could be made out on the path leading to the shelter trench. They walked over, the dim beam from their torches directed downwards.

"All's well", came a voice in the darkness. "We'll see people in alright".

A man brushed past, "Hurry along now". "There's no time to dawdle", called Inspector Stuart.

The two policemen turned right and up Tynemouth Road.

. . . .

At 23 King Street, the siren woke up 13 year-old Jessie Dial. She was scared of air raids. She found her mum in the living room soothing her younger brother.

"Your dad's out on duty with the ARP. He said we needed to go to Wilkinson's if the sirens go off. Bugga that. The racket in there keeps me awake. We're staying here. Get your blankets and we'll make a camp under the table".

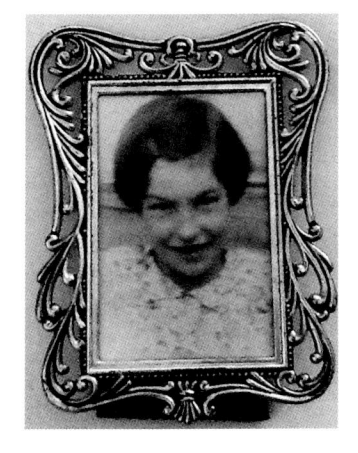

. . . .

Inside the shelter, people were settling for a long night. Who knew when the all-clear would sound? It was, however, unusually quiet. The accordion man hadn't started up and there had been no bingo, just a hubbub of chat and sporadic laughter and sing-song. Sandwiches were unwrapped and Thermos tea shared out.

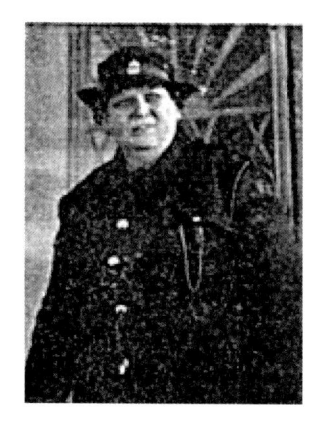

At about a quarter to midnight, Mrs Lee closed the entrance door. 190-odd inside tonight. A full house. She walked down the steps into Bay 1 and found Albert and Hilda on a nearby bunk. She put the notebook down and made a tour of the shelter. A quick look in Room 3. Packed. That smoke, she'd have to sort it out. "Nellie, come and have a chat". She turned back into Room 2. The accordion man was getting ready to play...

....

In George Street, the ARP Wardens stationed at Kettlewell School, told people hurrying now to the shelter, to go back to their homes. It was too late. The shelter was full.

....

It was close to midnight. The two policemen could hear an aircraft above.

"Heinkel?"

"No, Junkers 88", said Inspector Stuart. "You can tell by the engine drone".

"It's close. Very close."

The overcast sky meant they could see nothing, but the engine drone was getting louder.

And then a loud...THUD. Then, a deafening silence.

They began to run. Fast. Turning left into King Street, they saw a huge plume of dust and smoke. Brick, timber and glass littered the street. The clagging smell of demolished brick and wood and wall lime hit the back of their throats.

"Oh Jesus, the shelter, the shelter…"

Constable Layzell blew his police whistle as hard and as long as he could. Inspector Stuart ran back up King Street to the ARP warden's post.

"We're coming! I've rang it through. Help's coming now", someone shouted.

ARP men ran into King Street from George Street. They stopped at the corner and where the pop factory had once stood, there remained only the ghost of a building. Jagged debris seemingly suspended in mid-air, caught in the light of twenty torches. There was little left standing. Just rubble and debris. Some crates with intact bottles perched precariously on broken wooden beams. And thousands of white paper labels covered the pavements.

Constable Layzell picked one up.

"Smila", it read.

. . . .

Albert Lee remembered hearing only a loud "bonk". Then there was a blast of wind. The lights went out. Bricks and wooden spars fell around him. Chaos. And silence. Then the screaming started. Then silence again. He saw the bright glow of a match being lit and he shouted. "Put that bloody match out!". He checked himself over. He had a few scratches but that was all. His sister Hilda, next to him was in a bad way. She was moaning and crying. The woman who had been sitting opposite him was no longer there.

He heard his mother's voice from Room 2, calm and re-assuring.

"Can anyone see me light? If you can see me torch, come over to me and ah'll get you out".

Albert looked on, astonished, as he watched his mother shoulder charge a brick wall, over and over again, until it finally gave way. An escape route to the street.

"Come on then, Through the hole. Quickly before the rest comes down."

Albert was one of the first out, carrying his sister. Others followed. Lots of people followed.

Mrs Lee shouted across the street.

"Albert, get Hilda to Kettlewell. Then get home. Get me first aid kit and get me spare skirt. This one's burnt off. Hurry. Now!"

. . . .

"Davey, give me the keys. Ah'm driving tonight".

"What d'you mean? I'm the driver, you know that".

"Davey, don't argue. Wilkinson's shelter has been hit".

"Don't joke. The missus and bairns will be in there"

"I know Davey. Give me the keys."

The drive to the lemonade factory was the longest fifteen minutes of David Dial's life.

Jessie's mum heard the loud "thud" too. She opened the front door cautiously and took a few steps outside with Jessie. She looked down and saw her bare feet were bleeding. There was glass everywhere. Constable Layzell pulled them back.

"Get back inside now. The rest of it could go any minute".

When his ARP Rescue Squad lorry arrived at Wilkinson's, Davey Dial found men scurrying over a huge pile of masonry and shattered wood, thrown together and smashed as if by fighting giants. It didn't make sense. There was no chance for them, he thought. None.

Folk thronged along George Street and stood watching, dazed, from outside the old Pine Apple Inn. Wilkinson's lemonade factory was no longer there.

He glanced at his front door. Number 23, King Street. Still intact. Maybe, just maybe. He opened the door.

"Mam. Mam. It's dad. It's dad!" shouted Jessie..

Davey Dial sat on the stairs and wept.

. . . .

Outside Shrimplin's shop, ARP Heavy Squad Leader, George Newstead, found Constable Layzell,

"Bloody hell, how many?"

"We've counted 50 or so, outside. The walking wounded are being taken to Kettlewell. There's a few over there getting sorted in Webb's fish shop. Some completely untouched. Ambulances and cars are taking some of them to the Jubilee."

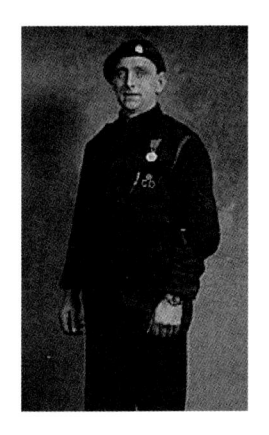

"How many still down there?"

"Mrs Lee reckons there was 190 or so in there tonight".

"I'll get the lads sorted with the kit. We'll get them out, don't worry. It's going to be a long night…."

4 Aftermath

ARP and Police personnel were at the scene almost immediately. A well-prepared Civil Defence response went into action.

The chain of command ensured effective communications. Alerted by the Warden centres at Kettlewell School and on Hamilton Terrace, ARP HQ at Cleveland Villa will have been directing the the three standing ARP Heavy Rescue and Demolition Squads within minutes. The hospitals were on stand-by.

As the scale of the incident became apparent, organisation and control of the rescue effort was essential. Such co-ordination of effort was not ad-hoc. ARP services had undergone training for such large incidents. It is known that the police and wardens first at the scene had to prevent desperate locals from digging amongst the debris in an effort to extricate those trapped. The scene was soon cordoned off.

The attempts at rescue went on all night and into the morning of the 4th. We meet some of the heroes of Wilkinson's later, but it is only fair to comment that many, many people across various rescue services, were involved. Their efforts, unstinting in the face of undoubtedly very grim scenes, tell us much about civilian determination when confronted by the horrors of war.

The right people, were at the right place at the right time. Lives were saved.

The Emergency Committee met in a special session the following morning.

Fred Egner, the Town Clerk, submitted a report to the Emergency Committee on May 14th detailing the response of the services under his remit that night. The Chief Constable's report, which would have had more detail of who, what and when, is unfortunately missing from the Tyne and Wear Archives.

Egner tells us that immediately after the 'Raiders Passed' signal had sounded on the morning of the 4th May, the Town Clerk's Office was opened as a General Information Centre, and information was supplied to all enquirers.

General Information Centre

At 9 a.m. the Tasker Hall (now a dance studio) on Howard Street was taken over for this purpose and kept open until 6 p.m. on each day until Thursday, the 8th May.

The approximate number of enquiries dealt with during this period amounted to 600.

Lists were prepared of persons requiring repairs to their properties, and these were forwarded to the Borough Surveyor for his attention. Similar lists in respect of furniture which required salving or removal were forwarded to the Salvage and Removal Officer.

Casualty Information Bureau

The Casualty Information Bureau obtained the necessary particulars relating to injured and dead from hospitals and mortuaries and lists were published outside the Town Clerk's Office, Tasker Hall and Police Station.

Relatives of dead persons were traced and notified by post or messenger.

North Shields 173

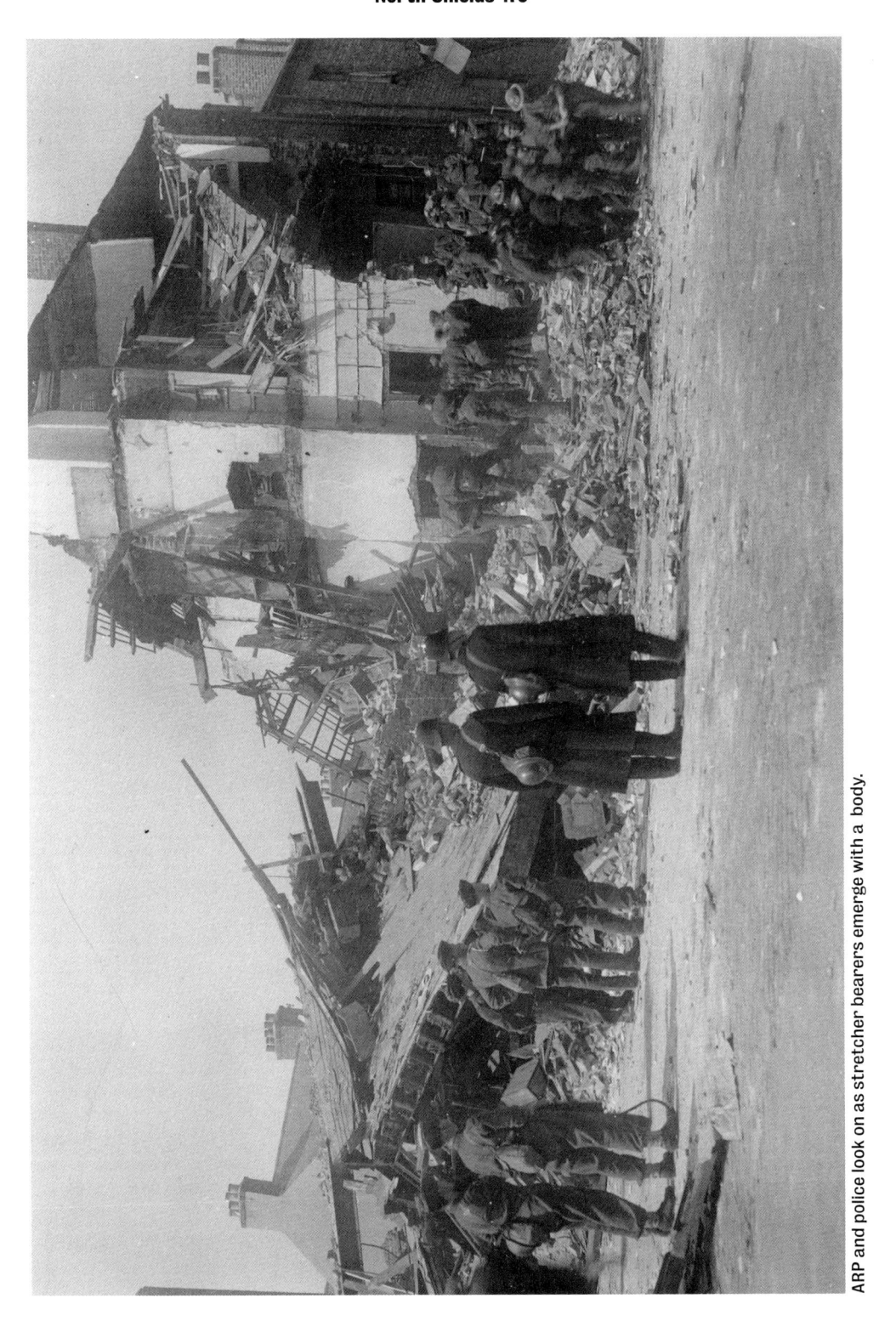

ARP and police look on as stretcher bearers emerge with a body.

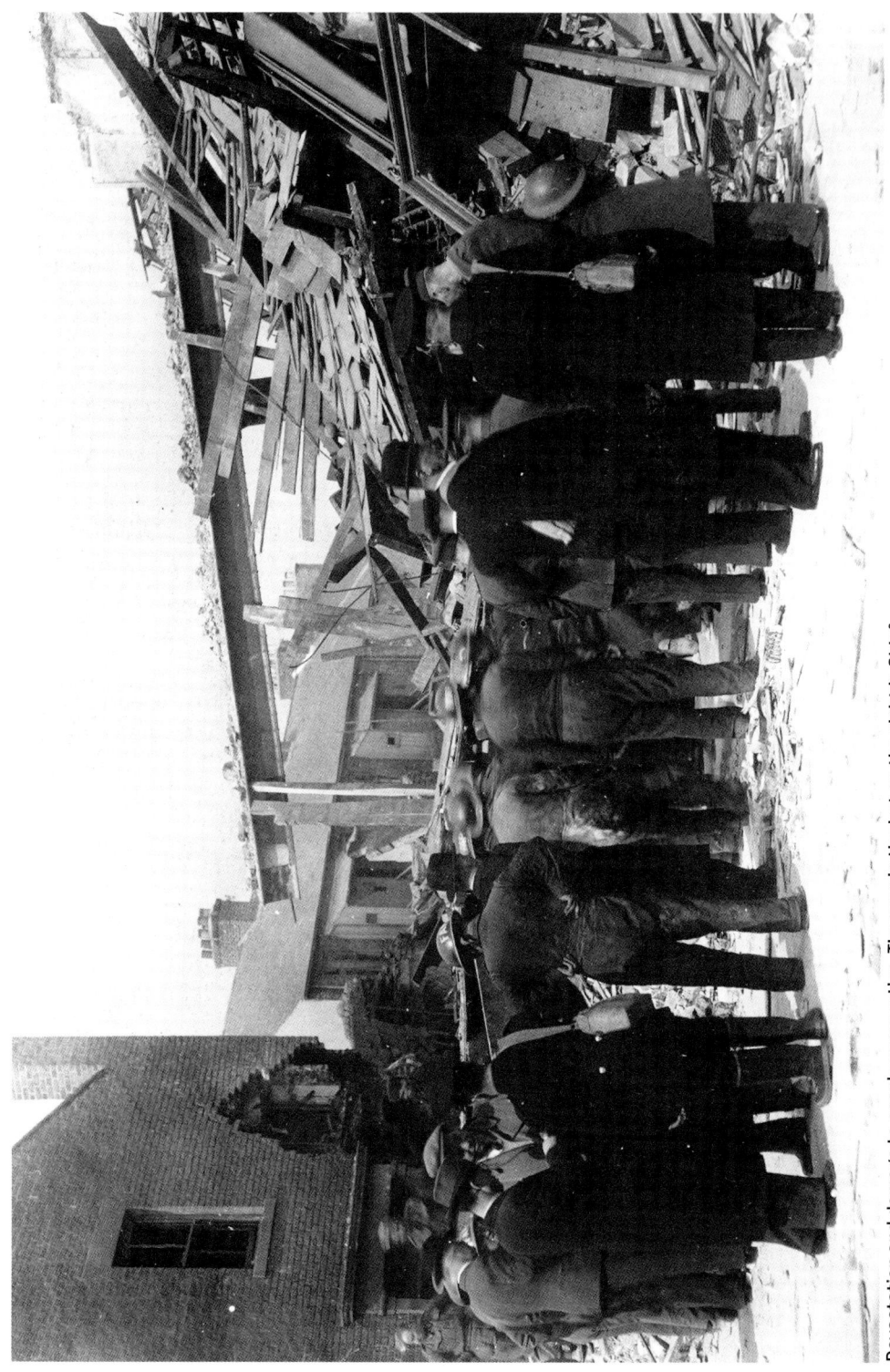

Devastation and damage to nearby properties. The man in the hat on the right is Chief Constable, Tom Blackburn. He appears in many of the Borough Bomb photos.

North Shields 173

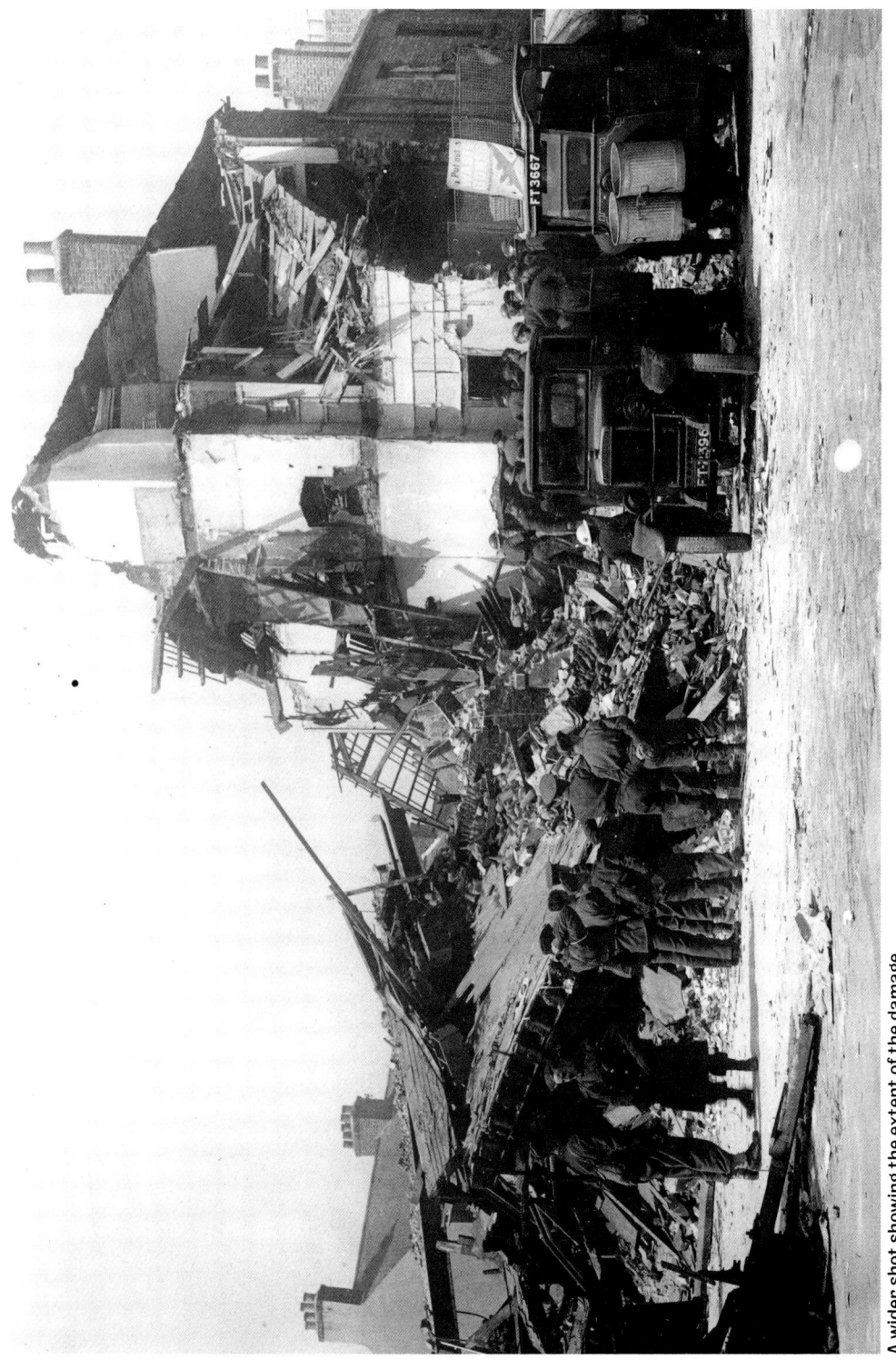

A wider shot showing the extent of the damage.

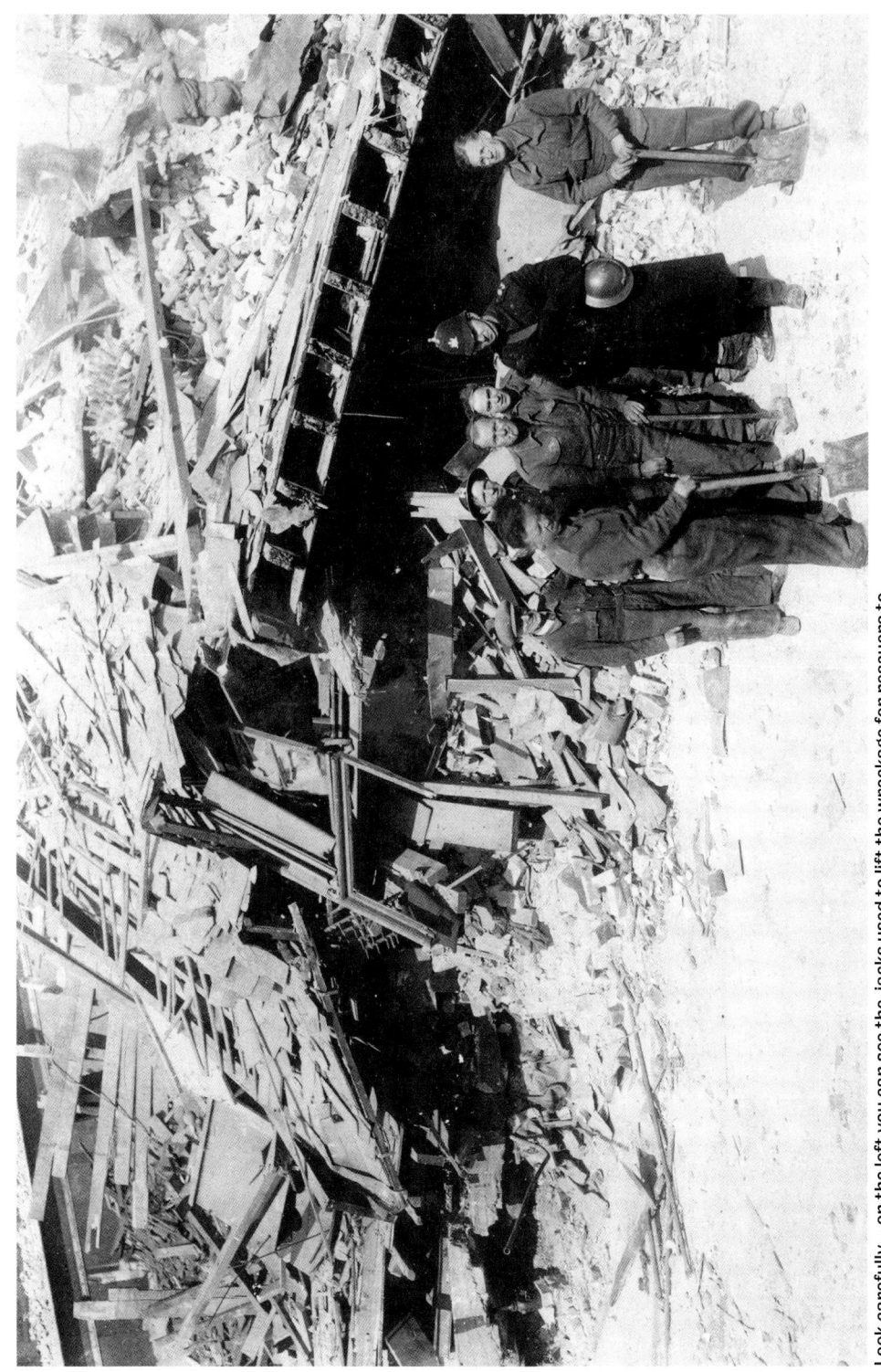

Look carefully – on the left you can see the jacks used to lift the wreckage for rescuers to crawl under. Unbelievably dangerous!

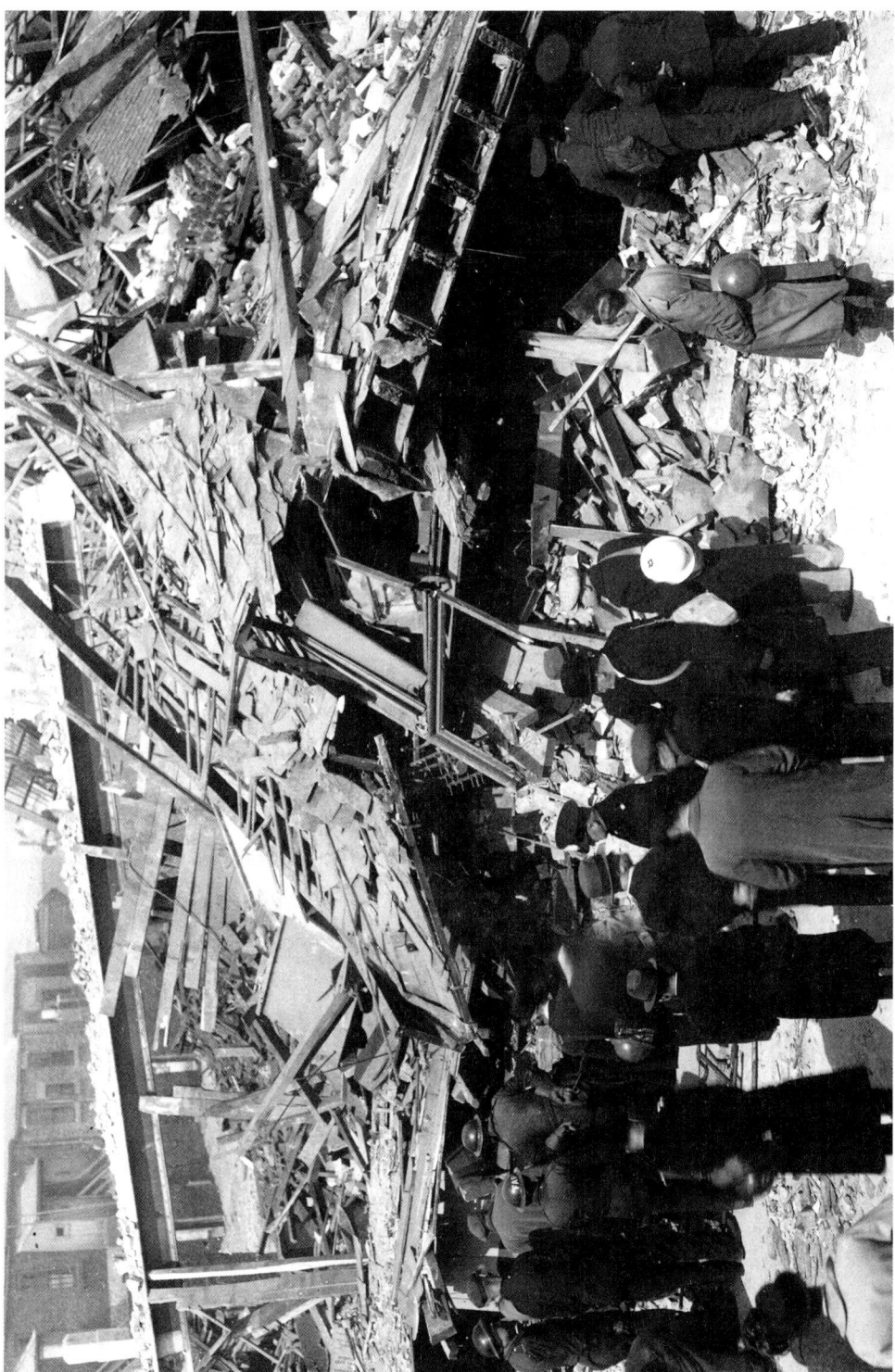

Further evidence of the dangerous conditions the Rescue Squads faced at Wilkinson's.

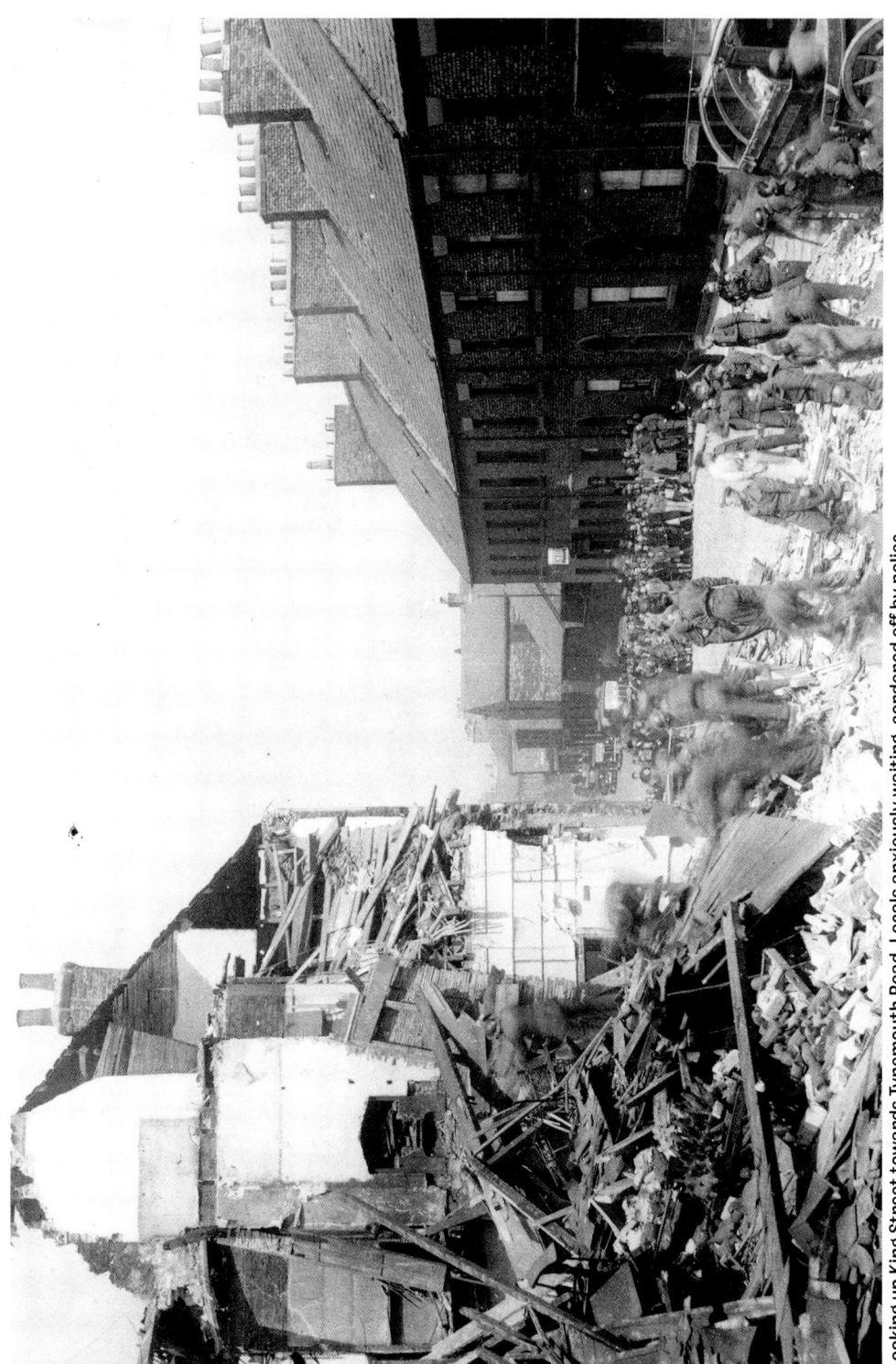

Looking up King Street towards Tynemouth Road. Locals anxiously waiting, cordoned off by police. Note the vehicles parked outside Wilkinson's yard. The CIU sign marks the former Phoenix House.

The total number of casualties recorded, in respect of the raid on the 3/4th May, was as follows:

Dead – 107
Admitted to hospital – 36
Treated at First Aid Posts – 16

Mortuary

Immediately after the raid, the Church Way Mortuary (old Bath House building) was opened and bodies continued to be admitted throughout the day. 102 bodies were received, and by Thursday, the 8th, all had been identified.

In many cases the victims were in a terrible condition but the Honorary Mortuary Superintendent (Mr A. Cragg) and his volunteer staff, drawn from E. Turnbull & Sons Ltd, worked with amazing energy and endurance from midnight on the 3rd until Thursday, the 8th with very short intervals for sleep only.

The Emergency Committee minutes show detailed planning for ARP Mortuary provision. On the 31 October 1939, expenditure on 250 aluminium ID tags and 12 dozen "Atlas" and calico body bags was approved. Sadly, they would be needed.

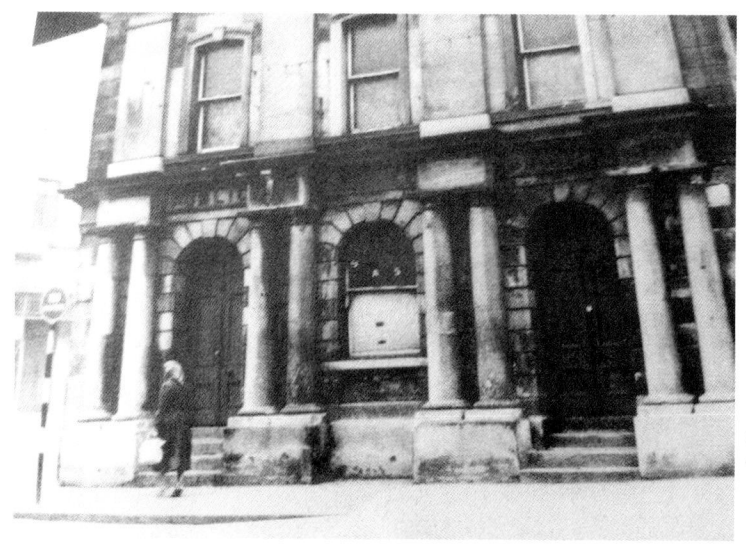

Church Way ARP Mortuary at the former public Bath House.

The maintenance of the Mortuary records was carried out by Town Clerk staff, who also assisted in the identification of the dead, and in the giving of advice to bereaved relatives. Egner drew particular attention to the outstanding work carried out by Messrs. J. Armstrong, R.L. Bradbeer and V.C. Marshall.

All relatives were informed that the Corporation would make arrangements for the burial, but in many cases the persons concerned desired the bodies to be buried privately.

The total number of burials carried out by the Corporation and under private arrangements, was as follows:

Date	Private Burials	Corporation Burials
Wednesday 7 May	8	11
Thursday 8 May	16	50
Friday 9 May	9	3
Saturday 10 May	31	1
Monday 12 May	1	7
Totals	37	79

Note: these figures also include those killed in raids on the 5th/6th May.

Preston Cemetery

Most of those killed at Wilkinson's are buried at Preston Cemetery, North Shields.

Their headstones are located throughout this beautiful cemetery according to denomination.

However, there is a communal area for most of the victims buried at the Corporation's expense. This can be found in Section C in the western part of the cemetery.

Walk up the main drive from the cemetery office. After the roundabout, continue past the section of Victorian/Edwardian graves on your left. When the hedge disappears, walk another 30m and you will see among

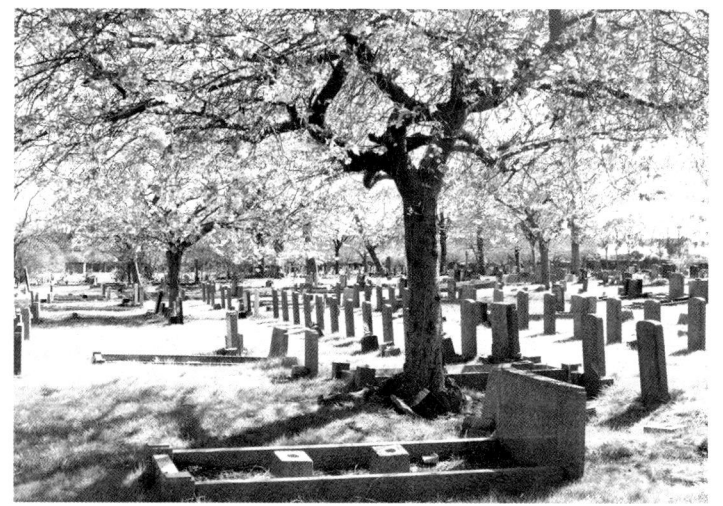

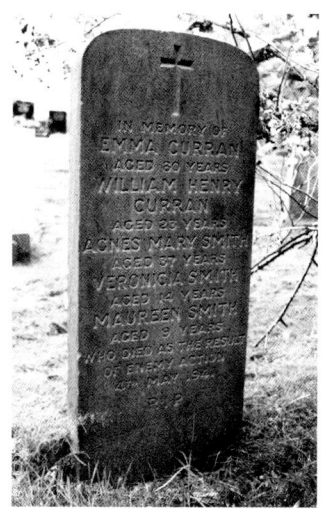

Preston Cemetery. Headstone photo courtesy of Brian Chandler.

the graves on the left, a double row of uniform headstones. The Wilkinson's graves are on either side of the cherry blossom tree. The headstones are very simple. Based on the Commonwealth War Grave design, the format was used for all civilian casualties in the Borough during the War.

There are of course, many buried in family plots. It can be quite a task to hunt them down.

There remain about 10 graves/headstones which I have been unable to locate.

There is a hugely ironic postscript to the location of these graves.

Preston Cemetery had its own air raid shelter. It is first mentioned as being under construction in September 1938. It was a trench shelter, timbered internally with a concrete roof. It had a capacity for 138 people - intended for folk caught in an air raid when visiting the cemetery or attending funerals. The shelter however was unpopular as it regularly flooded. Despite rectification work, it was deemed unusable by November 1940, filled in and sealed.

You can imagine my reaction when I was informed, almost as an aside, by cemetery office staff, that the location of this air raid shelter was where the Wilkinson's victims are buried. You really couldn't make that up, could you? Unbelievable.

The story of Wilkinson's is full of twists and turns, full of surprises.

Shields Evening News 5th May 1941

The bombing was reported in the local press but, with wartime censorship, locations were not revealed. Locals would of course know exactly what was being written about. The heroic actions of the Rescue Squads are naturally emphasised for morale purposes. It is interesting that the report of a "terrific explosion" is not one related subsequently by survivors and eye-witnesses. They almost all recall a dull "thud" or "bonk".

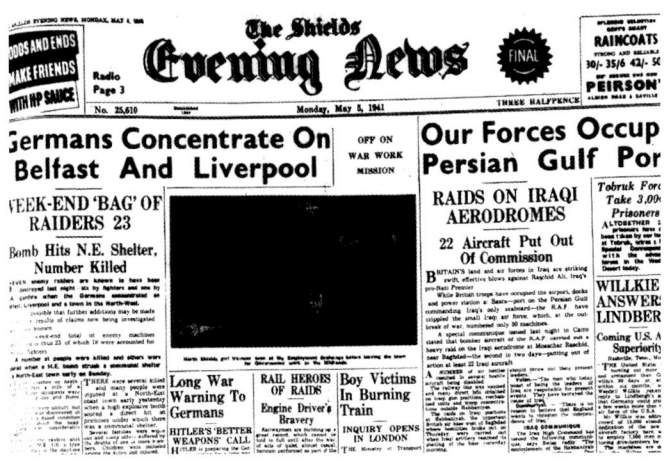

Bombing reported in the local press. Courtesy of the Shields Gazette/Johnston Press North East.

BOMB HITS N.E. SHELTER. NUMBER KILLED.

A number of people were killed and others were Injured when a H.E. bomb struck a communal shelter in a North-East town early on Sunday

There were several killed and many people were injured at a North-East coast town early yesterday when a high explosive bomb scored a direct hit on premises under which there was a communal shelter. Several families were wiped out and many others suffered by the deaths of one or more members. Children were included among the killed and injured. This shelter was extremely popular among residents of a working-class district on account of the fact that it had been heavily reinforced and was warm and comfortable. It is estimated that 200 people entered it after the sounding of the sirens and later the terrific explosion caused the collapse of the building and the shelter

SOLDIERS HELP

Some people near the exit were able to escape and others were brought out alive by members of the rescue and demolition squads who worked heroically for many hours. They received splendid assistance from soldiers. The task of ferreting among the debris for casualties proceeded all day yesterday. There were heartrending scenes of relatives inquiring after members of their family and there was agonising suspense while rescue work was going on. Practically all rescued alive needed hospital treatment and although the majority escaped with minor injuries there were some serious cases.

One man had a miraculous escape from losing a foot. Pinned down by a steel girder, rescue workers were unable to release him and a doctor went down the shelter and administered a sedative to relieve the man's agony. Strenuous efforts to release him failed and the doctor decided that the only way to save his life was to amputate the foot. When the doctor went for his instruments to carry out the operation, the rescue squad made a last bid to remove the obstruction and succeeded. The patient had been removed to hospital when the doctor returned.

Labels used by the firm on their bottles were scattered about the streets and by the irony of fate showed luscious fruit and bore the words "cheer up".

TWO WOMEN KILLED

Another bomb demolished property nearby and two women were killed.

People in a surface shelter close to this incident escaped injury. A third bomb dropped on the beach and did no damage. A.R.P. services worked magnificently throughout the night and day and ignored the danger of wrecked parts of buildings collapsing in their frantic 'efforts to save as many people as possible. It is feared that there is no hope of other entombed people being brought out alive. The raid was not a heavy one but it was unfortunate that a large shelter should have been struck.

RESCUERS' HEROISM

Grave risk of losing their lives was run by several members of rescue and first-aid parties and also soldiers. High tribute has been paid in all quarters to the resource and heroism of these men who laboured unceasingly to extricate casualties. Many of them refused to be relieved and carried on until acute weariness forced them to stop. One man, a member of the First-Aid Party, worked under extremely dangerous conditions and refused to come out when requested. As a result of his work, at least two lives were saved. This man remained in the shelter for 9 hours and was exhausted after his ordeal.

A large slab of concrete had to be jacked-up to facilitate rescue operations and despite the great danger of it collapsing, a soldier crawled underneath and entered the shelter to see if he could find anyone alive. All the time he was in the place his life was in jeopardy, but this did not deter him and it was unfortunate that his bravery was not rewarded by being able to save life.

Briefing

Wrong building, right place

At the time, the Wilkinson's disaster was considered an incident of war and filed away.

But there are serious questions to be asked, which should have been posed at the time. I can find no evidence that they ever were.

There are 2 key questions.

1. Why did they decide to locate a public air raid shelter in a building with obvious inherent dangers?
2. Did over-crowding, partly caused by over-provision of bunk-beds, contribute to the high death toll?

The wrong building in the right place?

The decision to requisition the basement at Wilkinson's for use as a public air raid shelter was taken after a survey of potential host buildings undertaken by the Borough Surveyor (Mr D.M. O'Herlihy) and his staff. ARP Committee minutes tell us this survey was begun in July 1939.

Wilkinson's was one of several buildings across the Borough under consideration. The survey must have included compliance with Home Office standards because we discover that in February 1940, a proposal to use the basement at the Park Hotel in Tynemouth was rejected because the basement walls were judged not thick enough to protect against blast and splinter.

Wilkinson's basement must have passed these Home Office standards. Two months later, in April 1940, the Home Office approved its use and allowed a grant of £95 for conversion works (installation of blast walls). On the 15th of May, the Corporation agreed a nominal rent of 5s per annum with W. A. Wilkinson Ltd for the use of their basement. The shelter opened in early Summer 1940.

One cannot imagine that there would NOT have been a discussion within the Borough Surveyor's team about the dangers posed by the machinery and material stored on the floors above the basement in the event of a direct hit. There is no evidence that the floors in this 140 year-old building were reinforced. Indeed, there are witness reports to the contrary that the floors above were wooden.

The Borough Surveyor's team were no doubt under intense pressure to ensure air raid shelter provision matched need….and quickly. There was a key requirement under the Civil Defence Act (1939) that Local Authorities had to provide free air raid shelter provision for those residents who had none or who were caught in the streets at the time of a raid.

This had particular resonance for the residents in the streets around Wilkinson's. In October 1939, residents of Church Street complained to the local paper about the lack of shelters in the surrounding area. Later complaints identified the problems with flooding in local trench shelters (especially Dockwray Square).

Tynemouth Corporation had toyed with the idea of "deep shelter" provision for its residents. It had considered huge, bomb-proof, shelters capable of protecting thousands. Ideas included the use of the local sewer system and the ambitious Kearney tube proposal for a railway under the Tyne to South Shields, whose tunnel could be used by both populations in times of air attack. In the end, Tynemouth preferred a "dispersal" provision via multiple smaller shelters which reduced the risk of catastrophic loss of life.

Later, in November 1940, the *Shields Evening News* carried Hastie D. Burton's (Chair of the Emergency Committee) avowal that "maximum effort would be given to building brick surface shelters with the dispersal of the population being a priority. Then attention would be given to further shelters in different parts of the town".

The East End of town was problematic. It was an area of back yards and lanes. There were few suitable buildings with basements large enough for a public air raid shelter. Pub basements (and there were lots of those) were prohibited for use as air raid shelters for obvious reasons. It was a heavily built up area with Luftwaffe targets immediately adjacent. Shelters were desperately needed for residents and workers.

The factory was in exactly the place where need was greatest. And, as luck would have it, Wilkinson's bordered Tynemouth Road, a key motor and pedestrian artery into and out of North Shields.

Was Wilkinson's then, simply too good an opportunity for officials to ignore, whatever the inherent dangers?

We will never know what really informed the decision to requisition that basement. Today it would not have cleared the proposal stage. 192 local residents trusted official judgement that night in May 1941, over a hundred would not see the morning. Nobody faced censure for this decision, which even in wartime can best be described as expedient.

Over-crowding and the Bunk Bed Problem

Another reason for official embarrassment over Wilkinson's is the strong probability that the shelter was over-crowded.

The number of people in the shelter was officially given as 192. Assuming it to be correct, then the occupancy slightly exceeded the Home Office designation of 188. In the photo, an external wall sign next to the shelter door clearly shows the figure of 210. The occupancy limit for the shelter may well have been increased since it was originally approved in 1940, but I can find no reference to this change in any of the available records.

The occupancy limit is important when combined with the issue of the bunk beds.

A Home Office circular instructed that bunk beds be installed in all public air raid shelters excluding trench shelters.

The *Shields Evening News* reported on 11th November 1940 that,

> *it is the intention of the Emergency Committee to make the shelters as comfortable as possible. The bunk system is to be introduced and measurements are now being taken. Basement shelters In the Borough are excellent and perfectly dry and bunks will be placed in these wherever possible.*

The Emergency Committee on 27th December 1940, instructed the Borough Surveyor to

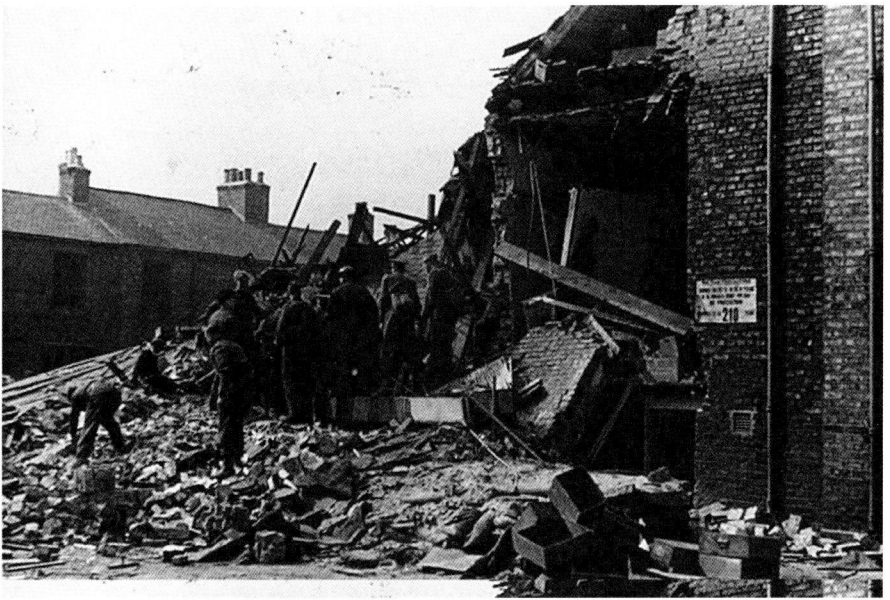

The entrance to basement shelter on King Street. Note the figure on the occupancy number sign – 210.

request and install enough bunks for a population of 39,364 persons.

So, just a few months before the disaster, the shelter on King Street was fitted with double bunks.

The installation of the bunks in the Borough's shelters, with the resultant reduction of space for people inside clearly raised a few red flags. The Chief Constable reported on the bunk bed situation to the Emergency Committee on 3rd April 1941. We do not know what was said in that report. It was resolved however, that the Borough Surveyor be instructed to:

a) reduce the numbers of bunks already erected in public air raid shelters with the reduction to be at the discretion of the Chief Constable and the Chief Air Raid Warden.

b) refrain from erecting any further.

This instruction was given a month before the shelter suffered a direct hit. Did the Borough Surveyor comply with this instruction so that the bunk provision at Wilkinson's was reduced before the bombing? Or did they agree only on a minimal reduction at Wilkinson's? .

The suspicion is that the bunks were not removed in time. One of the first instructions from the Emergency Committee on the 5th May (second meeting after the bombing) was that 50% of bunks were to be removed from public air raid shelters. The Borough Surveyor was also instructed to enquire from the Home Office, the number of bunk beds deemed essential in Public Air Raid Shelters. Clearly, there was something amiss.

The response from the Home Office caused the Emergency Committee to immediately restrict the maximum occupancy of all public air raid shelters in Tynemouth Borough to 50 people, with the number of bunks in such shelters in numerical relation to the capacity.

Was Wilkinson's overcrowded? Perhaps not in terms of its actual occupancy license, but in terms of reduced internal space, one can only conclude that it was. The installation of bunks meant that the occupancy limit was far too generous. The double bunk beds along each wall in the 3 rooms of the shelter will have reduced space and possibly contributed to the death toll from splinter injuries and the hampering of rescue attempts.

It can be imagined that the Emergency Committee received verbal reports from the Chief Constable and others immediately after the bombing and up to that second meeting. If the smashed wooden bunk beds had been discovered to be a contributory factor to the death toll, then it would come as a shattering blow to members. The Committee's resolutions seem to suggest there was no doubt.

Again, nobody was held to account.

Illumination

On 4th May, the morning after the disaster, the Emergency Committee (first meeting after the bombing) directed the Borough Surveyor to take such steps as may be necessary for diminishing the intensity of the illuminated direction signs at certain public air raid shelters.

One can detect a sense of "having to be seen to do something". The implicit suggestion that somehow an illuminated sign was a contributing factor to the disaster is absurd. The idea that the pilot of a Junkers Ju. 88 travelling at 250mph at maybe 10,000ft would be guided to a target by a wall sign is stretching it somewhat.

Wilkinson's is never referred to by name in the various minutes. After May 1941 it does not feature at all. There was a War to fight after all. Life moved on.

Forgotten?

It comes as no surprise then, that for decades, the disaster at Wilkinson's Lemonade Factory was written out of the town's history.

It must be remembered that the death toll at Wilkinson's makes it of national importance in the history of the wider Blitz. Until the digitisation of archival records and the rise of the Internet, national awareness of the disaster was negligible.

The bombing and its wider local context was covered in Dr Craig Armstrong's superb *Tyneside in the Second World War* (2007). It is also mentioned in Joshua Levine's *The Secret History of the Blitz* (2015). The **northshields173.org** website has of course explored the incident since 2000.

The disaster was never forgotten by those involved – many, many families were affected by the events of that evening. Following a memorial service at St Augustin's Church in the week following the disaster and after five days of mass burials, the community was left to get on with it. And this they did, seeing out the war with fortitude and dignity.

The East End community around what was Wilkinson's began to fragment and disperse with the slum clearances in the area during the 1950s and 1960s. Whilst a few families remained, there was no collective remembrance of the bombing event.

In the 1980s and with a new vogue for local and family history, North Tyneside Libraries began to mark anniversaries of the bombing with small scale reminiscence projects. Occasionally articles and letters about the disaster would appear in the local press.

A campaign led by ex-Servicemen groups prompted North Tyneside Council to finally mark the disaster officially. In 2003, a rather underwhelming plaque was erected with some ceremony, in the town's shopping mall.

In 2013, myself and a group of 5 shelter survivors took part in the BBC2 documentary series "How We Won the War".

The 75th anniversary of the disaster in 2016, was marked by a Memorial Service, appropriately held at St Augustin's Church. This attracted 200 locals, survivors and families of those killed, and was featured on TV and local radio. Members of the Wilkinson family commissioned a new memorial plaque which was unveiled by the Mayor of North Tyneside, Norma Redfearn, at the East End Youth and Community Centre, next door to the site of the factory.

Now, the purpose of this book, as a companion to the **northshields173.org** website, is to contribute to keeping the memory of the disaster alive. Although a tragic event, it is part of our town's story and it deserves to be remembered for those who lost their lives and those whose bravery rescued so many.

5 Wilkinson Heroes

With what remained of the factory likely to collapse at any moment, the number of those working amongst the debris was kept to a minimum. This caused disquiet amongst the local men and women, desperate to help, but cordoned off from the site by ARP personnel.

It was the Rescue Squads, First Aid Parties and doctors, now on scene, that would work through the long night and into the morning. It was their dedication and skill that would undoubtedly reduce the death toll.

As Craig Armstrong explains in *Tyneside in the Second World War,* the Rescue Squads had received extensive training in their work. This training and the evaluation of previous incidents led to growing expertise and the deployment of specific techniques. "For example, it was quickly discovered that it was safer to dig trapped people out from the side rather than the top of a pile of debris."

The aftermath photos show Rescue Squad personnel still on site, including stretcher bearers removing a victim. Theirs was a prolonged effort, exhausting and without doubt, emotional. For some, they were attempting to rescue friends and neighbours.

Many of those who worked to rescue victims that night remain unknown and unrecognised.

However, it was an endeavour that revealed true heroism, where individuals repeatedly risked their own lives to rescue those trapped.

Three ARP personnel would receive official recognition for their efforts.

One, remembered by many and whose determination and courage, saved 32 people from the basement. Her efforts went unrewarded.

Wilkinson's had a heavy death toll, but it also had its heroes of whom the town can be rightly proud.

There were 2 recipients of the George Medal and one recipient of the British Empire Medal.

The existing awards open to civilians at the start of the War were not judged suitable to meet the new situation, eg the Blitz. It was decided in 1940 that the George Cross and the George Medal would be instituted to recognise both civilian gallantry in the face of enemy bombing and brave deeds more generally. The George Medal would be awarded for gallantry "not in the face of the enemy".

Announcing the new awards, the King said:

> In order that they should be worthily and promptly recognised, I have decided to create, at once, a new mark of honour for men and women in all walks of civilian life. I propose to give my name to this new distinction, which will consist of the George Cross which will rank next to the Victoria Cross and the George Medal for wider distribution

The British Empire Medal was instituted in 1917 for meritorious service, but from the beginning some awards were for acts of gallantry. There were an increased number of cases in the Second World War for service personnel and civilians including the merchant marine, police and emergency services and civil defence. From 1940, the BEM was awarded for acts of gallantry that did not reach the standard of the George Medal.

Clarence Burdis GM

Mr Burdis – Leader, ARP Rescue Party, Tynemouth, was awarded the George Medal.

From the medal citation: *The London Gazette*, issue 35226, 22nd July 1941.

> *Burdis cut through a thick wall and entered another room in the basement in which a number of casualties were lying interlaced with timber from bunks which had collapsed. In spite of the great confusion Burdis extricated these casualties one by one, passing them through the small hole to other members of the Squad. He worked unaided in a confined space for nearly four hours until he partially collapsed through exhaustion. On recovery, he insisted on returning to the basement and, by his gallant efforts, saved a number of lives.*

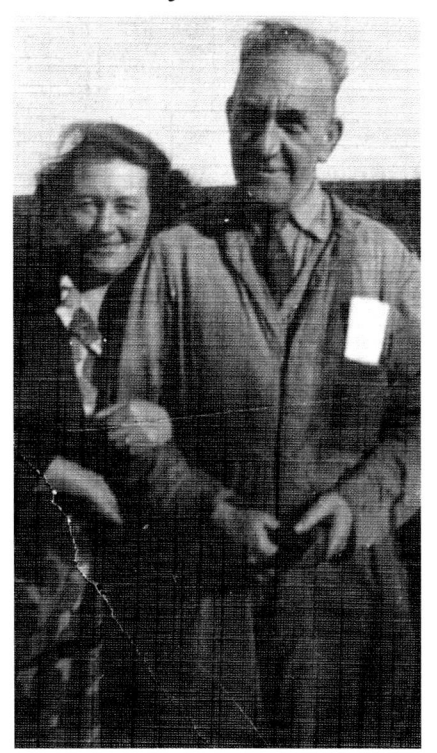

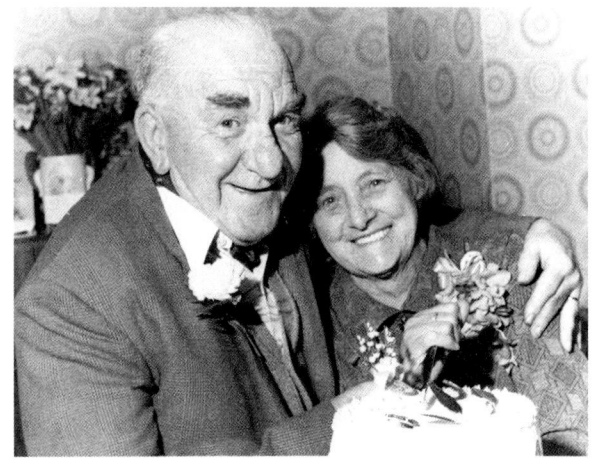

(Left) Clarence Burdis and his wife Charlotte. (Above) on their Gold Wedding.

Clarence Burdis died in June 1974. Born in 1901, he worked as a builder and labourer. These were prized skillsets for ARP Heavy Squad personnel.

George Newstead GM

Mr Newstead – Leader, ARP Rescue Party, Tynemouth – was awarded the George Medal.

From the medal citation: *The London Gazette*, issue 35226, 22nd July 1941.

> *A building suffered a direct hit and people were trapped in the basement. Newstead cut a hole through the wall to a room containing a number of casualties and arranged for their removal. One man was trapped by his leg under tons of debris. Medical assistance was called ctime Newstead, at great risk to his life, succeeded in getting into position a small jack and relieved the pressure on the man's foot. By cutting away the boot he succeeded in dragging the man to comparative safety. Newstead, who was aware that at any moment during the rescue operation the building might have collapsed, showed outstanding courage.*

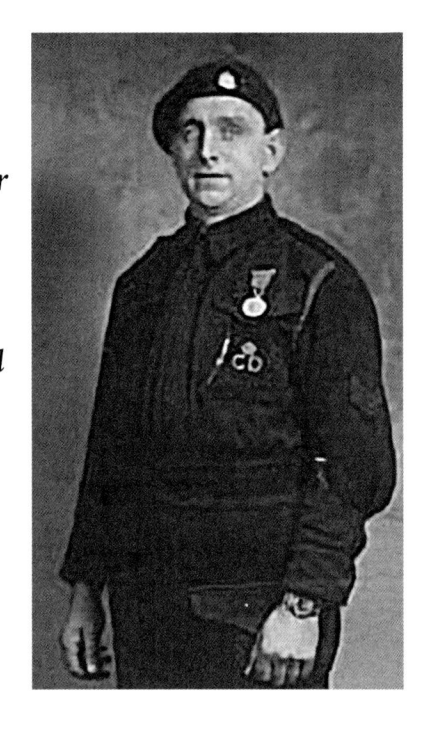

The following information was kindly provided by Mrs Patricia Lydon, granddaughter of George Newstead.

> My Grandfather never really mentioned Wilkinson's to us. He was a modest man and I suppose the War was just something he wanted to forget. He was a very active man, always busy providing for his family. I'm very proud of him and what he did.
>
> My Grandfather would've been about 40 years old at the time of Wilkinson's. He wasn't originally from North Shields – he was a miner from Langley Park in County Durham.
>
> When he came up here, he was a mason for Tynemouth Corporation

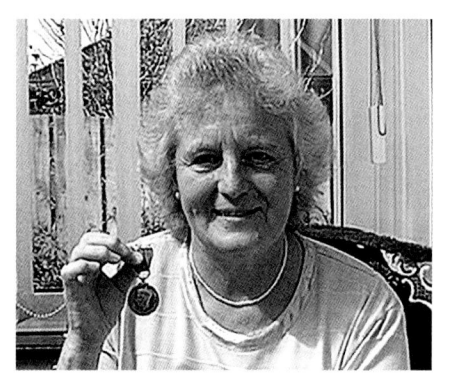

from 1931–1939. He was always good at making money though. He opened a General Dealer's shop in Grey Street next to Davies Dairy and lived above the shop. In the summer he used to have a candy floss machine and sold it to the day-trippers in Tynemouth. He also sold ice-cream at the Coast.

When the War broke out, he would make and give away pea soup and broth to the poor at his shop. He joined the Civil Defence and became a Sergeant. Perhaps he was on duty that night. Certainly, his mining background helped him get to the trapped man where others would have given up.

He presented his George Medal to Tynemouth Borough (this was later returned to him when he emigrated). After the War he kept the shop on and did more building work until the early 60's. In 1963 he and his wife Rachel emigrated to Australia to join their daughter Edith in Adelaide. Returning to North Shields briefly in 1969, George died in Australia in 1987.

Mr Burdis and Mr Newstead travelled to the Investiture at Buckingham Palace on Thursday November 6th, 1941. The *Shields Evening News* reported on the event. Note the censorship in the article.

North Shields Air Raid Heroes Decorated

For their gallantry and devotion to duty during air raids in May last, two members of Tynemouth ARP Rescue and Demolition Service, Mr George Newstead of 32 Waterloo Place, North Shields and Mr Clarence Burdis of 55 Roseberry Avenue, Preston were decorated with the George Medal by the King at an Investiture held at Buckingham Palace last night.

Both men displayed exceptional courage, endurance and resourcefulness in carrying out rescue work at a building which had been directly hit by a bomb and were instrumental in saving life.

Mr Newstead was accompanied by his wife and daughter, Edith and Mr Burdis by his wife, baby girl and his mother, Mrs T Dobing. They travelled together to London on Thursday, spent the afternoon and night in the city and attended the Palace yesterday morning.

Returning home by the night train, they arrived back at North Shields at 6 o'clock this morning.

"It was an outstanding experience in our lives", Mr Newstead told an *Evening News* reporter, "and apart from the object for which we went there, well worth the trouble of the journey to London.

Our wives and other relatives were placed in seats in the Investiture Hall and had a splendid view of the proceedings. Everyone was very kind to us after our arrival at the Palace and we felt quite at home.

Although very impromptu, it was a very homely ceremony, and everybody appeared to be quite at ease. There were about 200 recipients of the decoration altogether and we walked from the waiting room at the rear of the Palace to the Investiture Hall in single file.

Burdis was just in front of me. When my turn came, the King said, "Congratulations", shook me by the hand and hung the medal on my left breast. I felt very proud and said "Thank you, sir", and passed on to the band room looking into the Hall from which I had a good view of the rest of the proceedings."

Burdis agreed with Newstead that the ceremony was simple and homely and said that he also felt at ease.

"When my turn came the King asked me when the raid took place. I told him it was in May and the King remarked, "Oh yes, I recall it". The King then congratulated me shook my hand and hung the medal on my breast. My wife and my mother who saw the ceremony from beginning to end thought it was a grand sight"

(*Evening News,* Saturday 8th November 1941

Norman Darling Black BEM

Mr Black – First Aid Party, Tynemouth, was awarded the British Empire Medal.

From the medal citation: *The London Gazette*, issue 35226, 22nd July 1941.

> Black made sustained and strenuous efforts to free injured persons from the debris and rendered first aid. He displayed courage and devotion to duty with complete disregard of his own safety.

The following information was supplied by Norman Darling Black's son, George, (aged 72 at time of interview in 2000).

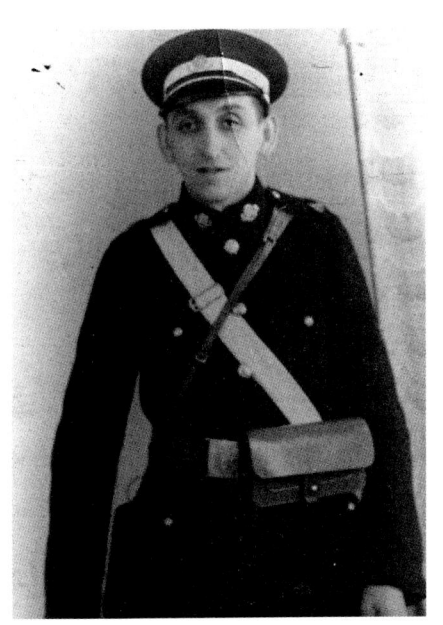

When the air raid sounded that night, my mother and I went to the nearest air raid shelter. My father was an ARP Warden and was on duty with the rest of the team members. At the time of the raid we were living in the caretaker's quarters of the Salvation Army in Prudhoe Street, North Shields.

During this air raid there was a bomb dropped which hit Wilkinson's lemonade factory. The basement of this factory was used as an air raid shelter for both day and night raids. Many families, amongst them friends and relatives went to this shelter. It held over 200 people. When the bomb hit, the factory machinery and everything came down trapping everyone in the shelter.

When the ARP team arrived, also the Police and Fire Brigade, they all realised what had happened and started straight away knowing the dangerous situation of all those trapped in the basement. After hours of working together with doctors getting the people out, one false move could have brought any heavy object down including machinery. The ARP team had to work on their backs, sides and fronts, inch by inch jacking masonry and machinery up very slowly to make it safe, so they could get people out. One story is of a man who was trapped. My father, working with a doctor, cut the man's laces to remove his boots and only then was he able to drag the man free.

My father was trained as a first-aider and seeing the seriousness of the situation was prepared to work until everyone was out. He did this for many hours in very dangerous conditions until everyone, injured or dead was taken from the basement.

For his bravery he was awarded the British Empire Medal. Two other men were awarded the George Cross. My father's friends and colleagues thought that he deserved further recognition for his actions, so they presented him with a gold watch.

On December 1st, 1941, my father, mother and I travelled down to London. On December 2nd at Buckingham Palace, His Majesty King George VI awarded ARP Warden, Norman Darling Black with the British Empire Medal. It was a proud and wonderful day for the family.

Whilst we were in London, we stayed at the Salvation Army Hostel, Hoxton Goodwill Centre and were escorted around by Captain Giles who was an Australian.

After the War, my father became a psychiatric nurse at St. Nicholas Hospital in Gosforth. Before he retired he became Deputy Chief Male Nurse.

Following the disaster numerous children were evacuated to safer locations. The day of the evacuation we all met at the school we attended which was Queen Victoria. Our mums and dads were there to see us off with a parcel of food, big hugs, kisses and a lot of love and tears.

EMPIRE MEDALLIST

At Buckingham Palace on December 2nd H.M. the King pinned the British Empire Medal to the breast of Colour-Sergeant Gordon D. Black, of North Shields Corps, and said, 'I congratulate you.'

A bomb struck a public shelter under a factory and many tons of debris and machinery collapsed upon it. Brother Black, serving with a First-Aid unit, struggled through a narrow opening, risking his life to find living people buried under the debris.

For four hours he worked at great hazard to extricate a child imprisoned by many tons of masonry. He was advised to rest after this dangerous feat but returned to rescue an imprisoned man. With a 'jack' Brother Black began to prise up the crashed roof, knowing that four high walls and about 40 tons of machinery were suspended insecurely over his head.

A doctor crawled in and handed anesthetic to Brother Black, who administered it to the imprisoned man. He then cut the victim's boots away and pulled the man out of his boots to freedom.

He does not know the names of the two whose lives he saved.

Brother Black has studied First-Aid for eight years. When his duties allow his joy is to carry the Army Colours. While in London for the presentation Brother Black, his wife and son were entertained at the Heaton Goodwill Centre.

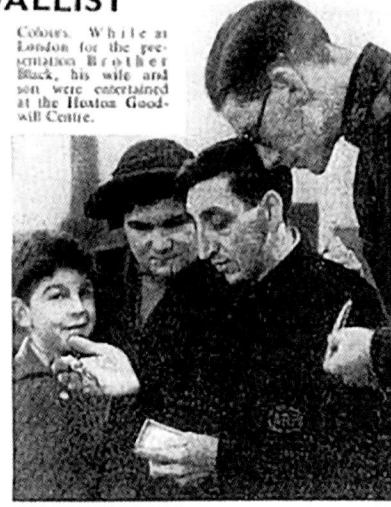

From War Cry, December 27, 1941.

My placement was at Horsley Vicarage near Otterburn, with the vicar, his wife and housemaid. There was another boy who stayed there with me. We went to Otterburn school. I'd like to say a big thank you to the people who looked after the boys when we were evacuated.

When my father and mother moved away from North Shields to a village called New York, about three miles away, I was allowed to go back to my parents. I lost contact with the boy who I became friends with when I was evacuated

I went to several local schools: Queen Victoria and King Edward's in North Shields, New York Junior School and Shiremoor Secondary Modern (?). Perhaps someone remembers me?. I left North Shields and joined the RAF as a musician. I then became a psychiatric nurse, just as my father had been.

Whilst writing this and remembering those times, Psalm 23 has been going through my mind…"the Lord is my Shepherd…". God bless.

Ellen Lee – Wilkinson's Shelter Warden

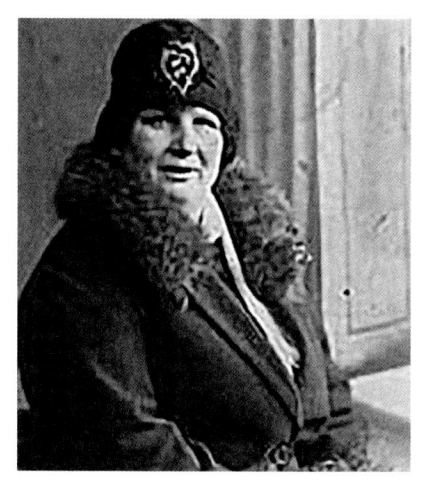

The person whom many survivors recalled vividly was the shelter Warden, Mrs Ellen Lee. She is thought to have seen 32 people to safety despite her own injuries which included acid burns from the chemicals stored in the factory.

At the time of the bombing, Mrs Lee lived at 2 Hamilton Terrace in North Shields, just around the corner from Wilkinson's factory.

She stood 6ft tall and weighed close to 18 stone. She was, as everyone recalled, a large lady with a big heart – she would do anything for anyone. She was known locally as Nellie.

Mrs Lee was the ARP Warden in charge of Wilkinson's Shelter. It was her job to open the shelter when the sirens sounded, counting people coming in and ensuring good order. As part of the wider ARP Warden network, she was trained in first aid and had an in-depth knowledge of the local streets, who lived where, the shelter arrangements of each family and where key emergency resources were located. Mrs Lee would have spent much time, to-ing and fro-ing between the ARP Warden centres at Kettlewell School and on Tynemouth Road.

Mrs Lee was inside the shelter in No. 2 Room. When the bomb hit, everything went dark and then the screams and shouts started. Mrs Lee called for everyone to keep quiet. Switching on her torch, she shouted: "See me light, I'll get you out". Moving through to No 1 Room, Mrs Lee found the exit door blocked with fallen rubble and bricks. Using her strength and weight she shoulder-charged the wall repeatedly until it gave way enough to make an opening onto the street. She stood at this escape route until 32 people had managed to get out.

Ellen Lee

Born: 24/3/1894
Ellen was one of 11 children.
Parents: Sarah Bell Parker (Dodds) and Joseph Parker
Married: Albert Lee 13/1/1916
Albert came from Bradford and was in the Duke of Wellington's Regiment. He died in 1965 at his daughter Hilda's home in Redditch.
Children: Albert and Hilda.
Residences: 1939: Coburg Terrace. 1941: 2 Hamilton Terrace. 1951: 155 Tynemouth Road.
Died: 24/4/1951, aged 56. Ellen was cremated at West Road Crematorium in Newcastle on 27/4/1951.

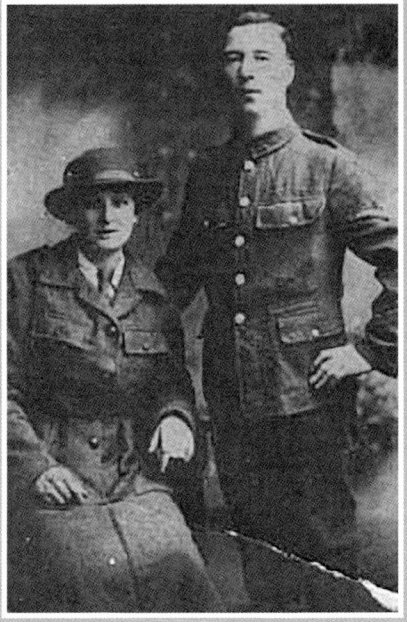

Ellen and Albert Lee during the First World War.

With thanks to Julie Simpson, the great, great niece of Ellen Lee for sharing her family tree research.

Mrs Lee suffered cuts and bruises and had extensive acid burns to her face Nevertheless she remained at her duty. Her son Albert and daughter Hilda were both in No 1 Room. Albert was unharmed but Hilda had bad injuries: a wound the size of her head in her side and a broken arm and leg.

Once she had guided the survivors to the street outside, Mrs Lee instructed Albert to run home to fetch a first aid kit and to bring her a new skirt – it had been blown off in the explosion! Mrs Lee then made her way to Kettlewell School and helped First Aid Parties tend to the injured.

Her husband, himself a full time first aider, rushed from his post in Albion Road to the school. When he got to Kettlewell, he didn't recognise his daughter Hilda as her injuries were so severe.

On Wednesday 18th June, during the visit of King George VI and Queen Elizabeth to Tynemouth, She was introduced to the King and Queen with the blue chemical residue from Wilkinson's still marking her face. The Queen shook her hand and expressed her admiration saying; "You were very brave indeed".

Mrs Lee continued as an ARP Warden until the end of the war. She built a close relationship with the soldiers of the Third Regiment Maritime R.A. billeted at Kettlewell School. She washed, darned and sewed for them, advised them on personal and general problems and did everything she could to make their stay comfortable.

At the end of the war, Mrs Lee received a letter from Major S. Horne enclosing a cheque in recognition of her services to the men.

Mr's Lee's lack of official decoration seems a strange oversight. She was widely admired for her actions that night and received universal praise. She was injured herself in the bombing and remained in the shelter at some personal risk, until over 30 people had escaped using a route she had fashioned. Furthermore, she spent the rest of the night, tending to the injured. Without doubt, she demonstrated outstanding courage, leadership and determination.

Was Mrs Lee overlooked because of her gender? Or was it because she was simply an ARP Warden and not part of the Officers' Club?

The injustice rankles still. Recently, attempts have been made to rectify the situation. North Tyneside Council has made approaches to see if she can be posthumously recognised. Apparently, this is unlikely, unless substantial new evidence supporting her case can be submitted. One hopes that some official memorial or honour can be organised for this remarkable lady.

Out of the debris then, amazing stories of courage, endurance and resourcefulness. A different breed perhaps, a different generation. How would we cope today?

6
The Victims A-Z

The following 107 people were killed as a result of enemy action at Wilkinson's Air Raid Shelter: May 3rd and 4th 1941.

Details of each victim killed in the shelter and taken to the temporary mortuary at the old Public Bath House in North Shields were recorded on official Mortuary Forms. These are available to view at Tyne and Wear Archives at the Discovery Museum, Blandford Square, Newcastle upon Tyne. Forms do not exist for those who died later in hospital from their injuries.

The information is edited from the original Mortuary Forms. The clothing and personal effects information is similarly edited. This was often all that allowed individuals to be identified, such were the injuries suffered. It is a starkly poignant and sad read.

Mortuary Form.

Entire families and households were lost. The Chater family lost all 6 members. The Hall family lost a mother and 5 children, the Kays, a mother and 4 children. The 3 related families living at 66 North King Street (a 5 bed-roomed flat above what was Atkinson's The Fruiterers), lost 7 members. The bombing was a community disaster by any standards. Many of the victims were related to each other or were friends and neighbours. For those who survived and those who were bereaved, life was never the same again

The Mortuary Forms confirm the working-class background of the shelter victims. There are no lawyers, doctors or accountants listed among the victims. This was a poor, working class, area of town. It did not attract "strangers", as would perhaps a shelter in the centre of town.

To date, there are no confirmed Wilkinson employees among those lost. We can surmise also that the shelter was cold inside – check the amount of clothing worn by many, prepared for a long night ahead. Sadly, the long night ahead never came.

Additional notes have been informed by the 1939 Register and from information supplied by visitors to **northshields173.org**.

Male Victims	51	41–65 year olds	21
Female Victims	56	66+ year olds	6
Died in Shelter	100	Number at school	22
Died in Hospital	7	Youngest Victim	6 months
Number of Military Personnel	4	Oldest Victim	80 years old
Number of ARP Personnel	4	**Burials at Preston Cemetery**	
Number in Reserved Occupations	7	Wednesday 7/5/41	13
Average Age of Victims	27	Thursday 8/5/41	66
0–4 year olds	15	Friday 9/5/41	9
5–17 year olds	29	Saturday 10/5/41	11
18–40 year olds	36	Monday 12/5/41	1

Beavers   35 Whitby Street, North Shield   1 dead

Name	Occupation	Age	Clothing & Effects	Mortuary Form
Clarence Beavers	Confectioner (Cake Maker)	25	Pawn Ticket Number 549 issued by Middleton Dixon Driver, 186 Linskill Street, North Shields to Herbert Beavers of 30 Whitby Street. Grey jacket. Pyjamas, white with red stripe. Woollen muffler. 2 grey pullovers. Cufflinks. Black shoes.	67

Notes
Identified by J. T. Hart (friend).
The 1939 Register shows him resident at this property along with his parents Robert and Nora and 2 others. Buried at Preston Cemetery: 8/5/41. Plot Number: 1718.

Bennett   68 Camperdown Street, Gateshead   1 dead

Name	Occupation	Age	Clothing & Effects	Mortuary Form
John Cowen Bennett	Soldier	34		79

Notes
Rank: Gunner. *Regiment/Service:* Royal Artillery. *Service No:* 1739327.
Probably stationed at Tynemouth Castle and billeted at Kettlewell School on George Street.
Identified by Capt J.W. Phillips. Buried at Gateshead East Cemetery.

Brown   73 Hudson Street, North Shields   1 dead

Name	Occupation	Age	Clothing & Effects	Mortuary Form
William Henry (Billy) Brown	General Timber Labourer	19	Plated cigarette case with W.B. monogram. Gold signet ring. 14/- in silver. Torch. Key. Brown overcoat. Blue overcoat with grey belt. Sweater. Blue cotton shirt. Blue signet ring.	7

Notes
Identified by Stanley Brown (brother).
In 1939, Mr Brown resided at 3 Lily Gardens with his parents, Adam and Ann E. and two siblings.
Buried at Preston Cemetery: 12/5/41. Plot Number: 12057.

Burgess   105 Plane Street, Anlaby Road, Hull   1 dead

Name	Occupation	Age	Clothing & Effects	Mortuary Form
John (aka Jack) Burgess	Soldier	25		Not known

Notes
Rank: Gunner. *Regiment/Service:* Royal Artillery. *Service No:* 984302.
Probably stationed at Tynemouth Castle and billeted at Kettlewell School on George Street.
Identified by Capt J. W. Phillips. Buried at Gateshead East Cemetery.

Chater 110 Church Street, North Shields 6 dead

Name	Occupation	Age	Clothing & Effects	Mortuary Form
Alfred Chater	Lorry Diver/ARP Rescue	42		80
Henrietta Chater	Household Duties	35		98
Henrietta Chater	At school	11		94
Mary Chater	At school	9		103
Edith Chater	At school	7		104
John Chater	Under school age	4	Green Jersey – red border on collar. White vest. Grey pullover. White shirt. Black stockings. Grey herringbone trousers.	46

Notes
The highest family death toll. Equal with the **Hall** family. However, NONE of this household survived. Mother, father and 4 children killed.
Bodies identified by J. H. Chater (uncle), Stanley Chater (uncle), T. Rackham (aunt) and Camelia Hardy (aunt).
The 1939 Register shows this property also housed the Luke family. Unknown if they went to the shelter and survived but they are not listed among the victims.
Buried at Preston Cemetery: 8/5/41. Plot Number: 12996.

Craig 10 (Back) George Street, North Shields 3 dead

Name	Occupation	Age	Clothing & Effects	Mortuary Form
John Craig	Cart man	37	Wallet – 7/4d cash. Cigarettes. Grey overcoat. Blue double breasted coat. Brown waistcoat. Sleeveless pullover. Striped trousers. Grey socks. White shirt with black stripe. Grey tie with red diamond. Black shoes.	43
Ethel Craig	Household duties	31	Blouse. Apron. Black Dress. Camisole. One shoe. Tweed Coat. Toy Watch. Two half pennies.	28
Audrey Craig	At school	11	Grey flannel shorts. White vest. White socks – green band on top. Coloured cotton jumper – floral pink, White cardigan.	51

Notes
Mother, Father and 1 daughter. 2 siblings of Audrey survived.
John Craig identified by W. Craig (brother). It is now known that this W. Craig was Billy Craig, featured elsewhere in the book. It is unknown if Billy was in the shelter with his brother. We understand he worked for the ARP during the War.
Buried at Preston Cemetery: 8/5/41. Plot Number: 12994.

Cummings 5 Tynemouth Road, North Shields 3 dead

Name	Occupation	Age	Clothing & Effects	Mortuary Form
George Cummings	Horse Driver / ARP Decontamination Squad	50		95
George Cummings	At school	13	Identity Card GBAO 250/3. Brown Jacket. Navy scarf Grey jersey. White shirt with blue stripes. White vest. Brown trousers. Khaki collar. Wool helmet. Fawn socks.	28
Roland Cummings	At school	11		51

Notes
Father and 2 sons. Husband of Ethel Cummings.
Identified by G. Hornsby (friend).
Buried at Preston Cemetery: 8/5/41. Plot number: 13008.

Curran 66 North King Street, North Shields 2 dead

Name	Occupation	Age	Clothing & Effects	Mortuary Form
Emma Curran	Household Duties	80	Brown cardigan. Fur coat. Fawn underskirt. Blue jacket. Dressing jacket. Black dress. Overall. Underskirt, Vest. One shoe. Black stockings. Wedding ring.	34
William Henry (Billy) Curran	Shipyard Painter	23	Cash – £1 14s. Wrist watch (Medana with expanding strap). Leather purse. Smiths Dock badge – Yard No 347. Brown pullover – zip. Khaki shirt. White vest. Grey trousers. Dungaree trousers. Leather belt. Black socks. Pocket knife.	52

Notes
Emma Curran was the oldest victim of the bombing, aged 80. Wife of late William Henry Curran. Daughter of the late George and Joan Peversley of Gateshead.
Billy Curran is thought to have been the shelter accordionist, mentioned by many who used the shelter.
Bodies identified by W. H. Curran (son/father).
Emma's daughter Agnes May **Smith** and her 2 children also killed in shelter.
66 North King Street was a 5-bedroomed flat above Atkinson's The Fruiterer.
The Curran's shared this address with relations – the **Smith** household (3 victims) and the **Glynn** household
(2 victims). There were 7 deaths from this one address – the highest death toll for a single address.
Buried at Preston Cemetery: 7/5/41. Plot number: 1731. Shared headstone with **Smith** victims.

Dale 33 Park Crescent, North Shields 1 dead

Name	Occupation	Age	Clothing & Effects	Mortuary Form
Henry Medcalf Dale	Butcher	60	Grey overcoat. Tie (striped). Shirt. Wool vest. Packet of Birdseed. Blue Jacket. Wallet containing £9. Blue waistcoat. Screwdriver. 5 farthings and 2 foreign coins. Trousers. Wallet with wages packet. Identity card and 4/11d cash. Socks.	72

Notes
Husband of Catherine Dale.
Identified by A. R. Morrison (son-in-law).
Buried at Preston Cemetery: 10/5/41. Plot number: 1105.

Dickson 31 Upper Queen Street, North Shields 1 dead

Name	Occupation	Age	Clothing & Effects	Mortuary Form
Mary Elizabeth Dickson	Household Duties	54		N/A (see Notes)

Notes
Died 15/5/1941 at Shotley Bridge Emergency Hospital.
Wife of Samuel Dickson. Daughter of late Adam and Mary Jane Craig.
Buried at Preston Cemetery. Plot number: 1737.

Donkin 5 Ponton's Buildings, King Street, North Shields 2 dead

Name	Occupation	Age	Clothing & Effects	Mortuary Form
Elizabeth Lindores Donkin	Household Duties	22	Identity card, NU Seaman Card – J.W. Donkin. Marriage Certificate. Ration Books. Papers. Brown leather purse – 1/2d cash. Yale key. Matches. Red Cotton Blouse. Skirt. Vest.	60
Elizabeth Ann Donkin		11 mths	Black patent shoes. White socks. Sleeping suit. Red bonnet. Pink wool coat. Vest. Red blanket. White and Green bed cover	48

Notes
Mother and daughter. Wife of James William Donkin, Merchant Navy.
Identified by O. A. Smith (brother) and Flora Smith (mother).
Buried at Preston Cemetery: 8/5/41. Plot number: 13610. Shared headstone with **Ward**..

Elliott   58 (Back) George Street, North Shields   2 dead

Name	Occupation	Age	Clothing & Effects	Mortuary Form
Anthony Elliott	Street Lamp Attendant / ARP Demolition Squad	42		101
Anthony Elliott	Slater's Labourer	17		97

Notes
Father and son. Identified by T. H. Mullen (brother-in-law).
Buried at Preston Cemetery: 8/5/41. Plot number: 13018.

Ferguson   58 George Street, North Shields   1 dead

Name	Occupation	Age	Clothing & Effects	Mortuary Form
Mary Jane Ferguson	Domestic duties	56		N/A (see Notes)

Notes
Died 5/5/1941 at Preston Hospital, North Shields.
Wife of Thomas Ferguson.
Buried at Preston Cemetery: 8/5/41. Plot number: 12056.

Frankland   36 Upper Queen Street, North Shields   1 dead

Name	Occupation	Age	Clothing & Effects	Mortuary Form
Alexander "Sandy" Frankland	Pit boy	15		69

Notes
Body identified by Edwin F. Frankland (father).
Household of 6 in 1939, including father above, Nellie B (mother) and siblings, Nora Sturrock, William J (Billy) and Arthur E.
William and Arthur were both rescued from the shelter. Nora had decided not to go that night.
Buried at Preston Cemetery: 9/5/41. Plot number: 11046.

Germain 25 Reed Street, North Shields 4 dead

Name	Occupation	Age	Clothing & Effects	Mortuary Form
Robert Germain	Street Sweeper	56		N/A (see Notes)
Ivy Germain	At school	10	Black shoes. Brown socks. White vest. Blue flowered frock. Green and black scarf. Blue jumper (zip). Tweed coat – green lining. Hair slide. Earrings and beads.	49
Edwin Germain	At school		White Shirt. Vest. Wool Shawl. Green Sweater. Grey Pullover. Blue stockings.	29
Ethel Germain	Under school age		Woollen vest. Brown sandals. Tartan skirt. Blue jumper. Wool scarf. Petticoat. Black Coat.	18

Notes
Father and 3 children. Husband of Eva Germain.
Robert Germain died from injuries at Victoria Jubilee Infirmary on 4/5/41.
Bodies identified by G. Chessher (uncle) and Albert Prest (uncle).
Buried at Preston Cemetery: 8/5/41. Plot number: 13006. Family surname is misspelt on headstone.

Gibson 96 Church Street, North Shields 2 dead

Name	Occupation	Age	Clothing & Effects	Mortuary Form
Elizabeth Gibson	Household duties	60	Dark coloured coat. Grey skirt. Red Woollen Jumper. Blue woollen jumper. White vest. Grey Vest. Scarf. Blue apron. Purse – Bell Bros. Token. Keys.	68
Ethel Maud Gibson	Household duties	32	Flowered cotton dress, Purse –12s 2 1/2d cash. Blue coat belted at back. Vest. Pink cardigan. Navy scarf. Brown silk scarf.	54

Notes
Wife and daughter of J Gibson.
Identified by G. W. Horn (brother)
Buried at Preston Cemetery: 10/5/41. Plot number: 13040.

Glynn 66 North King Street, North Shields 2 dead

Name	Occupation	Age	Clothing & Effects	Mortuary Form
John Thomas Glynn	General Labourer	58	Glasses. Prayer book in case. Snuff box. Purse. Cash – 3/8.25d. Keys and ring. Identity card. Personal papers. Rosary – cross, silver chain. Trousers. Scarf. Grey pullover. Vest. Waistcoat. Shirt. Braces.	58
Margaret Glynn	Domestic duties	29	Black boots size 5. Corset. Cardigan (Yellow Flowers). Two pairs of stockings. Blue coat with fur collar. Vest. Slip. Blue skirt. Blue dress – white collar.	35

Notes
Father and daughter. Bodies identified by J. C. Glynn (son/brother)
Shared address with **Smith** household (3 victims) and **Curran** household (2 victims), totalling 7 deaths from this one address.
Buried at Preston Cemetery: 7/5/41. Plot number: 1733.

Goodwill 7 North Church Street, North Shields 3 dead

Name	Occupation	Age	Clothing & Effects	Mortuary Form
Joseph Goodwill	Confectioner (cakes)/ARP Stretcher Bearer	30	Identity Card GBAD 252/1. Infirmary Card issued to Joseph Goodwill. Leather Wallet. Notes – £5 10/s – cash 5s/6d. War Savings certificate for 15/-. Burberry Macintosh. Grey Flannel trousers. Brown shoes. Black socks. Blue shirt. Grey pullover. Light blue scarf. Stretcher Bearer badge.	65
Edward Brown Goodwill	At school	8		45
John William Goodwill	Under school age	4	Blue overcoat. Grey short trousers. Grey and Red jersey. Grey shirt. Red sleeveless pullover. White vest. Grey stockings. Identity disk.	N/A (see Notes)

Notes
Father and 2 sons. Husband and children of Elizabeth Goodwill.
Identified by N. Goodwill (brother).
John William died at Shotley Bridge Emergency Hospital 14/6/41. No burial records found for Joseph and Edward.

Gray 70 Linskill Street, North Shields 3 dead

Name	Occupation	Age	Clothing & Effects	Mortuary Form
Joseph Henry Gray	Labourer Building Trade	53	Blue overcoat. Blue wool gloves. 1s 5d cash. Yale key. Wallet with misc. papers. War ribbons. Spectacles in case. Boots, Navy leather belt.	90
Margaret Gray	Domestic duties	50	Wedding ring. Dark blue heavy coat. Brown flowered dress. Green cardigan. Pale Blue cardigan. Pink wool vest. White vest. Black skirt. Flowered pinafore.	86
Mary Gray	Not known	21	Blue coat – light grey fur collar. Blue wool coat – zip. Blue dress. Blue socks. Shoes.	93

Notes
Husband, wife and daughter. Identified by J. H. Gray (son).
Buried at Preston Cemetery: 10/5/41. Plot number: 13038.

Haggerty 103 High Street, Kidlington, Oxford 1 dead

Name	Occupation	Age	Clothing & Effects	Mortuary Form
Charles Henry Haggerty	Soldier	22		77

Notes
Rank: Signalman. *Regiment/Service:* Royal Corps of Signals. *Service No:* 869892
Stationed at Tynemouth Castle and probably billeted at Kettlewell School on George Street.
Identified by Capt J. W. Phillips.
Buried at Preston Cemetery: 8/5/41. Plot number: 14441 (Forces).

Hall 65 George Street, North Shields 6 dead

Name	Occupation	Age	Clothing & Effects	Mortuary Form
Martha Hall	Domestic duties	31		70
John Hall	At School	9	Khaki shirt. Grey pullover. Red jersey. Sandshoes. Blue stockings. Grey dressing gown.	10
Sydney Hall	At school	7	Blue trousers and braces. Khaki shirt. Brown jersey. Grey pullover. Vest.	14
James William Hall	At school	5	Helio pullover. Vest shirt. Wool sweater. Fawn wool pants. White socks. Blue balaclava. Helmet braces.	13
Shirley Hall	Under school age	4	Black and white checked coat – velvet collar. Knitted frock – blue silk. Light coloured shoes. Brown socks. White vest.	53
Alfred Hall	Under school age	2	Red coat – belted. Red bonnet. Green trousers. Blue jumper. White cardigan. White vest. Grey socks. One sandshoe.	50

Notes
Mother and 5 children.
Equal highest family death toll with **Chater**.
Family of John A Hall, trawler fisherman.
Bodies identified by J. B. Taylor (brother of Martha Hall) and Jane Richardson (aunt).
The Halls lived over the road from Wilkinson's. In 1939 the family lived at 44 Little Bedford Street.
Buried at Preston Cemetery: 8/5/41. Plot number: 12998.

Harman 26 Reed Street, North Shields 4 dead

Name	Occupation	Age	Clothing & Effects	Mortuary Form
Mary Ellen Harman	Domestic duties	38		N/A (see Notes)
Thomas Harman	At school	7	Tin with buttons inside. Red penknife. Three marbles. Empty cartridge case. Toy submarine. Anchor. Black boots. Brown stockings. Wool scarf. Blue trousers and braces. Blue coat. Grey pullover. Wool vest. Check shirt.	26
Joan Harman	At school	5	Green coat. Mauve Jumper. Pink and green wool bonnet. Liberty silk petticoat. Wool vest. Blue wool coat. White socks. 1 black patent shoe. Metal ring.	15
Richard Harman	Under school age	3	Blue overcoat. Orange wool coat. Fawn shirt. Pink wool coat. White shirt – blue stripe. Blue trousers with braces. Cloth scarf.	4

Notes
Mother and 3 children. Family of the late Thomas William Henry Harman.
Children identified by Matilda Harman (grandmother).
Mary Ellen Harman died from injuries at Tynemouth Victoria Jubilee Infirmary, North Shields, 4/5/41.
Buried at Preston Cemetery: 8/5/41. Plot number: 13004.

Henderson 60 (Back) George Street, North Shields 2 dead

Name	Occupation	Age	Clothing & Effects	Mortuary Form
Phyllis Henderson	Domestic duties	61		91
James Henderson	Fireman	60		83

Notes
Husband and wife.
Identified by T. W. Hogarth (son-in-law).
Daughter, Hilda **Shearer** and her 2 children also killed in shelter.
Buried at Preston Cemetery: 8/5/41. Plot number: 13002. Shared headstone with **Shearer**.

Herrett — 27 Upper Queen Street, North Shields   1 dead

Name	Occupation	Age	Clothing & Effects	Mortuary Form
Lillian Margaret Herrett	Under school age	4	Blue coat. Siren Suit. Vest. Yellow dress. Blue petticoat. Wool Bonnet. Sandshoes. White silk scarf.	27

Notes
Identified by Stoker A.C. Herrett RN (father). It is believed the Herretts were from Scarborough and were staying with the Cook family. They went to the shelter together. John Herrett, aged 10, survived but had acid burn injuries.
Lillian Herret was killed on her birthday. Buried at Preston Cemetery: 8/5/41. Plot number: 13026.

Hewson — 44 Stanley Street West, North Shields   1 dead

Name	Occupation	Age	Clothing & Effects	Mortuary Form
David Venture Hewson	Shipyard Joiner	24		64

Notes
Identified by W. M. Hewson (brother). Buried at Preston Cemetery: 7/5/41. Plot number: 3779.

Hodgson — 21 Upper Queen Street, North Shields   4 dead

Name	Occupation	Age	Clothing & Effects	Mortuary Form
Alexina Hodgson	Domestic duties	28	Blue Coat. Green Cardigan. Flowered skirt. Leatherette Belt. Wedding ring. Engagement ring.	10
Violet Hodgson	Domestic Servant	19		41
Elizabeth Hodgson	At school	5	Blanket. Pyjamas. Vest. Grey Wool Coat. Siren suit.	30
Henry Henderson Hodgson	Under school age	2	Sleeping Suit. Red Wool Jacket. White Sandals. Vest. Siren Suit (Purple).	24

Notes
Mother and 2 children.
Identified by Henry Henderson Hodgson, Royal Northumberland Fusiliers (husband).
Violet Hodgson resident at 10 East George Street. Identified by James Albert Hodgson (brother).
Buried at Preston Cemetery: 7/5/41. Plot number: 11803.

Howard   27 Church Street, North Shields   1 dead

Name	Occupation	Age	Clothing & Effects	Mortuary Form
John George Howard	Labourer	18	Long overcoat – half belt. Black shoes. Brown jacket. Brown trousers. Blue shirt. Black socks. Grey pullover. Green pullover. Purse – empty. Identity card – GBAY 135/3	66

Notes
Identified by J.T. Kirkham (uncle). Son of Rosella Howard and John S. Howard.
Buried at Preston Cemetery: 9/5/41. Plot number: 12580.

Hull   16 North King Street, North Shields   2 dead

Name	Occupation	Age	Clothing & Effects	Mortuary Form
Samuel Hull	Soldier	29	Army uniform. Army pay book and 7s 4d cash. 10 razor blades. Comb. Broken fountain pen.	56
Evelyn Hull	Canning Factory Worker	17	Light blue coat – fur edged. Yellow jumper. Blue silk jumper. Blue slacks (zip). White slip. Dark brown scarf. Blue ankle socks.	44

Notes
Children of Samuel and Alice May Hull.
Samuel Hull, Gunner, Royal Artillery 72 Anti-Tank Regt, Service No 6214905, believed to be on leave.
Identified by T. Barton (uncle). Evelyn and Ernest identified by L/Cpl Luke (friend).
Buried at Preston Cemetery: 8/5/41. Plot number: 13030.

Kay   95 Church Street, North Shields   5 dead

Name	Occupation	Age	Clothing & Effects	Mortuary Form
Doreen Robina Bilton Jackson Kay	Domestic duties	33		57
Ernest William Kay	At school/part-time delivery driver	14	Paper. Pencils. Jacket. Waistcoat. Flannel trousers. Flannel shirt. Flannel vest. Wool pullover	59
Hylton Stewart Kay	At school	11		57
Sydney Jackson Kay	At school	7	1 marble. 1 diary. 1939 foreign stamps. Blue trousers – braces. Brown waistcoat. Blue jersey – zip. Vest. Khaki shirt. Blue overcoat.	12
George Alan Kay	Under school age	2	Fawn pullover. Siren suit (fawn). Vest blanket.	11

Notes
Mother and 4 children. Second highest death toll.
Identified by Private Ernest Kay, The Durham Light Infantry (father).
Buried at Preston Cemetery: 8/5/41. Plot number: 13000.

Kirby 1 Hackworth Street, Dean Bank, Ferryhill 1 dead

Name	Occupation	Age	Clothing & Effects	Mortuary Form
Amy Kirby	Independent Means	56		81

Notes
Identified by S. Urwin (Brother-in-law). No burial details found.

Livesley 11½ Back George Street 1 dead

Name	Occupation	Age	Clothing & Effects	Mortuary Form
Ethel Livesley	Domestic duties	55	Wedding ring. Blue silk dress (spotted). Cotton petticoat. Woollen vest. Black stockings. Cotton slip. Green jumper – half sleeves. Blue rain coat – belted. Three keys. Green jumper. Green and white bonnet.	36

Notes
Wife of Albert Livesley. Identified by M. T. Livesley (brother-in-law).
Buried at Preston Cemetery: 8/5/41. Plot number: 13024.

Liddle 10 George Street, North Shields 2 dead

Name	Occupation	Age	Clothing & Effects	Mortuary Form
Margaret Adelaide Liddle	Domestic duties	35	Flowered print dress. Silk slip. Vest. Brown silk stockings. One black shoe. Blue tweed coat. Wedding ring.	42
Jean Liddle	Under school age	1	White nightgown. Salmon overcoat – Belted. Blue shoes. Green Pixie cap. White vest. Napkin. Knitted shawl	47

Notes
Mother and daughter. Identified by Charles Liddle (husband).
Buried at Preston Cemetery: 8/5/41. Plot number: 1233.

Logie 55 George Street, North Shields 1 dead

Name	Occupation	Age	Clothing & Effects	Mortuary Form
Margaret Logie	Domestic duties	73	Blue serge coat. Brown overcoat. Black apron.	99
Margaret Thomson Logie	Dressmaker	40	Wedding ring. Light coloured Macintosh. Tweed costume jacket. Fawn cardigan. Blue coat. Grey Jumper. Dark Skirt. White Flannel vest. Wool skirt. White pinafore.	63

Notes
Widow and daughter of late Robert Logie. Bodies identified by A. Kell (friend) and J. Henderson (cousin). Buried at Preston Cemetery: 10/5/41. Plot number: 13042.

Lough 23 Upper Queen Street, North Shields 2 dead

Name	Occupation	Age	Clothing & Effects	Mortuary Form
William Robert Lough	Motor Driver (Fish Trade)	32		102
Margaret Ann Lough	At school	10	Vest. Green Jumper. Brown boots. Ribbed stockings. Blue knitted dress. Print dress. Petticoat. Liberty bodice.	32

Notes
Father and daughter. Husband of Margaret Lough. Bodies identified by Robert Lough (father/grandfather).
Buried at Preston Cemetery: 9/5/41. Plot number: 13034.

Mather 258 Church Street, North Shields 1 dead

Name	Occupation	Age	Clothing & Effects	Mortuary Form
William Mather	Labourer	19		96

Notes
Identified by J. W. Mather (brother). Buried at Preston Cemetery: 8/5/41. Plot number: 13014.

Mavin   96 Church Street, North Shields   3 dead

Name	Occupation	Age	Clothing & Effects	Mortuary Form
Marguerite Ada Mavin	Domestic duties	30		71
James Mavin	At school	9		61
Rosalie Mavin	Baby	1	Brown sleeping bag. White slippers. White vest. Woollen vest. Coat. Bangle with word "Baby"..	40

Notes
Mother and 2 children. Identified by James William Mavin (husband).
Buried at Preston Cemetery: 8/5/41. Plot number: 13012.

McGuire   55 King Street, North Shields   1 dead

Name	Occupation	Age	Clothing & Effects	Mortuary Form
Mary Ann McGuire	Domestic duties	48	Brooch. Gold chain. Wedding ring. Signet ring. Dress ring – centre stone missing. Black dress. Blue wool jacket. Brown wool jacket. Raincoat. Apron. One shoe.	21

Notes
Wife of Thomas Matthew McGuire. Identified by W. E. Ogle (father-in-law).
Daughter of Margaret and late John Southern.
Buried at Preston Cemetery: 8/5/41. Plot number: 11815.

McPhillips   50 Upper Queen Street, North Shields   1 dead

Name	Occupation	Age	Clothing & Effects	Mortuary Form
John Andrew McPhillips	Stevedore	42		N/A (see Notes)

Notes
Husband of Gladys May McPhillips.
Died at Victoria Jubilee Hospital 4/5/41.
Buried at Preston Cemetery: 8/5/41. Plot number: 13183.

Nesbitt 105a Church Street, North Shields 2 dead

Name	Occupation	Age	Clothing & Effects	Mortuary Form
John Robert Nesbitt	Retired Labourer	76		76
Eliza Ann Nesbitt	Domestic duties	65		75

Notes
Husband and wife. Bodies identified by E. J. Marshall (niece) and T. Brown (nephew).
Daughter of late J. R. Nesbitt.
Buried at Preston Cemetery: 8/5/41. Plot number: 13016.

Nicholson 148 Grey Street, North Shields 3 dead

Name	Occupation	Age	Clothing & Effects	Mortuary Form
Edward Nicholson	Ship's Plumber	34	Driving Licence. Army Registration Card. Cheque for £4 signed by R.S. Driver. Diary 1939. Ring – white metal. Wallet with photographs. 1 door key. 9/- silver, 3d copper, seven £1 notes. Handkerchief.	39
Emily Nicholson	Domestic Duties	34		N/A (see Notes)
Ivy Hastie Nicholson	At school		Green coat with velvet collar. Blue gym dress. Green jumper. Green cardigan	88

Notes
Husband, wife and 1 child.
Edward identified by R. Nicholson (brother). Ivy Hastie identified by E. Hastie (uncle).
Emily Nicholson died at Preston Emergency Hospital 4/5/41. She was the daughter of Mr W. H. Hastie.
Buried at Preston Cemetery: 9/5/41. Plot number: 10568.

Nicholson 95 Church Street, North Shields 1 dead

Name	Occupation	Age	Clothing & Effects	Mortuary Form
Mary Nicholson	Domestic duties	57		73

Notes
Identified by Richard W. Nicholson (husband).
Buried at Preston Cemetery: 8/5/41. Plot number: 13020.

Oliver   148 Grey Street, North Shields   1 dead

Name	Occupation	Age	Clothing & Effects	Mortuary Form
Christina Oliver	Domestic duties	45	Wedding ring. Blue Mackintosh. Blue wool cardigan. Blue flowered dress. Silk scarf. Coloured pinafore. Black skirt. One shoe.	62

Notes
Wife of William John Oliver. Identified by J. T. Downie (brother).
Buried at Preston Cemetery: 8/5/41. Plot number: 13032. Headstone removed by family c1960 and replaced without commemoration of victim.

Patterson   70 George Street, North Shields   1 dead

Name	Occupation	Age	Clothing & Effects	Mortuary Form
Elizabeth Ann Hyde Patterson	School Cleaner	52	Dark coloured heavy coat (belted). Green coat – Isaac Walton Ltd. Blue jumper. White bands. Green cardigan. Black silk dress. One shoe. Wedding ring.	87

Notes
Widow of Robert Patterson. Identified by Jennie Robson (niece).
Shared headstone with **Mather** and **Ribson**.
Buried at Preston Cemetery: 8/5/41. Plot number: 13014.

Phillips   159 Linskill Street, North Shields   1 dead

Name	Occupation	Age	Clothing & Effects	Mortuary Form
Edith Louvaine Phillips	Shop Assistant	14		74

Notes
Daughter of John W. S. Phillips and Alice E. Phillips. Identified by father.
Buried at Preston Cemetery: 9/5/41. Plot number: 13028.

Potts   9 East Percy Street, North Shields   1 dead

Name	Occupation	Age	Clothing & Effects	Mortuary Form
Richard Potts	Labourer	63	Dark suit. Grey silk scarf. Heavy leather belt. One penny.	84

Notes
Husband of Margaret T. Potts. Identified by G. Dixon (friend).
Buried at Preston Cemetery: 10/5/41. Plot number: 13043.

Robson   4 Oakwood Avenue, North Shields   1 dead

Name	Occupation	Age	Clothing & Effects	Mortuary Form
Isabella Robson	At school	8		3

Notes
Daughter of Robert William and Isabella Robson. Identified by father.
Isabella was in the shelter with her twin sisters Jennie and Margaret both of whom survived.
Buried at Preston Cemetery: 8/5/41. Plot number: 13014. Shared headstone with **Mather** and **Patterson**.

Rowntree   4 Beacon Street, North Shields   1 dead

Name	Occupation	Age	Clothing & Effects	Mortuary Form
Margaret Rowntree	At school	12	Vest. Liberty bodice. Green dress. Petticoat. Green bonnet. Brown ankle socks. Brown shoes. Blue blazer.	33

Notes
Identified by L. Walker (sister).
Daughter of late A. H. Rowntree.
Buried at Preston Cemetery: 8/5/41. Plot number: 12457.

Sanderson   16 Albert Terrace, North Shields   1 dead

Name	Occupation	Age	Clothing & Effects	Mortuary Form
James Sanderson	Apprentice Carpenter	20		100

Notes
Identified by M. Krauble (aunt).
Buried at Preston Cemetery: 10/5/41. Plot number: 12507.

Shearer 12 King Street, North Shields 3 dead

Name	Occupation	Age	Clothing & Effects	Mortuary Form
Hilda Shearer	Domestic duties	22	Wedding ring. Signet ring. White raincoat. Dummy teat. Child's socks. Bracelet (child's). Blue flowered dress. Grey pullover. Black suede shoes. Purse containing: £1 note, 10/- note, 7s silver, 1s/7d copper. Milk registration coupon in the name of Miss Hilda Shearer.	37
Norma Shearer	Under school age	2	Wool coat. Vest. Liberty bodice. Petticoat. Red dressing jacket. White socks. Red tablecloth. 1 red slipper.	31
Robert Shearer	Baby	3m		89

Notes
Mother and 2 children. Wife of Robert Collins Shearer, Merchant Navy. Identified by T. W. Hogarth (brother-in-law).
Daughter of James and Phyllis Henderson both also killed in shelter.
Robert Shearer was the youngest victim of the disaster.
Shared headstone with **Henderson**. Buried at Preston Cemetery: 9/5/41. Plot number: 13002.

Smith 66 North King Street, North Shields 3 dead

Name	Occupation	Age	Clothing & Effects	Mortuary Form
Agnes May Smith	Domestic duties	37	Gold wedding ring. Blue coat – fur trimmed. Grey dress. Blue wool cardigan. Grey wool cardigan. Grey wool Hug-me-tight. Blue slip. Grey scarf Brown shoes.	6
Veronica Smith	At school	13	Blue coat. Brown cardigan. Cotton dress (flowered). Blue cotton dress. Black sandals. 4 half pennies Comb Small Catholic medallions. Tartan handkerchief.	9
Maureen Smith	At school	9	Catholic medallion. Blouse Blue skirt. Liberty bodice Blue wool scarf. Pink jumper. One black patent shoe Green coat.	20

Notes
Mother and 2 children.
Wife of David Smith. Daughter of Agnes May Smith. Identified by W. H. Curran (brother).
Mother Emma **Curran** and brother also killed in shelter.
A total of 7 people (**Curran, Smith, Glynn** households) residing at this address were killed.
Buried at Preston Cemetery: 7/5/41. Plot number: 1731.

Sutherst 24 Upper Queen Street, North Shields 1 dead

Name	Occupation	Age	Clothing & Effects	Mortuary Form
Kathleen Sutherst	Domestic duties	32		92

Notes
Identified by Private Robert Sutherst, The Gordon Highlanders, (husband).
Kathleen's niece Edith Louvaine **Phillips** was also killed in the shelter.
Buried at Preston Cemetery: 9/5/41. Plot number: 13028.

Ward 27 Lawson Street, North Shields 1 dead

Name	Occupation	Age	Clothing & Effects	Mortuary Form
Maureen Ward		6m		23

Notes
Daughter of William Ward, Merchant Navy and Lillian May Ward. Identified by father.
Shared headstone with **Donkin**.
Buried at Preston Cemetery: 8/5/41. Plot number: 13010.

Weldon 46 King Street, North Shields 1 dead

Name	Occupation	Age	Clothing & Effects	Mortuary Form
James Wallace Weldon	Builder's Labourer	50		82

Notes
Identified by James Weldon (father).
Buried at Preston Cemetery: 8/5/41. Plot number: 13022.

Woolford 27 Lawson Street, North Shields 1 dead

Name	Occupation	Age	Clothing & Effects	Mortuary Form
William George Woolford	Ship's Painter/ Sergeant, Home Guard	35		78

Notes
Husband of Margaret Woolford. Identified by Mrs E Dempsey (friend).
Buried at Preston Cemetery: 8/5/41. Plot number: 13050.

7 The Victims by Street

Unsurprisingly, the streets in closest vicinity to Wilkinson's bore the highest number of victims. The basement shelter was an easy option for those living close by.

It is worth remembering, however, that Wilkinson's was not a universally popular shelter and that locals had other options for protection during air raids. These will have included yard shelters and cellars, if available, or a walk along to the basement shelter on East Percy Street or the police dwellings on Stephenson Street.

With hindsight, if only everyone had decided to stay at home that night…

Streets not within North Shields are not included in the list below.

Where multiple households share one address, it is assumed the buildings are divided into flats and bedsits.

Map of the immediate area around Wilkinson's, showing the streets where the Air Raid Shelter victims lived.

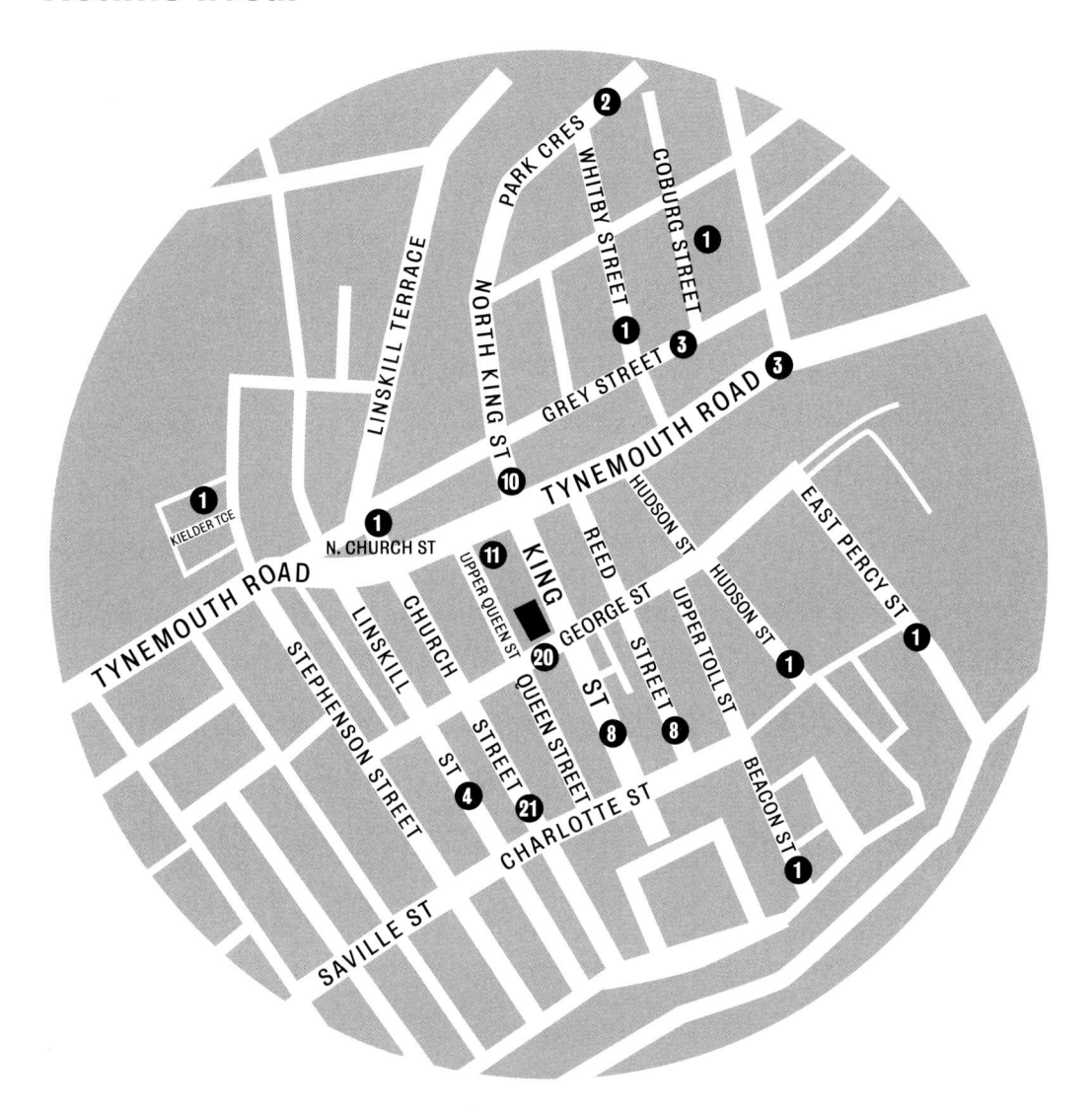

The numbers in black circles represent the fatalities on that street. Wilkinson's is the black rectangle at the junction of King Street and George Street.

NOTE: Not all victims lived in the streets shown in the map – Maureen Ward lived in Lawson Street, in the west of the town, while eight-year-old Isabella Robson lived in Chirton, to the north west of the area shown above.

Street	Family	Fatalities	Street Total
Albert Terrace			
16 Albert Terrace	SANDERSON		
Back Coburg Street			
12 Back Coburg Street	LAWSON	1	1
Beacon Street			
4 Beacon Street	ROWNTREE	1	1
Church Street			
27 Church Street	HOWARD	1	
58 Church Street	MATHER	1	
95 Church Street	KAY	5	
95 Church Street	NICHOLSON	1	
96 Church Street	GIBSON	2	
96 Church Street	MAVIN	3	
105a Church Street	NESBITT	2	
110 Church Street	CHATER	6	21
East Percy Street			
9 East Percy Street	POTTS	1	1
George Street			
10 George Street	CRAIG	3	
10 George Street	LIDDLE	2	
11½ George Street	LIVESLEY	1	
55 George Street	LOGIE	2	
58 (Back) George Street	ELLIOTT	2	
58 George Street	FERGUSON	1	
60 (Back) George Street	HENDERSON	2	
65 George Street	HALL	6	
70 George Street	PATTERSON	1	20
Grey Street			
148 Grey Street	NICHOLSON	3	3

North Shields 173

Street	Family	Fatalities	Street Total
Hudson Street			
73 Hudson Street	BROWN	1	1
Kielder Terrace			
10 Kielder Terrace	OLIVER	1	1
King Street			
5 Ponton's Buildings, King Street	DONKIN	2	
12 King Street	SHEARER	3	
45 King Street	WOOLFORD	1	
46 King Street	WELDON	1	
55 King Street	McGUIRE	1	8
Lawson Street			
27 Lawson Street	WARD	1	1
Linskill Street			
70 Linskill Street	GRAY	3	
159 Linskill Street	PHILLIPS	1	4
North Church Street			
7 North Church Street	GOODWILL	1	1
North King Street			
16 North King Street	HULL	3	
66 North King Street	CURRAN	2	
66 North King Street	GLYNN	2	
66 North King Street	SMITH	3	10
Oakwood Avenue, Chirton			
4 Oakwood Avenue	ROBSON	1	1
Park Crescent			
1 Park Crescent	PEARSON	1	
33 Park Crescent	DALE	1	2

North Shields 173

Street	Family	Fatalities	Street Total
Reed Street			
25 Reed Street	GERMAIN	4	
26 Reed Street	HARMAN	4	8
Stanley Street West			
44 Stanley Street West	HEWSON	1	1
Tynemouth Road			
5 Tynemouth Road	CUMMINGS	3	3
Upper Queen Street			
21 Upper Queen Street	HODGSON	4	
23 Upper Queen Street	LOUGH	2	
24 Upper Queen Street	SUTHERST	1	
27 Upper Queen Street	HERRETT	1	
31 Upper Queen Street	DICKSON	1	
36 Upper Queen Street	FRANKLAND	1	
50 Upper Queen Street	McPHILLIPS	1	11
Whitby Street			
35 Whitby Street	BEAVERS	1	1

8 The Injured

The true number of injured at Wilkinson's will probably never be fully known.

Some "walking wounded" were treated immediately at the First Aid Centre at Kettlewell School. 16 were patched up and sent home. Some 36 injured were taken directly to Tynemouth Victoria Jubilee Infirmary and Preston Emergency Hospital according to the Town Clerk's Report. Several of those admitted locally were later transferred to other locations including Shotley Bridge Hospital.

Assuming 192 (given in official figures) people in the shelter, it would appear then that about 30 people walked away from Wilkinson's physically unharmed. A minor miracle.

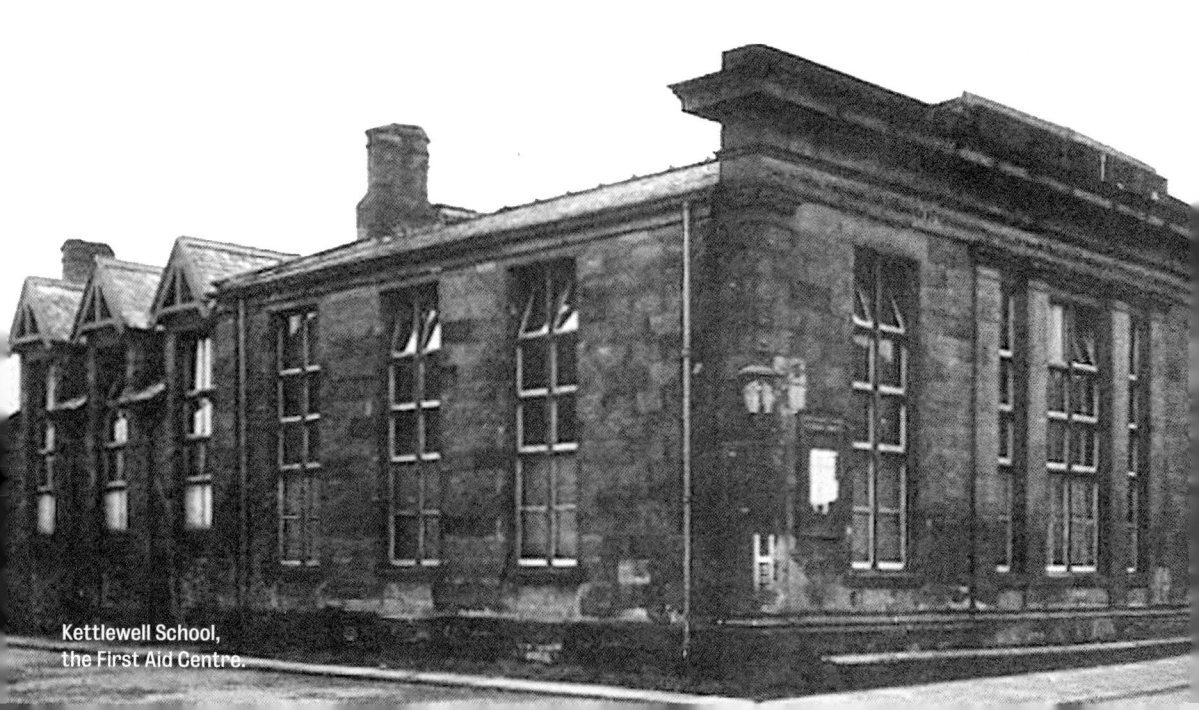

Kettlewell School, the First Aid Centre.

Name	Address	Apparent age	Condition
ATKINSON, Margaret Annie	5 King St, North Shields	57	Slight
BROWN, Janet	25 King Street, North Shields	19	Slight
BROWN, Raymond	81 Charlotte St, North Shields	29	Slight
CHATTERTON, Dorothy	90 Church St, North Shields	44	Serious
COOK, Stanley	166 Linskill St, North Shields	9	Slight
CUMMINGS, Ethel	5 Tynemouth Rd, North Shields	47	Slight
CURRAN, Evelyn	66 North King St, North Shields	39	Slight
DICKSON, Elizabeth Mary	31 Upper Queen St, North Shield	54	Serious
DOUGAL, Henry	10 Charlotte St, North Shields	44	Slight – outpatient
FERGUSON, Mary Jane	38 George St, North Shields	56	DIED 5/5/41
FRANKLAND, Arthur	36 Upper Queen St, North Shields	6	Slight
GLENN, Annie	66 North King St, North Shields	66	Slight
GODFREY, Annie	7 George St, North Shields		As evacuee, house down
GOODWILL, Elizabeth	North Church St, North Shields	30	Serious
GOODWILL, Jack	North Church St, North Shields	5	Dangerous
GRIFFITHS, William L/Cpl; 44447572	Durham LI/Apparent Age	33	Slight – On Duty
HERRETT, John	27 Upper Queen St, North Shields	12	Slight
HERRETT, Annie	27 Upper Queen St, North Shields	34	Slight
HOGILL, Mary	7 Upper Pearson St, North Shields	6	Slight
LEE, Hilda Mary	2 Hamilton Tce, North Shields	21	Slight
LANE, Elizabeth	24 Upper Queen St, North Shields	48	Slight
LIVESLEY, Albert	11½ Back George Street, North Shields	57	Slight
LOUGH, Margaret	23 Upper Queen St, North Shields	31	Serious
MAIN, Kathleen	28 Upper Queen St, North Shields	4	Slight
MASON, Elizabeth	60 George St, North Shields	66	Serious
NICHOLSON, Emily	Church St, North Shields	34	DIED 4/4/41
PESCOD, Joseph James	4 George St, North Shields	76	Slight
PREST, Joan	22 Reed St, North Shields	13	Serious
ROBSON, Margaret	4 Oakwood Ave, North Shields	18	Slight

Name	Address	Apparent age	Condition
ROBSON, Martha	4 Oakwood Ave, North Shields	64	Slight
ROBSON, Thomas	4 Oakwood Ave, North Shields	6	Slight
SANDERS, Ann	16 Albert Tce, North Shields	23	Serious
SANDERSON, Jennie	16 Albert Tce, North Shields	53	Slight
SUTHERST, Robert	24 Upper Queen St, North Shields	66	Slight
SUTHERST, Martha	24 Upper Queen St, North Shields	64	Slight y
SUTHERST, Thomas	24 Upper Queen St, North Shields	6	Slight
WARD, Lilian	27 Lawson St, North Shields	2	Slight
WARD, Lilian	27 Lawson St, North Shields	27	Serious

Admitted to Tynemouth Victoria Jubilee Infirmary on May 4th 1941

Name	Address	Apparent age	Condition
CHARLTON, George	98 Church Street, North Shields	17	Poor
GERMAIN, Eva	25 Upper Reed Street, North Shields	39	Poor
GERMAIN, Robert Lomas	25 Upper Reed Street, North Shields	56	DIED 4/5/41
HARMAN, Nellie	25 Upper Reed Street, North Shields	37	DIED 4/5/41
McPHILLIPS, John	50 Upper Queen Street, North Shields	33	DIED 4/5/41

Out Patients at Tynemouth Victoria Jubilee Infirmary on May 5th 1941

Name	Address	Apparent age	Condition
COOK, Mona	166 Linskill Street, North Shields	7	Awaiting x-ray result
DAWSON, Annie	9 George Street, North Shields	28	Slightly Injured
LOUGH, Raymond	23 Upper Queen Street, North Shields	8	Slightly injured
NICHOLSON, Alice	91 Church Street, North Shields	53	Satisfactory
SURREY, Robert	158 Stephenson Street, North Shields	41	Slightly Injured

Briefing

Casualties controversy

The casualty figure at Wilkinson's changes depending on whose account you are reading or which person you are listening to. It ranges from 96 to 105. In wilder flights of fancy, hundreds died.

It is important that we get the number correct to both recognise all those lost and to appreciate the scale of the disaster.

For many years it was accepted that, officially, 105 people were killed in the Wilkinson's bombing disaster.

Having become confused myself by the varying figures, I began to research the casualty numbers.

As a result, the death toll can be finalised, I hope, with some certainty at 107.

Here's how:

The Official Air Raid Figures issued by the Borough, states that 105 people were killed in the Wilkinson's disaster. This has long been accepted as fact.

However....

The Mortuary Records for this incident lists 102 victims. Of these, 2 people did not die at Wilkinson's. (Ethel Ada HUNTER, aged 49 and Margaret KING, aged 61, were killed when a bomb hit 3 George Street.) They died in the same raid and were processed at the same time.

So, we have 100 Mortuary Forms for those certified dead in the basement shelter.

But this count does not include the 7 people who died from their injuries later in hospital.

The total of deaths from this perspective is therefore 107.

Confusion is further caused when using the Civilian War Dead Roll of Honour. This resource gives 96 deaths in the shelter plus the 7 who died later. It omits 4 of the known dead recorded by mortuary forms because they were military personnel and not civilian casualties.

The total of deaths here is also 96+7+4 = 107.

There is also the grim local myth that many people were too difficult to extract from the debris and were simply left there and the basement filled in. This did not happen. All bodies were retrieved. There are no records of missing persons following the incident.

Briefing

Forgotten victims

Of the four bombs dropped by the enemy plane, 2 caused no casualties. One bomb hit the high water mark on The Flatts on the river and another hit the railway embankment on Stephenson Street. This bomb failed to explode. We have read about the direct hit at Wilkinson's Lemonade Factory.

Another of the bombs destroyed No 3 George Street, just along the road from Wilkinson's between Church Street and Queen Street, killing the 2 occupants inside, Ethel Ada HUNTER (aged 49) and Margaret KING (aged 61).

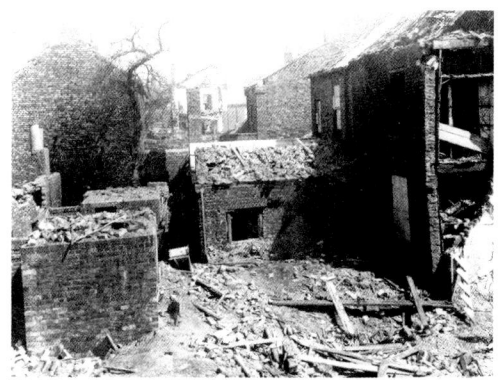

Number 3 George Street, front.

Number 3 George Street, rear.

9 Shelter Stories

Over the years I've had the great pleasure to meet and speak with many locals involved to a greater or lesser extent in the events of that terrible night in May 1941.

These are their stories. I have not amended any for accuracy, although in some cases, memory does not tie in with the known facts. The accounts are valuable, nonetheless.

Thanks are due to Joyce Marti and staff at North Shields Central Library for rediscovering an audio recording of survivor accounts, recorded at a reminiscence event at the library in 1994. Thanks also to librarian Val White who recorded the session.

What comes across to us today is the sense that this was a "different generation". What they went through as individuals, families and as a wider community deserves our respect.

BBC 2 – How We Won The War

On 11th May 2012, following a local newspaper appeal, survivors of the disaster and myself were invited to the Tyneside Cinema to be interviewed for the BBC2 documentary series, "How We Won The War".

At the time there were known to be six survivors still alive. Five of them met for the TV recording. The programme has a 10 minute segment on Wilkinson's in which several of the survivors speak movingly of their experiences. The programme is regularly repeated and is worth a watch.

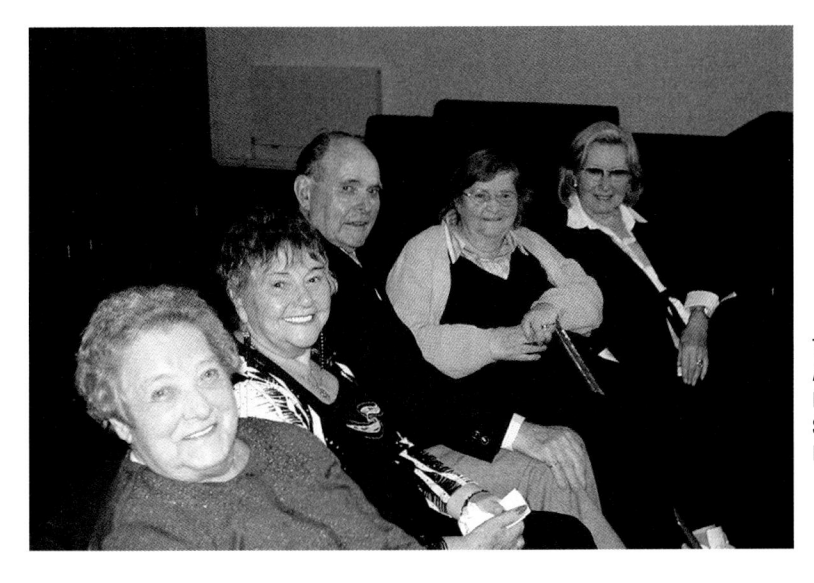

The last five. (left to right) Alma Chatterton, Millie Matthews, Robert Sutherst, Kathleen Main, Maureen Saunders

Albert Lee – shelter survivor

Albert Lee aged 17, was in the shelter and survived the disaster.

My mother (Ellen Lee) was the ARP warden in charge of Wilkinson's air raid shelter. So, naturally we used the shelter every time there was a raid on. That night I was in the shelter with Hilda, my sister.

We were sitting on the bunks in Room No 1. The shelter had a lot of people in it, but it was fairly quiet, some singing, just people chatting. When the bomb hit, I heard a dull 'bonk' sound. Then everything went black and people started screaming. I saw a match flicker somewhere, so I shouted 'Put that bloody match out' – I was thinking there might have been a gas leak.

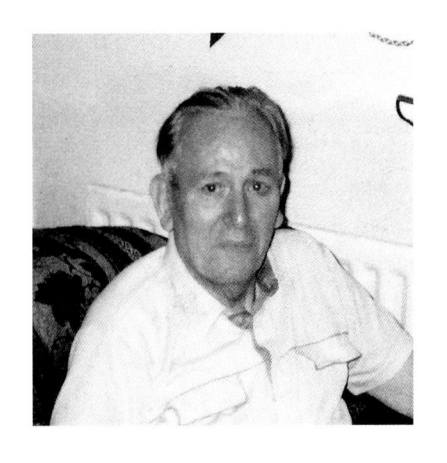

And then my mother told everyone to follow her torch light. The exit was blocked but she just shoulder charged the wall until it gave

way. She got over 30 people out. I was unharmed but my sister was in a bad way: she had a big wound in her side and a broken arm and leg. My father didn't even recognise her when he came to Kettlewell School where the injured were taken. The woman sitting opposite me…well, there wasn't much left of her."

Once we got outside my mother told me to run home and fetch her first aid box and some clothes – her dress had been burned off in the explosion. She was incredible, she didn't think about herself, she just worried about the injured and those still in the shelter. She stayed at her duty from the start to the end, despite her own injuries.

Even after 60 years I am immensely proud of what she did that night. I can't understand why she didn't win a medal for her bravery – she deserved one.

Robert Sutherst – shelter survivor

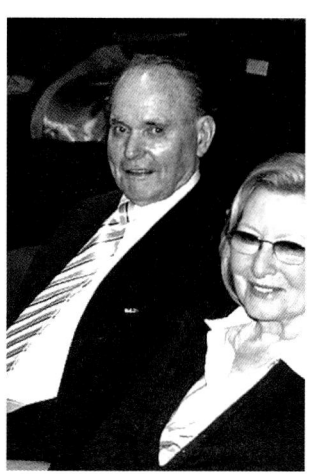

We did have a brick shelter in the back lane but it was deplorable and damp. That's why we had taken to going to Wilkinson's. People were friendly and there was an accordionist. People could forget the troubles of that particular time.

I was in the shelter with my mother, my brother and my cousin Edith. We were in the front bay. I remember I was on the top bunk. The shelter had 3 bays. The factory machinery was on the floors above the middle and rear sections.

I don't remember a "bang". It was more a "thud" sound. The blast was on one side. For some reason I could only hear my brother Tommy shouting. I told him to stand up and that we'd get out together. He said he couldn't stand or walk. So I shuttled him along.

There was a big hole on the King Street side with an ARP warden and a couple of army lads. They were shouting "give me your hand". I was curious as to why Tommy couldn't walk so I reached down and touched his leg and shuddered. Tommy had lost part of his leg and ear.

I was taken to Webb's fish shop, got cleaned up and consoled with the people there and then I went to Preston Hospital. I went off to stay with my Aunty Mona, she had a public house, The Borough Arms, on Camden Street. After the blast, my 2 year old sister was missing. The Marshall family found her crawling up King Street in the rubble. They took her in and looked after her.

Some days later my father came home on compassionate leave. He had to identify my mother, Kathleen Sutherst down at the old Wash House on Saville Street. She had a piece of white heather in her coat. My cousin Edith Louvaine Philips who was with us, also died.

I remember it all as if it was yesterday. It never goes away.

Emily Brooks – shelter regular

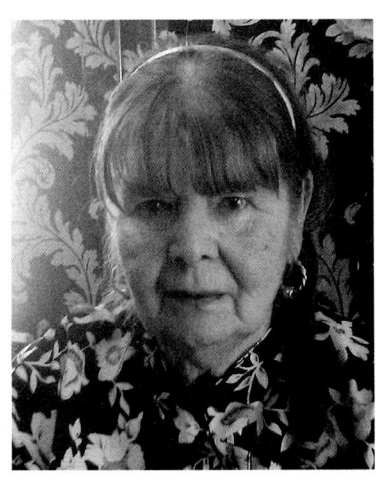

Emily Brooks was 12 at the time of the Wilkinson's bombing. She went to Linskill School. With her mother, sister and brother, she was a regular user of the basement air raid shelter. The shelter warden, Mrs Lee was her aunt.

Emily remembers using the shelter almost every evening. It was a safe place to be, especially since her home on Church Street had no external or internal shelter. She remembers the stone floor and the benches around the walls. She recalls it being cold inside.

With her friends, she would wait for the shelter to open at 5.30pm. They would gather at Tucker Crow's sweet shop opposite the factory on George Street. Then, a quick dash over the road and entry to the shelter via a dark grey, heavy metal door. Opening the door would turn off the internal light, closing it would turn the light on – a familiar precaution in the Black Out.

Emily is convinced that the earlier death of her older brother Harry, saved the family from the Wilkinson's bombing. She remembers that one night, Mrs Lee told her mother, Ethel, that she had better go back home as there was a telegram for her. Ethel left the shelter with her children. Sadly, she discovered that her eldest son had been lost in the sinking of the "Empire Brigade". The ship sank on the 19.10.1940.

From that date the family never used Wilkinson's shelter. Emily believed that, with Harry gone, it was pointless trying to make them safe and that they would take the risks that came. Shortly afterwards the family moved to Howdon Road.

The day after the Wilkinson's bombing, Emily and her mother went back to the site of the factory. It was a scene of great activity; men and ARP workers pulling away the rubble and debris. Ethel had thought that perhaps her husband Jack, an ARP worker had been in the shelter. Fortunately, he had been on duty down in the harbour. Emily remembers talking with her aunt, Mrs Lee at the scene. She can still see the grime and soot etched into the wrinkles of her face…and her tiredness.

Emily lost one of her school friends in the shelter.

Mrs Marshall (Sanderson) – shelter survivor

I lost my brother James Sanderson, aged 20, in the shelter.

I was 13 then. I was dragged to the shelter every time. I couldn't get out of bed. I was a lazy girl. Me mother used to stand over me, pull the clothes off and at the finish used to say, 'I'm going out for the Polis'. And he used to yank me out. He used to say, 'You're the only one around here who won't get out of bed.' I didn't get dressed (to go to the shelter) I had my pyjamas on all the time.

Me mother never took me to the shelter. It was the Polis. She used to go mad. We lived a block up from Wilkinson's, in Church Street. We hadn't got a shelter in our house. Nothing. We went to the shelter with my aunt and her family. One of her daughters, her fiancé was with my brother in the smoker's room. He was killed as well. Nice young man about 22. We'd been in the shelter for a couple of hours or so. Me Mother and Aunt were talking across me when all of a sudden, I said 'Be Quiet'. I heard the whistle. Didn't know what it was. That was it. I was in the corner…with my mother and auntie either side. I never even had a scratch. They had bricks on their back, everything. Wound up in hospital. My brother was in the smoker's room, where half the men went.

I can't remember a lot about the rescue. Mrs Lee (an ARP warden) she was there everywhere, helping everybody. She was outside all the time when the bombs were dropping to see everyone was all right. She was great, better than the men. She saw everybody in. I don't think that woman had a nerve in her body. I was trapped for six or seven hours. It was the next morning. There was a hand in front of us, pulled us out. That was it. I just wandered away. I was in a stupor through it all. Not unconscious. I was awake. I wandered off a mile away down to where the Royal Quays are now. A policeman found me and took me home. My mother and auntie were in hospital, so I went in to an empty house. Of course, they were out the next day with back injuries. She was ill a long time me mother. I had to stay off school to look after her.

Afterwards, when I worked in a shop, I started to stutter. I was so shy. My mother used to call me 'Gob' until it happened. But I was never frightened of anything until I was 17 and a half and joined the WRENS and you know the barracks – the black out and everything – I went berserk. I went screaming. I thought I was still in the shelter, but I knew I wasn't. I went stupid. It told on me then. I mean I'd lost a brother, but it just didn't sink deep enough. But when I joined up, I had to see a psychiatrist. Got over that. I think with the blackout and everything I just went off it.

Later, I got me confidence back. I was posted as an officer's stewardess to a little country place near Newcastle under Lyme. Well, as we were going on the train, I met up with this Liverpool girl and we got friends. I said to her 'Look out there. Look at all those cows. We're going to have an awful time'. Oh boy. It was great. Yanks! I used to get cups for jiving.

You know even now I've got to sleep in a bedroom where I can see daylight. That's how it tells on me. You don't realise. It tells on you in some way.

Billy Curran – shelter accordionist

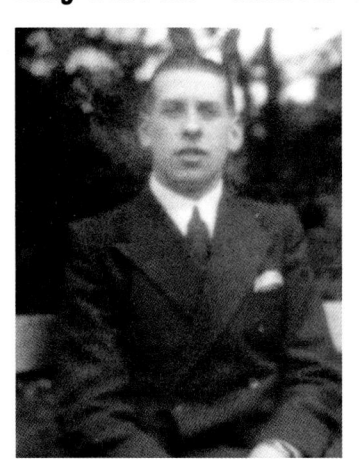

Many survivors and shelter users mentioned with affection, a musician who would regularly entertain those in the shelter.

Thanks to Bill Atkinson, we have been able to identify him as Billy Curran, who died in the shelter aged 23.

Billy was with his grandmother Emma Curran, who also lost her life, aged 80. Emma was the oldest victim of the bombing.

Bill Atkinson's mother, Lillian Atkinson (née Curran) lost seven of her dearest relatives in the shelter bombing. Amongst them were her grandmother, Emma, who's life she had saved days before by pushing her into the cupboard under the stairs, just before much of the house came down. Lillian's brother was Billy the accordionist.

Amanda Mills - Maureen Saunders – the youngest survivor

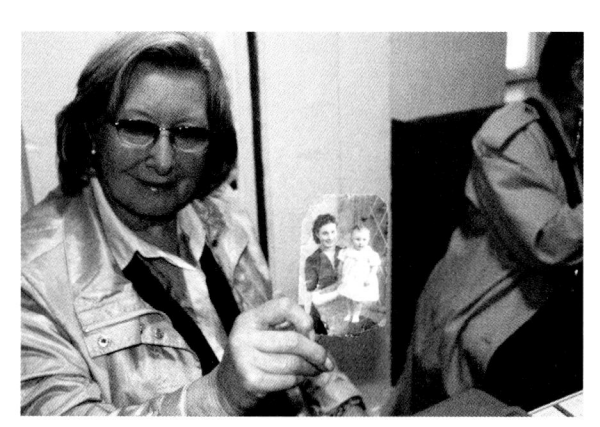

My mum Maureen Saunders is one of only very few survivors left from that terrible night. At the time, my mum was a tiny baby. My mum survived the bombing as her mum Nancy Saunders courageously lay across her baby daughter to protect her.

Nancy suffered severe injuries from the bombing including a broken spine, she had treatment at Hexham Spinal Unit. Nancy and Maureen were evacuated to Allendale in Northumberland.

Another member of the family was killed in the Wilkinson's shelter that night – Clarence Beavers was my great aunt's fiancé.

Mrs Dean, Mrs Dixon, Mrs Allcock (Kay) – mother's lucky escape

We were in our own shelter in the backyard and we could hear the "thud".

We lived on George Street in the caretaker's house at Kettlewell School. We had soldiers and ARP wardens stationed in the school.

I remember vividly Mrs Lee. We heard this child crying, "I've lost me shoe. I want me mammy". And Mrs Lee had her in her arms. Then somebody in charge, an officer rushed in and shouted, "Bring everything you can, blankets, bandages, whatever, Wilkinson's shelter's been hit!".

We could hear the heavy, running, footfall of people, soldiers, on the pavement outside.

Can I tell you though, fate took a hand. My mother was heavily pregnant. But you didn't know in those days that your mother was pregnant. Well, you didn't, did you?

My father had always said Wilkinson's was a death trap. But my mother had said, "I'll feel safer in the shelter".

"Well, if you want to go to the shelter, get yourself away to the shelter," he told her.

She went to the door and there was a soldier on guard. And she asked him to take her to the shelter, which was just over the road, around the corner. And he said, "It's more than my life's worth. I'll be court-martialled for leaving my post. You're safer in your own shelter. Go back in."

We were all in the shelter, the whole family, 5 or 6 of us. And my mother came in and just shortly after that, we felt our shelter lift, up and back down again.

The memory of the running feet and the child crying, that stays with you.

We lost an aunt, Doreen Kay and her four boys, Ernest, Hylton, Sydney and George. Our father's brother's family. It was terrible.

Ethel May Shaw – the Hall family

I was aged 14 and I was at home with my mother Maria Binks and my seventeen year old sister, Sheila and my baby brother Jimmy, who was 18 months old.

When the sirens went off, my mother tried to get us off to the shelter. Sheila wouldn't get up out of bed and said she wouldn't go

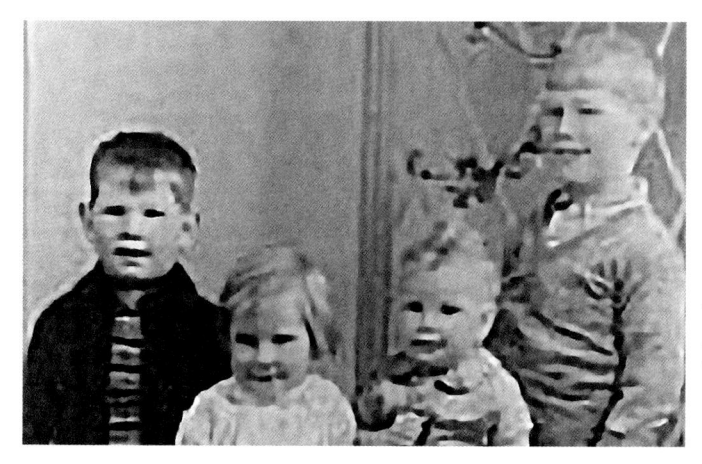

The Hall children. James, Shirley Anne, Alfred and John. Sydney wouldn't have his photo taken!

to Wilkinson's. As a result, none of us went and we stayed in the backyard shelter in Norfolk Street.

My Aunt, Martha Hall and her five children, our cousins, John Alfred, Sydney, James, Shirley and Alfred were all killed in Wilkinson's shelter.

Their father, my uncle, John Alfred Hall was at sea at the time with the Royal Navy. He never recovered from the shock. He never remarried and never had any more children.

I personally never went into the shelter, but my Aunt Martha was in the musical section which is where she always went as there was an accordion player there.

Wilkinson's had a shop on Albion Road where they sold lemonade.

People thought that the shelter would be safe because it had a concrete ceiling, but I know there was a lot of heavy machinery on the floor above.

Mrs Tennison – the Harman family

Mrs Tennison lost her sister in law, Mary Ellen Harman and her 3 children, Thomas, Joan and Richard in the shelter.

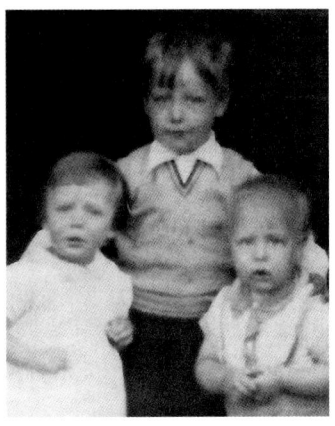

Mrs Tennison was in the WRAF and was at home on leave that night. Mary Ellen (Nellie) and the children had started off for the shelter but changed their minds and had tried to go back to their home, just around the corner, at 25 Reed Street. The ARP wardens along George Street said there wasn't enough time and pushed them back towards the shelter.

Nellie had been baking bread when the sirens went. When Mrs Tennison went around to the house after the bombing, the loaves had risen perfectly.

Mary Ellen died from her injuries on Sunday 4th May at Jubilee Infirmary.

The children's grandmother, Matilda Harman, identified their bodies at the Bath House Mortuary. They had mauve acid burns from the chemicals stored on the upper floors at Wilkinson's.

(Photo courtesy of Steve Robinson).

Millie Matthews (Cook) – shelter survivor

I was Mildred Cook then. We, me sister aged 5, me brother 7, and I was 14, we had to go up and stay with me mother's twin sisters in Queen Street, while me mother was away. We stayed in Queen Street, the next street to Wilkinson's.

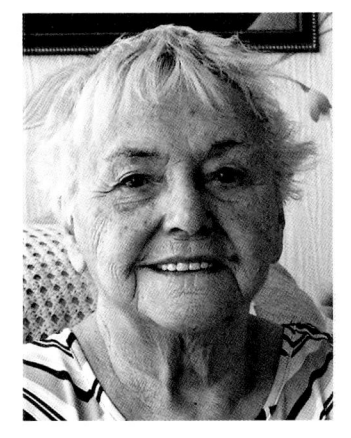

My mother and I didn't usually go to this shelter because we lived down Linskill Street. We just went there an odd time – just to see her sisters. My aunties had a strong shelter in their back yard, but they used to go to Wilkinson's because it was an entertaining evening. They used to play bingo or cards. There was sort of like 3 bays in the shelter. There was a place where people went to smoke, a place for the young 'uns and a part for sing-alongs. There was a guy who used to play the accordion

A friend of mine was called Frances Chatterson. We both went to school together. We used to play with the children. As I recall, I had just gone on top of a bunk – then all of a sudden it was dead silent and black. I had no warning. I couldn't tell what was going on outside. It just went…like putting the light out. Frances shouted 'Millie' and dragged me off the bunk and just then the bunk collapsed. She still jokes about it, 'Millie I saved your life'."

It was probably seconds later before people began crying, yelling and screaming…it was awful. One bloke was striking matches and someone shouts 'Put that bloody match out!' They must have been frightened, maybe about gas.

We had a little lad staying with us from Scarborough, an evacuee. He was blinded by the gas from the lemonade. A lot of people turned blue. He was called John Herrett, about 10 years old. It was his sister Lillian Herrett's birthday and my aunty Kathleen Sutherst had been baking all day. We were going to have a party at Harbottle's Field. Lillian sadly didn't make it. Everybody came out blue from the acid. Their skin was coloured. John was blinded by it. He got over it, but it took a long time.

The next thing I knew was this air raid warden. Mrs Lee. I heard her voice from outside. 'Can anybody hear us?' she was yelling. I said 'Yes' and she asked, 'Can you see a light?' I saw the light of her torch through a tiny hole. She said, 'Can you try and show us where it is?' I must have climbed up somewhere. I don't know on what…but I climbed up and put my finger through this little hole where I could see the light. I can always remember her getting hold of my hand and making the hole bigger.

I was pushing these children out of the hole, maybe's two or whatever. And then I heard my brother, who was 7, shouting, 'Millie, Millie, Millie'. Then I felt all this blood on him. As I recall I was quite calm mesell, until I got hold of me brother. That seemed to click something in me and I got me brother out. He was shouting for me to get out, so I went with him.

We got out with some other children and we were taken to the fish and chip shop over the road. Then an ambulance came and we were taken to the Boys Club opposite the Infirmary. We saw Robert Sutherst's brother, Tommy, come in on a stretcher and we thought he was dead as there was a white sheet over him. He was alive but he had a very serious leg injury.

My aunty, Kathy Sutherst died. She was 32. Her twin sister Nora survived but she had a fractured skull and concussion and had a silver plate put in her head.

They had a sort of mortuary in an old wash-house. Her husband, me uncle Bobby, was sent home from the army. He was at the police station all the time. That was where they used to put the names of those who had been killed outside on a list.

He went to the Mortuary and there was a bag with a piece of my aunty Kathy's coat - a grey, astrakhan coat - it had a piece of white heather in the lapel…and that was draped over the bag. Whether they found her or not we never knew. She was killed with Edith Louvaine Phillips, her niece.

I wasn't physically hurt, but mentally I was in a bad way. I was going to join the Land Army, but the doctor exempted me. If the weather was thundery, I would hide under the bed or in cupboards. I used to hang on to my mother all the time. I couldn't be left alone at all. I still suffer from claustrophobia.

Jessie Lorrison (Dial) – lucky escape

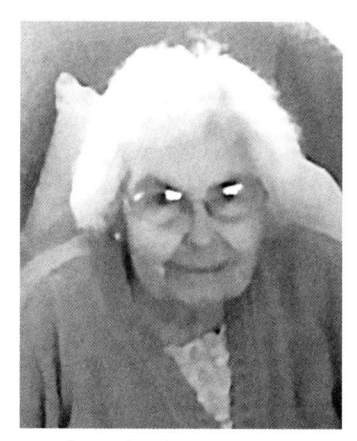

I was 13 at the time and we lived at 23 King Street. Wilkinson's was just over the road. We used the shelter often but very luckily, not that night.

My father worked for the gas company. He also worked as a driver for the ARP. I remember he told my mother that if there was a raid that night, she was to take us into Wilkinson's for safety. When the sirens went my mother decided to stay in the house. She didn't want to go to the shelter because with it being a Saturday night, she knew there would be music on. She didn't like the accordion music. It kept her awake.

Instead we hid under a table in one of the bedrooms. Right after the bomb hit, we ran over to the shelter, but the doors wouldn't open. We knew straight away that it was a disaster. A policeman told us to get back indoors as there was a chance of more of the walls collapsing. Our feet were bleeding from all the glass on the road. We hadn't noticed!

I remember Mrs Lee, the ARP woman. She was a big, nice lady. We called her Tessie O'Shea. I think she got a medal. The soldiers at Kettlewell School came to help.

Harry Rose – the Franklands

I was born on March 2nd 1935, so one can say that I was a child of the Depression. I cannot recall much of that time but I do know that my father was directed by the labour exchange to dig two deep underground shelters in Dockwray Square. This must have been late 1939 because I was old enough to be sent with Dad's sandwiches for him at lunch-time so I was not yet at school.

I remember this in particular because Dad gave me a bite of his sandwich and of course it had mustard on it. Dad was soon called up into the Army which upset him as he was an experienced trawler man. Still, as I eventually found out myself, one does not argue with the armed forces. He was a soldier in the Worcester Regiment.

At this time we were living in a rented house in Hamilton Terrace which is part of Tynemouth Road and it was a two storied corner house with a haberdashery next door.

While Dad was away in the army, we were told that the house was to be requisitioned as an Air Raid Warden Centre and we would have to move. Mother was upset to say the least, especially when she was told that we would have to move to Dockwray Square. This was a poorer area of town and not very desirable. Then she was told that it was a newly converted house with indoor toilet, kitchen and bathroom. Suddenly all was smiles and she was eager to move. I went to school from Dockwray Square and had all of the adventures that boys then had.

Sometime in 1940 I was evacuated to Rothbury, together with many of my school mates . We went to school there and for the most part had a reasonable time. As there was little or no bombing my mother took me back home. The German High command must have heard that I had returned to North Shields because in 1941 they began bombing us.

The War affected everyone because men were away. Everything was rationed and tragedy happened to someone every day. Somehow, as kids we did not grasp the enormity of the situation which is just as well for our unformed minds.

Mother was frightened as we had already lost her brother, my uncle Bob who was lost 8th March 1941 aboard the steamship Togston.

Uncle Bob had already survived a sinking when aboard the Goodwood which was sunk 10th Sept 1939 in the North Sea. Uncle Bob was awarded the British Empire Medal and Lloyds Gallantry Medal. (see "In Peril on the Sea" by D Masters – The Cresset Press 1960)

The War was exciting to me in my childish innocence and I happily gathered shrapnel with my school friends after an air raid. We grew quite expert so we thought at estimating where the spent bullets or shrapnel would be from the scars on the buildings. Some of the lads found all kinds of wonderful things such as the fins from incendiary bombs and bits of planes. Trouble started when some fellows found a load of unfired bullets that must have fallen from a damaged aeroplane. They fired these by wedging them in fence planks and hitting the base with a brick. One can imagine the row that caused in the schools. We would be "frisked" in the morning for "goodies" and various important people went around the schools telling us of the dangers. I cannot say that it stopped it going on really. School kids are experts at deception when they wish to be and the "code of the closed mouth" ruled.

My father was on leave on the 3rd of May 1941 when Wilkinson's factory shelter was hit, killing my cousin Sandy Frankland and damaging his brother Arthur, as well as lots of people I knew. During the raid the bombers were very close to our house which was in line with the tankers in the Tyne and Dad decided we should leave for somewhere safer, preferably deeper. We all set off for Wilkinson's to arrive not long after it was hit. Mother and I with Mrs Talantyre and daughter Marjory were sent to Northumberland Street Mission while Dad started helping to dig for survivors hoping that this would mean his sister Nellie and her family. We were lucky in that Aunt Nellie and cousin Sephie had stayed at home in their own shelter.

Tragically Arthur and Sandy had gone to Wilkinson's for the "fun". Sandy was among the dead and Arthur was never really the same again. He had been buried with Sandy for about a day. There were 107 people killed and 43 injured that night in Wilkinson's Mineral Water factory shelter. The largest loss of life in a single raid that North Shields suffered.

Dad wanted to stay to be with Aunt Nellie but was told to return to his unit. Mother and I eventually left Shields when mother got a position in Cumberland.

Kathleen Alderson – the Ward family

Obviously before I was born (1950) back in 1941, my aunt Lilian May Ward went to a photographer together with my cousins Lilian and Maureen Ward. She got her 6 week old daughter's photograph taken – first and only photo. Little did she know.

After visiting the photographer, she went to see some relative of her husband's, I think, who lived near King Street in North Shields. Normally she would never have been along that end of the town. Whilst she was in that area the sirens went to alert folks that German bombers were on their way to bomb the shipyards by the Tyne. They all had to go to the nearest shelter, so she took her two children and they went into Wilkinson's shelter. Not sure if the bomb was a rogue bomb accidentally dropped or if it was jettisoned out as the German planes were finished and due to go back to Germany. Anyway, the bomb exploded when it hit the pop factory and the shelter was blown up.

My aunt Lilian May Ward (about 27/28 years old) was injured and was on crutches following the blast. My cousin Lilian Ward (about 3/4 years old) was found standing next to her mother totally unharmed and Maureen Ward (6 weeks old) was blown off my aunt's knee and was killed.

My mother Amy Knowles (nee Conaty) was asked to identify the baby. She told me that the only way she could identify Maureen was by her clothes (I think she wore a blue dress) as she had seen her that morning. She was buried in a small grave in Preston cemetery.

My cousin Lilian appeared safe and sound but years later she was diagnosed with schizophrenia and it was thought that this experience she went through as a child could have had something to with her illness in later years. She suffered with her nerves in adult life and awful mood swings. All terribly sad for this family.

(This was all told to me by my mum Amy who died age 95 years and 7 months old in October 2011.) Hope I have recalled everything correctly.

Olive Seddon – the Wears family – stayed at home

My mam (Sarah Ann Wears (Bertram)) used to go into Wilkinson's shelter.

The night it was bombed she was under the stairs at home with my nana (Edith Wears) and my sister Ann. My nana used to go under the stairs as she was scared of the thunder and lightning. So, when the bombs came, under the stairs she went. She didn't like my mam going into Wilkinson's shelter. I'm pleased she didn't go to the shelter that night as we wouldn't be here!

My nana lived in Coburg Street and Dockwray Square in those days. She wouldn't go in the shelter. My mam said it wasn't nice in there. My mam's sister, May, is still alive, she's 92 and she said that as youngsters they would go outside to watch the bombs. No fear eh!

Ruth Mather & David Hodgson – the Gray family

We lost our grandparents and aunt at Wilkinson's.

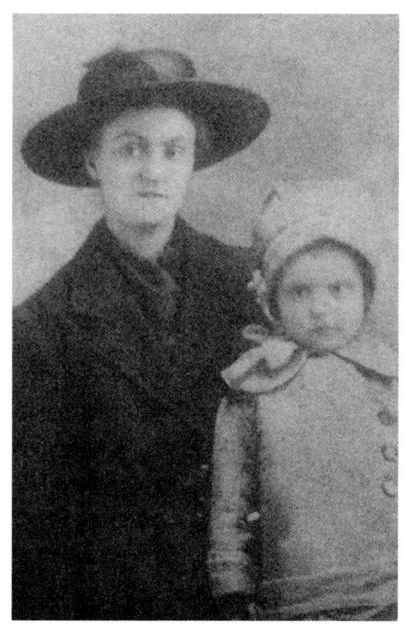

We don't actually have a lot of information about our family members as it clearly had a very traumatic effect on our mother and appeared to leave her almost devoid of a sense of humour or ability to have fun. She had been in service as a housekeeper/cook from the age of 15 to a Jewish family in Newcastle and, as such had been away from home for a number of years before the tragedy with only a few home visits to her mother and sister while her father was at work as a builder's labourer. She appeared to feel some guilt about the lack of contact with her family according to our father.

Margaret and Elsie Gray. (Courtesy of Ruth Mather/David Hodgson)

Our mother Elsie Gray, born 15th September 1915, was away from home, having trained as a Salvation Army officer and was posted to a children's home in Portsmouth when she received the news about the Wilkinson's disaster. Her only brother, 6 years her junior, was a submariner in the Royal Navy and was away on active service at that time. She was called home to deal with her parents and sister's funerals – Joseph Henry Gray, Margaret Gray and Mary Gray. The family lived at 70 Linskill Street at the time of their deaths.

Our father Chris Hodgson, born 28th October 1902, was an Air Raid Warden who was part of the team who retrieved the bodies from the air raid shelter and said that the Gray family were among the last bodies to be removed from the debris. Dad actually knew the family as Mam had been a pupil in his Sunday School class at the Town

Mission where Dad was a lay preacher and a friend of Pastor Ross during his time at the Mission. Dad's first wife had died in childbirth along with the baby in 1938, leaving him with a 9 year old daughter.

Our father used to tell the story that he was walking on Tynemouth Pier with two lady friends on a Sunday afternoon following the air raid and saw our mother walking towards them and introduced them as "Miss Brown, Miss Green, meet Miss Gray". They continued their afternoon stroll together. He attended the family funeral and they stayed in touch and began corresponding when she returned to her post in the children's home.

I'm not sure exactly when she returned to the North-East but they were married on 23rd March 1946.

Maureen Rumfitt – the Franklands – Internet discovery

Maureen Rumfitt had never used the internet before when she logged on for the first time. But within seconds of entering her father's name into a search engine she had found the clues to help solve a family mystery that had haunted her for nearly 50 years.

Maureen was nine when her mother and father died within six months of each other in 1955. Split up from her brothers and sisters, Maureen spent several years in foster care at Hillcrest in North Shields, filled with questions about her family that she never thought would be answered.

Maureen's online search led her to northshields173.org. Through the site Maureen found out that her father William Frankland was injured in the raid (smoking at the entrance, Billy was flung clear). His brother Arthur was buried up to the neck in rubble but was taken to hospital and survived. However, sadly, another brother Alexander (Sandy) Frankland was killed. She also discovered the full name of her grandfather, which she had never known and learned of relatives who she never knew existed.

"I'm just so grateful to the site for giving me answers to questions I had about my family, particularly my father", Maureen says. "It's been amazing being able to find out the truth after all these years."

Bill Atkinson – the Glynn family

The guests at my parents' wedding. The little lady on the left (as we look at it) of the front row is Ann Glynn.

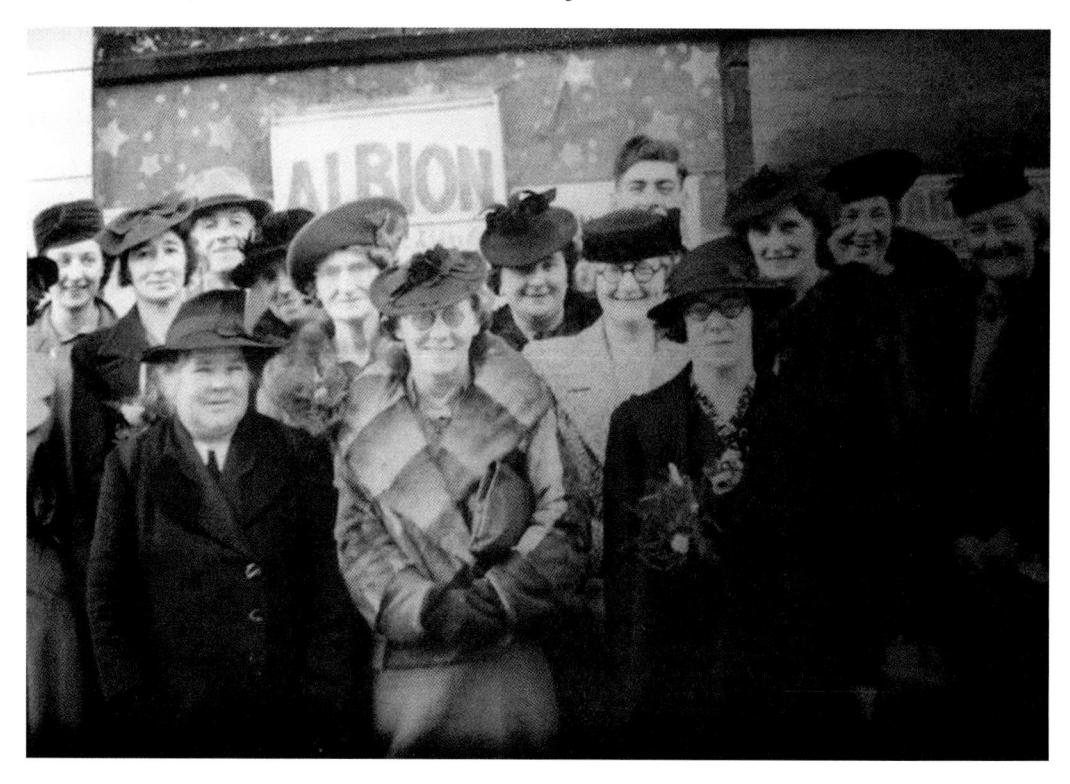

Aunty Ann lost her husband (John Thomas Glynn), daughter (Margaret Glynn) and mother (Emma Curran) in the shelter. She spent the rest of her life living at 66 North King Street, as did her daughter Annie.

As children, my brother and I went to Auntie Anne's to watch the FA cup final, as she had a telly and we didn't. She was always a kind and cheerful woman.

On the right of the front row is Mum's aunt Eveline. She was a shelter survivor. Jilted as a young woman, she remained a spinster until later life when her ex-boyfriend, by then a widower, searched for and found her. They married and had a few happy years together.

Aunt Eveline looked after Billy Curran (now identified as the shelter accordionist) before this photo was taken. He was in fact living at her home at the time of the bombing. My Mum told me that her step-mother had gone to Eveline's soon after the bombing to see if there was an accordion there that she could take to sell! It takes all sorts, as they say!!

The tall chap at the back of the picture is we think, Aunty Ann's son. He may also have been a survivor. His name was Jack Glynn. I remember him, his wife Kathleen and son Tony. I think they lived on the Marden Estate.

James Robert Ward – the Donkin family and Maureen Ward

I am indebted to Philip Pattinson and his family for permission to publish the following extract from James Robert Ward's unpublished memoir "The Low Street Boy".

Mr Ward lost two cousins and a half-sister in the bombing disaster. Elizabeth Lindores Donkin, Elizabeth Ann Donkin and Maureen Ward.

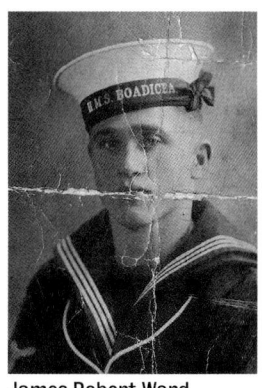

The last time I saw Mrs Gibson and Ethel was in the old Wash House on the corner of Church Way and Saville Street, opposite the Alnwick Castle pub, I was looking at their faces, but they could not look at mine; they were dead, victims of the bombing of Wilkinson's Air Raid Shelter. The Wash House was utilised for a Mortuary. I was in there with my brother Bill, looking for three of our family, they were there with many more we knew.

James Robert Ward

It seemed that somebody up there did not like our family. Then came that terrible night of the 4th of May 1941. I think that the "Repulse", "King George the Fifth" and the destroyer "Khandhar", had left the River before high-tide. At the time of the high-tide and with a "Bomber's Moon" the hordes of enemy planes came in. They dropped their incendiary bombs on Osbeck's Timber Yard and it was full of props at the time, and this blaze lit up the river. So that the bombers could drop death and destruction.

We got news that Wilkinson's Shelter had been hit. My sister and my two nieces died there.

My uncle Ossie Henderson was there helping to dig them out. If only my sister, sister-in-law and their three children had stayed in my sister's house. It was only twenty yards from the shelter and was undamaged.

My brother Bill and I went through the Wash-House, to identify our dead, we managed to get Bill's wife Lily out and their eldest daughter Lily. As we went into the Mortuary, the attendant offered us a cigarette, Bill took one, I don't smoke. The attendant had a cigarette case with a lighter attached, the first that I had seen. He could not keep his hands still as he tried to light Bill's cigarette. This man had the worst job in Shields at that moment. Bill steadied his hand and he took us around. The children and small adults were on the top bunks and the big people on the bottom bunks. It was like walking down "Memory Lane", there was everybody I knew by name or sight, Mr Gibson and Ethel, the Broans from Tyne Street, and one woman in particular, her big black eyes used to make me uncomfortable when I was a kid, and there they were staring at me as before.

I was going to go around the back of the bunks, when the attendant said, "Don't go around there, there is nothing there for you". He was wrong. I did go around and found my sister Lizzie. She had a black eye and I think that she had been pregnant at the time. The back of the shelter was like a butcher's shop, all of the corpses were wrapped in burlap, that kind of muslin that the butcher's used. Bill had found Ann, Lizzie's daughter, but could not find Maureen his own daughter. We climbed up the ladders to examine each child. One did look like her, but the attendant showed me, three chalk crosses on the side of the bunk. Three people had identified this child as their own. It was so hard to tell the difference.

We went home to find out what his daughter had on at the time of the raid. What had happened was that my sister, having been a "Fisher Lass" did a lot of crochet and that night she dressed my brother's daughter in some of her own daughter's clothes, they were dressed identical, but when we went back and further explained what outer garments she had on, the man showed us her siren suit and patent leather shoes. I won't explain further.

These attendants must have had a terrible and heart breaking job. I don't know the true statistics of that raid, but I was told there were 109 killed out of the 190 that were in the shelter. We went to the burials at Preston Cemetery, there is no need for me to describe the scene there. True to our family tradition, I went on duty that night.

Neil Hodgson – the Hodgson family

I am greatly indebted to Neil Hodgson, son of Sidney Hodgson, for the following information and photographs which are reproduced with his permission.

Four members of the Hodgson family were killed in the shelter. Violet Hodgson (sister of Sidney Hodgson), Alexina Dodgson (wife of Henry Henderson Hodgson) and her two children, Elizabeth and Henry Henderson Jr.

Sidney Hodgson was a firewatcher in North Shields. He had been out dancing and walked his sisters along to the shelter and then went on to his own house.

> As you can see from the photo , their ages must relate closely to the time of their death.
>
> I think that given the fact my father, Sidney, had a copy of this photo, it may have been the last photo taken of the family together

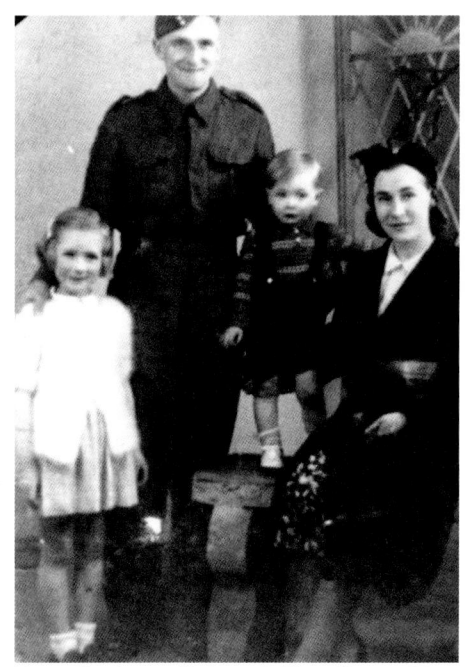

Henry Henderson Hodgson in his uniform, with his wife Alexina, his daughter Elizabeth and son Henry Henderson. As you can see from the photo, their ages must relate closely to the time of their death.to the time of their death.

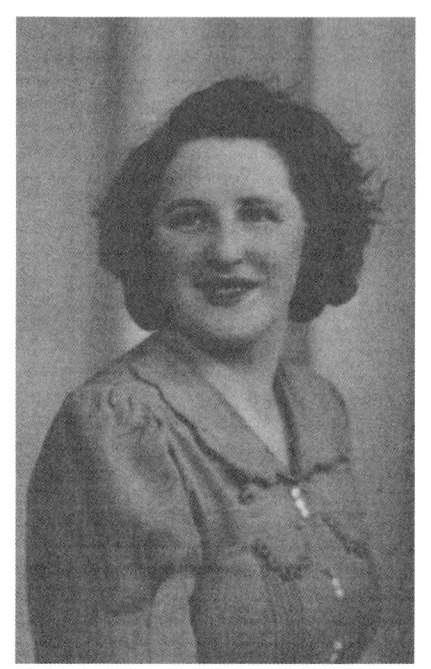

Violet Hodgson.

as a family, and the fact that Henry is in uniform may make its date very close to that of the Air Raid."

"The other photo is of my aunty Violet, my father's sister. I understand that my father who was then approaching 17 years old, had been out with his sister and that on their way home together, Violet had decided to go to the air raid shelter and my father continued on alone.

Judging by this photo, Violet, who was a Domestic Servant aged 19 at the time of the air raid, must have been about the age in this

George Sturrock – Nora Sturrock and Alexander "Sandy" Frankland

My mother, Nora Sturrock, lost her brother Alexander "Sandy" Frankland in the bombing.

Mrs Sturrock lived in Upper Queen Street. She and her boyfriend George (later husband) were standing in the doorway when the Wilkinson's bomb blast flung them both into the passageway covering them in lime dust.

Nora and George had decided not to go to the shelter that night because it got rowdy with people taking in their own drink which led to a lot of singing and carrying on.

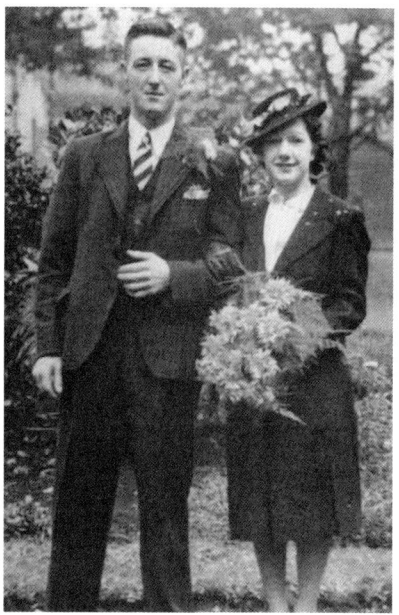

George and Norah Sturrock. Courtesy of George Sturrock

George was one of the first at the scene. They both knew that her brothers were in Wilkinson's. Alexander "Sandy" Frankland was killed. Arthur Frankland survived although he was buried up to the neck in rubble and Billy Frankland was flung clear smoking at the entrance.

My father also lost a brother who never returned to North Shields Fish Quay after the small fishing boat he was on was torpedoed.

My parents were lucky on another occasion when they were in a cinema in South Shields and decided to leave and go for the North Shields Ferry when they heard the air raid siren - the cinema was bombed during the air raid.

On another occasion they were machine gunned by a German airplane as they were going home down the back lane that was opposite the entrance of The Albion Cinema.

My father was a welder which was a reserved occupation and he was stationed at Tynemouth firing Anti-Aircraft Guns. I didn't realise how difficult it must have been to actually hit an aircraft. He used to joke about being awarded with one and a half hits for the whole of the War saying he didn't understand how he got half a hit. He used to put weld into the bullet & shrapnel holes in the large Gas Tanks at Howdon which were full of Gas at the time. They had to dive into a doorway to dodge the bullets.

Lily Holmes – Elizabeth Lindores Donkin and Maureen Ward

Mrs Holmes, whose aunt Elizabeth Lindores Donkin died in the bombing, contacted me with the following…

> These are a few lines about my aunt Lizzie, a victim of the Wilkinson's bomb disaster on May 3rd 1941, as told to me by my mother and her brother Sid.
>
> She was married to a soldier called William Donkin and had a young baby Elizabeth Ann. They lived at the Pontin buildings around the corner from the shelter. William had just gone back to the army after being on leave. Auntie Lizzie, as we knew her, had her sister-in-law Lily Ward staying with her that weekend and Lily's children, young Lily and Maureen who was a six month old baby.
>
> My mother's other brother Freddy should have been staying with her too but because of Lily and her family staying, Freddy was told not to go (luckily for him, as he also could have been a victim).
>
> But when the siren went Lizzie, Lily and the children went into the shelter. A witness account said that Lizzie was sitting with the baby on her knee and when she started crying, Lizzie began to walk back and forth so she gave up her seat to an old lady.
>
> After the bomb fell and the survivors came out, Lily Ward and her oldest child, Lily, were among them but sadly Lizzie and her daughter, Ann and baby Maureen were killed. Ironically the old lady

to whom she gave up her seat, survived.

Sid, a 12 year old paper boy at the time, was the one who told his mother about the tragedy. The whole family watched as they brought the bodies out and took them to the make-shift morgue at the old wash house buildings.

It was the sad duty of Ozzie, Lizzie's younger brother, to identify her body and her mother identified baby Ann. Maureen was identified by her father William Ward, but she was only recognizable by the dress she was wearing which had been given to her by Auntie Lizzie.

Her husband William was given compassionate leave for the funeral. Her younger brother Ozzie was lost at sea two years later in the Atlantic Crossing.

I feel proud and privileged to have been asked to write this small dedication to an aunt that I never knew in life. Her memory was kept alive by my mother who was her only sister. Now with her name in print she will be remembered always.

Mrs Oliver – Alice Nicholson – shelter survivor

Mrs Oliver's grandmother, Alice Nicholson, survived at Wilkinson's. She was saved because a door fell on her and sheltered her from the falling masonry. She was showered with money from a till from the factory shop which fell on her lap.

Her mother used the shelter regularly and apparently people were in the habit of booking a seat for the shelter if you went in the day time.

Mrs Heslop – mother survived

Mrs Heslop's mother survived the bombing of Wilkinson's shelter. She spent 5 hours buried in the shelter in the section where the children normally went. She recalls seeing her mother coming home to the back door of the house in a terrible state, covered in soot and brick dust.

Her father was an ARP Warden. Mr and Mrs Brannen, ARP Wardens in Whitby Street were family friends.

Mr Henderson – loss of grandparents

Mr Henderson lost his grandfather and grandmother: James Henderson and Phyllis Henderson.

For some reason his family did not go to Wilkinson's that night as they usually did. He recalls possibly being at the Boro cinema instead to watch Laurel and Hardy. When air raids were on the manager would come on to the stage and clear the house. Mr Henderson was later injured at home when a bomb fell on Addinson Street in the west end of the town.

Raymond Lough (survivor aged 8) – the Lough family

Mr Lough, aged 8, survived the air raid disaster. He lost his father, William Lough and sister Margaret at Wilkinson's.

He recalls being very nervous during air raids. That night he was trying to sleep in a top bunk when the bomb hit. He remembers being almost suspended in mid-air for a few seconds and then he started to crawl along the floor until he saw a flash light. He was taken to Kettlewell School by the ARP rescuers.

Haydon Sharp – Edith Louvaine Phillips

> I was 13 at the time and I lost my friend, Edith Louvaine Philips aged 14 at Wilkinson's.
>
> My uncle lived next door to the factory. He suffered from Parkinson's Disease and always used the shelter when there was a raid on. For some reason though, he didn't go that night. It saved his life.
>
> We lived in Linskill Street and that night I was standing with my father at the front door watching the 'fireworks' (i.e. the raid, searchlights, flak etc)

My father used to work on a dredger on the Tyne and I was wearing a soldier's tin hat he had dredged up from the river. After the bomb hit a policeman came up the street holding a little girl by the hand. He asked us to take her into the house. She was in a right state. When my mother undressed her, she was covered from head to toe in soot and brick dust. I remember that later, me, Dolly and Jenny Taylor took the girl along to the Hope Inn where we had been told her Aunt lived. The next morning, we went up to see the bomb site. It was cordoned off. A group of miners wanted to help clear the rubble but the Rescue people wouldn't let them. The atmosphere was very tense.

Kathleen Parkin (Bulman) – Wilkinson labels and debris

After the bombing of Wilkinson's, all the debris was used to fill in the burn which ran down Red Burn View, where we lived. I remember scrambling over the debris and finding lots of household items: knives, forks, spoons and also lipstick and rouge and millions of bottle labels. It seems like yesterday.

Jennie Ford (Forrest) – helping the survivors

I am 92 years old now (Jennie was interviewed in 2000). At the time we lived quite near the shelter. My mother, Mrs M Forrest was a volunteer and was on duty that night when the bomb fell on Wilkinson's shelter.

Her station at that time was at Northumberland Street Mission. She went to the shelter and gave help to the few who were alive. They were taken to the Mission, a bed was made and food was given to each one. When it was daylight, she took some of the survivors to their homes. One was an 11 year old boy. His mother and grandmother had slept through that bombing being drunk! They only lived a few doors higher up the street. It was amazing how anyone got out, as there was heavy machinery in the shelter.

I always felt that my mother and the other helpers should have had some recognition. But in those days we kept each other.

Henry P Rose – the Frankland family

I was six years old in the March of that year and my father came home on leave in the May, just in time for the bombing. When the sirens sounded, we went to our own shelter which was in the yard. Father was not happy with this because he felt that we were too near the river and that the bombers could be trying to get the shipping. He decided that we should move to a shelter away from the bank top and he chose Wilkinson's.

So, my parents and our neighbours set off for Wilkinson's shelter with my father carrying me. At the bottom of King Street, the air was full of dust and the smell of wall lime. Even today when I pass an old building being demolished that smell of lime dust takes me back. An air raid warden stopped father and told him that the shelter had received a direct hit about ten minutes before.

It had been the habit of my cousins, the Frankland's to go to Wilkinson's because it was more fun to be with a crowd than in their own shelter at home. Father and mother knew many of the people that used Wilkinson's and they at once feared the worst. Mother and I, together with our neighbours, were sent to Northumberland Street Mission Hall which was used as a collection point for the rescued. Father was in uniform and at once began digging for his sisters and nephews. I saw the injured come into the Hall covered in dust and shocked. Some were children I went to school with.

Cousins Arthur and 'Sandy' Frankland had been in the shelter. Sandy died and Arthur was saved but Arthur was never the same again.

I do not think that children of my age fully realised the horror because two or three days later I and my school friends were out again looking for shrapnel in the streets.

Rose Graham (Nutman) – acid burns

Rose was a 22 year old nurse working at Hexham Hospital. She recalls many survivors being brought in by ambulance, most of them with horrific acid burns caused by the chemicals used in the factory. She and other medical staff worked for days in treating the injured. Mr Rutherford was the Doctor/Surgeon in charge.

Karen Robinson (Watson) – the Watson family

My Dad, Dennis Lewis Watson was a survivor of the bombing of the factory along with his mother Ellen Watson and sister Maureen.

Dad lived in Reed Street, North Shields. He was only 3 years old at the time, so he passed on only vague recollections. I do remember Dad telling me that a man was killed instantly – he had swapped places with my Grandma and Dad giving them his bottom bunk bed, so that he could be next to his family. My dad remembers coughing up black soot for many days after the bombing. I guess many survivors experienced this too.

I often wonder if Mrs Lee helped my Dad and his family to safety, regardless, Mrs Lee deserves recognition for her bravery.

My Dad kept in touch with a childhood friend of his, Raymond Lough, who lost family members in the bombing. Ray still lives in North Shields.

My Dad brought us to New Zealand in 1973 when I was almost 6 years old. (Ironically we lived in George Square, North Shields prior to emigrating). Family history has always been very important to me. My Dad told me about the bombing and how he was lucky to

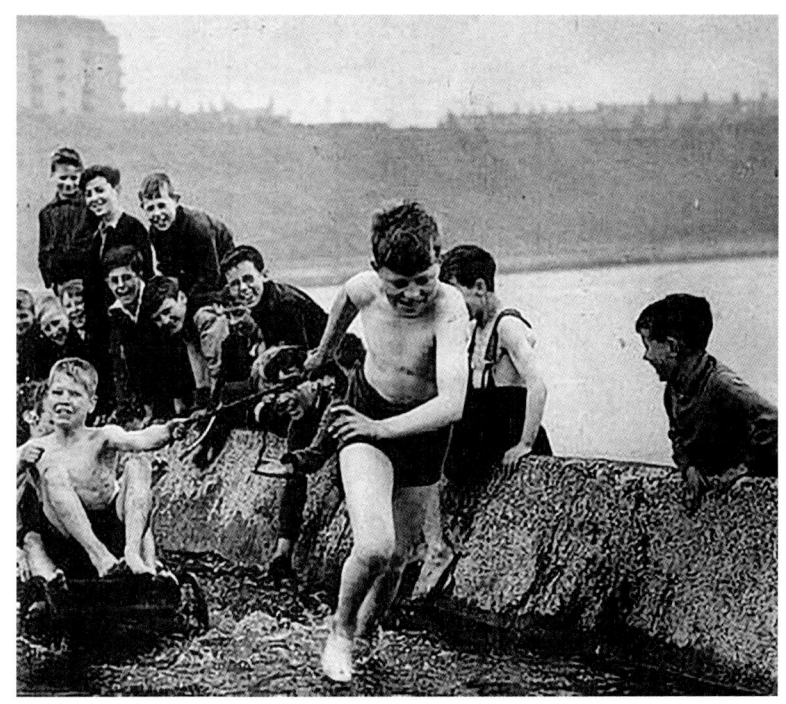

Boys having fun: Fish Quay Sands, North Shields c1943/4.

Dennis, aged 5–6, is pictured third from the left just above the boy (Jimmy Duck) being pulled along on the go-cart (bogey). The boy pulling the cart is William Taylor, aged about 8.

have survived when so many lost their lives. I only wish Dad had been able to see the web site. Dad passed away on 19th September 1998 after a long battle with lung cancer. Mam (Hilda) took Dad "home" to be buried at Preston Cemetery next to my Grandparents.

Thank you for providing the website. It has given my family an "insight" to part of our family history and that of so many other families in North Shields.

We are so lucky in this so called "peace time" and take so much for granted. It is important that we all acknowledge the devastation that war creates. May it continue to provide an insight for our children!

Mary Harrison – the Chater family

Let me try to put some thoughts down about life in North Shields during the War.

I was born in North Shields, an only child, my parents were Jane Henighan (nee Turner) and Joseph Henighan. My father was in the Royal Navy, so like for many other children, he was just a photograph on the wall. My mother was from a large family (one of nineteen). We lived on Little Bedford Street, as did my grandmother (maternal) and two of my mother's brothers and a sister. I attended St. Cuthbert's School on Albion Road.

1941 was not a very good year for our family – on February 18, 1941, my father's youngest brother Eddie (aged 22) was a casualty on board the S.S. Black Osp which was torpedoed off the Irish coast. Also on board was my mother's oldest brother, Bill (aged 45). The priest came to my grandparents' house to break the news. Then 11 days later on March 1, 1941, the priest came to visit again. My father's second youngest brother, Albert (aged 25) had met the same fate in the same place, on board the S.S. Eff. They were merchant seamen doing the North Atlantic run, Canada to the United Kingdom. They were in convoys bringing essential supplies back home. The Royal Naval vessel my father served on was torpedoed, but he was one of the lucky ones.

These memories are still quite vivid, even though I was only five, there are some things that stay with you always. I couldn't understand why everyone was so upset, but I knew it was something bad. Of course, with no bodies there were no funerals, which meant no closure and my relatives had a hard time dealing with this. As children, we were able to bounce back to normal within a couple of days.

Then came Wilkinson's shelter disaster.

The reason I remember it so clearly is because my aunt and uncle lived on Queen Street, with their three children, and the night of the disaster my uncle Peter (who worked at Tyne Dock, South Shields) was out at work, leaving his family at home. My two uncles (Albert and Alex) who lived next door to my mother were still at home (one worked at Smith's Dock and the other on one of the tugs on the Tyne). They were both ARP Wardens, and as soon as the siren sounded they were down on what we used to call the bank top at the end of Little Bedford Street, which overlooked Clive Street and the river.

From inside our shelters we heard the bomb explode, and I remember my grandmother saying it was very close, she thought it was down on one of the shipyards. Then my uncles came in and said there had been a direct hit on Wilkinson's Shelter, and they had been told to go over to help with casualties, the ironic part was they had forgotten that my aunt and her children used Wilkinson's shelter.

My two uncles described the scene as something they would never forget for the rest of their lives. They were lined up outside the shelter passing bodies, or in some cases pieces of bodies, as they were being dug out from the rubble. My uncle Peter was one of the lucky ones. His wife had arrived at Wilkinson's shelter and had been told it was full when she got there, so she left and headed to another shelter. My mother's relatives who were killed in the shelter were a family by the name of Chater. They were cousins of my mother's. I didn't know much about them. The feelings of my relatives after the disaster were hard to determine, as they went on about their business, as normal as possible, and kept things to themselves. Of course, it could be that the bad things about the War were not discussed in front of children. Most of the information I gleaned from the odd discussion I heard about the War, was when I was older. They just didn't talk about it.

The War carried on, it seemed like there was a raid every night, no sooner did we go to bed than the siren sounded. My mother tried to ignore it because she hated going into the shelters, but my uncle would come to the back door and bang on the door until she opened it. I remember him saying, "I don't care what you do, but give me that child," and I was wrapped up in a large tweed cape, which had belonged to my father's mother, and hauled down to the shelter, with my grandmother and my aunt. My mother used to turn up eventually. The street we lived on was just above the shipyards, so after each raid we used to go out on the street to look for shrapnel, because most of the bombing was targeting towards the shipyards. Not knowing how bad it really was, to a lot of children the War was like a big game.

I remember after the War was over, I was outside playing with friends when I saw a sailor walking down the street towards my house. He walked past us and then went into my house, I had no idea who this was, and obviously he didn't know who I was; when I went indoors, I found out he was my father, the person in the picture on the wall. It took a while to get used to him, but I was one of the lucky ones, my father came home from the War.

Emma Chapman – the Curran, Smith and Glynn families

I lost 7 members of my family that night at Wilkinson's. I was 23 at the time. I lived at 24 Hylton Street and during raids I would often use my mother's brick shelter at her house in Little Bedford Street. Fortunately, I never used the Wilkinson's shelter.

My relations had really bad luck. Their house had been damaged in a raid – the windows had been put out. They decided to move in with my uncle and aunt who had a five bedroomed flat above Atkinson's the Fruiterer at 66 North King Street.

When the alert sirens went my uncle said that they all had to use Wilkinson's as there was only enough room for 3 people in his yard shelter. It was their first time in that shelter. 9 people went and only 2 came out alive.

Mrs Lee, the ARP warden was my aunt. She was a lovely woman and we all called her Nellie. I remember she came to our house on the Sunday – she looked terrible. She told us that she had found my grandmother, Emma Curran, but that she hadn't suffered, she'd been killed instantly. And then the police came and we found out about the others. William Curran, Agnes Smith (daughter), Maureen Smith (grand-daughter, Veronica Smith (grand-daughter), John Glynn (son in law), Margaret Glynn (grand-daughter).

We just couldn't believe we wouldn't see them again. The two survivors (Evelyn Curran (daughter) and Anne Glynn (daughter)) were both taken to hospital at Hexham. My mother and brother went to organise the funeral.

I don't think Nellie got an official award (she helped rescue over 30 people) but I remember that the soldiers billeted at Kettlewell School made a presentation to her because of her bravery.

The mortuary was in the old Public Wash House opposite the Alnwick Castle pub.

I heard that when the alarm sounded, the police stopped a bus travelling from Tynemouth. They took everyone onboard to Wilkinson's. The bus was full of girls after a night out at the coast – I don't think many of them survived.

I had a funny 1941. I had been working in domestic service at a big house in Monkseaton (175 Holywell Avenue: 1934-41), in the February I got married, then Wilkinson's and then on the 30th September my own house was flattened in a raid.

After a lot of to-ing and fro-ing I managed to get a job at Holmes Farm at Sharperton near Rothbury (Northumberland). I got £1.00 per week and the use of a stone cottage. I took my mother and sister with me. My mother had never really got over Wilkinson's and it was good to get away from the raids. My father couldn't come with us and he went to stay at Mrs Lee's.

Georgina Frazer (Rose) – Alexander Frankland, the Goodwill family

Dad (Redvers James Rose) was born November 28, 1900. He was in the Royal Navy as a boy of 16 in World War I. Before that he was on the trawlers at 14 with his father.

> He served most of his life in the Merchant Navy. Owing to having a kidney removed he was not accepted in the forces in World War II. His age was also against him. He worked at the Tyne Brand factory cutting up frozen meat.
>
> When he got home he put on his ARP uniform and walked to his billets in Military Hall on Military Road in North Shields. Mum used to take him his tea in a can and something to eat. The hall was all bunk beds.
>
> Dad was almost on the doorstep when the factory was bombed. We heard the blast it was so close and lost a few windows.
>
> My cousins lived on Queen Street. Three young boys around 11 to 14. Dad worked non-stop looking for bodies hoping against hope our cousins had survived. Dad found Alexander Frankland (we called him Sandy) sitting up with not a mark on him. My other two cousins had head injuries.
>
> They lived to have a family but did not live a long life. The surname was Frankland.
>
> I remember there was not a sound while the men worked. All us relations were cordoned off just waiting for loved ones. They were brought out with a grey blanket over them.
>
> My husband's aunt, Mrs Goodwill, lost 2 sons and her husband. She was injured and lost an ear. That was common, one survivor out of a family.

All bodies were taken down to the low sands to what we called them days, the 'dead house' and washed. It was all very sad.

Stanley Hull – shelter survivor

I was nearly 19 at the time. I was sitting just inside as you go in from the door in King Street. You went down two or three steps. Suddenly there was a dull thud and a big gust of wind. The lights went out. The dirt and dust fell around me.

My first reaction was to get out. I saw a gap in the wall. I went for it and went straight out and just walked home to North King Street and told my mother and father. I came out again and stood at the corner at Shrimplin's. I stood watching them trying to get people out.

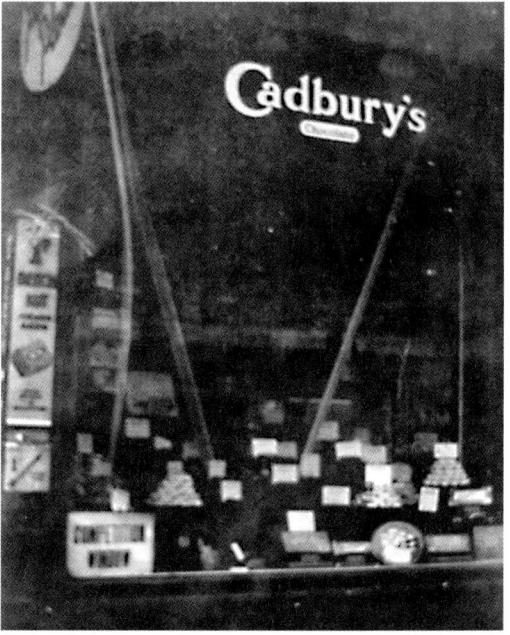

Shrimplin's sweet shop on corner, opposite Wilkinson's. Photo courtesy of Heather Dunkley.

I didn't know my eldest brother was in there. He'd come home on leave and was still in uniform.

I lost my 2 brothers Samuel Hull, Ernest Hull and my sister Evelyn Hull.

Mr Ronald Curran – the Curran family

Mr Curran lost 7 members of his family that night, including his grandmother, aunt and her two children, Veronica and Maureen who was buried on what would have been her ninth birthday.

We lived in Sidney Street at the time and I was only four. I knew there was something wrong. My father had lost his mother. He was dreadfully upset and was crying. It was the first time I had seen an adult cry. Until then, I thought only children cried. I was told my canny little grandma had gone.

One of our relatives had tried to persuade us to go to the shelter but my mother had said that if we were going to die then we'd die in our own home. So, we hid in the cupboard under the stairs.

The family was devastated. Even though I was just a child at the time it still touches me very deeply.

Ken Robson – Isabella Robson

Ken Robson lost his aunt Isabella Robson, aged 8, at Wilkinson's.

The family had lived at Back George Street but moved to Oakwood Avenue in Chirton.

They must have been visiting friends and family that day and they went into the shelter together.

Isabella was with Margaret and Jennie, her twin sisters. She was sitting on Margaret's knee. When the bomb hit, Isabella disappeared. The rest of the family survived. Isabella was identified by her father, Robert William Robson.

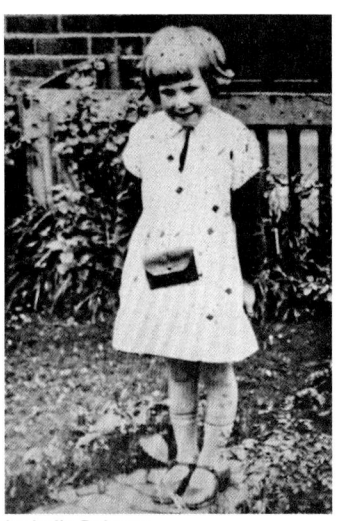

Isabella Robson.
Photo courtesy of Ken Robson.

Heather Dunkley – grandmother stayed at home

Heather tells us that her grandmother, Eleanor Mary Shrimplin (née Simpson), refused to use Wilkinson's shelter. She preferred to stay in the flat above the shop, "Shrimplins", which was situated directly opposite the factory on the corner of King Street and George Street.

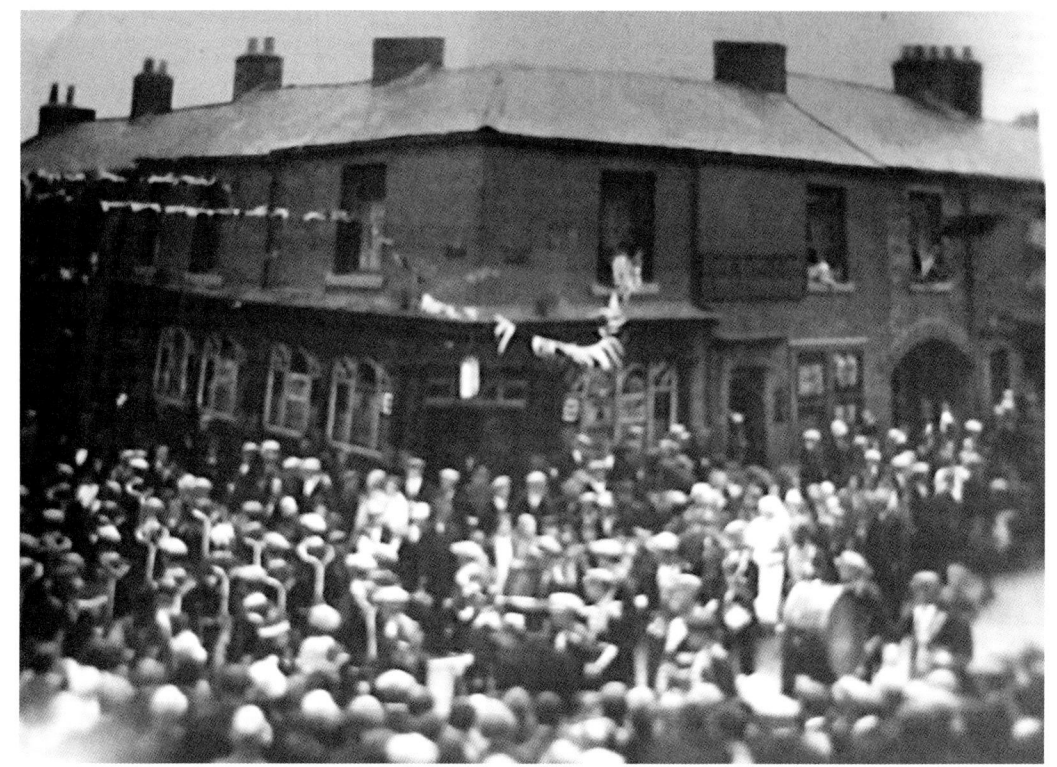

This photo, taken from the Shrimplin's upstairs flat, shows a celebration outside the Pine Apple Inn opposite Wilkinson's. It is possibly Empire Day. The Pine Apple pub was not trading in 1941. Photo courtesy of Heather Dunkley.

Pat Blakey and Jessie Dial – amazing coincidence

At the commemoration event at St Augustin's Church on May 3 2016, we spoke about Jessie Dial's lucky escape on the night of the air raid. Jessie was 13 at the time and lived directly opposite the factory on King Street. Her father had wanted her mother to take the family to the shelter. Her mother refused and stayed at home. Her father, an ARP worker, arrived at Wilkinson's thinking his family had been killed.

At the end of the event, Pat Blakey came up to us and told us she had been amazed by Jessie's story. "Why especially?" we asked. She told us that she was born in 1951 in one of the two council houses built on the site of Wilkinson's. And that her maiden name was… DIAL. She'd never heard of Jessie before but had no family living to ask if they were related.

An email next day brought confirmation from Jessie that Pat's mum and dad, Ella and George, were her aunt and uncle!

Jessie, her sister Maureen and Pat met up later that week and spent hours chin-wagging. So, a family reunited after 60 years!

Briefing

The worst air raid disaster?

The casualty toll at Wilkinson's was the highest in the North East of England during World War Two. It is thought only the disaster at Durning Road in Liverpool exceeded it outside of London. Wilkinson's was one of the worst single bomb civilian death tolls nationally during the entire War.

The following are believed to be the heaviest air raid shelter death tolls:

London – South Hallsville School Disaster – 10th September 1940 – Death Toll: 77 (official) / 600 (estimated actual)

The school was being used as an evacuation centre for locals who had lost their homes through earlier raids. It suffered a direct hit from a parachute mine which left a crater 20 feet deep and reduced the school to rubble.

The Government released figures showing 77 people had died in the raid. Local residents estimated that c600 people had actually been killed and that the official figures were a cover-up.

At the time the press was prevented from reporting on the incident and from publishing photos and disclosing the location. Papers in the National Archives released in 2010, appear to back up the local residents who believed that the government opted not to release full details of what had happened in order to preserve morale at a national and local level.

Liverpool – Durning Road Disaster – 29th November 1940 – Death Toll: 166

An estimated 300 people were sheltering in the basement of the three-storey Ernest Brown Junior Instructional College when a parachute mine hit the school. Among those sheltering were workers from nearby factories and passengers who had left trams during the air raid, in addition to local residents.

The building fell into the basement. The college furnaces exploded and those sheltering were killed by scalding, boiling water and steam. Burst gas pipes were set alight and fire raged amidst the bombed out building. Wardens, firemen and volunteers worked tirelessly to recover survivors and it two days to pull the bodies out from the shelter.

Prime Minister Winston Churchill described the tragedy as "the single worst civilian incident of the War."

London – Stoke Newington – 13th October 1940 – Death Toll: 160

The cellars under Coronation Avenue Flats were designated "Public Shelter No. 5". Over 300 people gathered there on the evening of October 13, 1940. A bomb ripped through the flats above. Masonry blocked the shelter exits and the water and gas pipes running through the basement were shattered. 160 people died, many from drowning.

The following incident is normally quoted as the highest civilian death toll caused by an air raid. However, it was not caused by enemy action.

London - The Bethnal Green Tube Disaster – 3rd March 1943 – Death Toll: 173

The Bethnal Green Tube Disaster of 1943 was, officially, the UK's largest single loss of civilian life during World War II.

When the sirens began at 20:17, locals hurried to the shelter. As the new anti-aircraft guns in nearby Victoria Park began test-firing, people mistakenly thought it to be enemy bombs and the crowd surged forward in panic. One woman fell at the shelter entrance causing others to fall, surging from the top of the stairs. Bodies quickly piled up. 173 people, mainly women and children were killed through asphyxiation and crush injuries.

10 The Mineral Water King

William Arthur Wilkinson arrived in North Shields in 1866, following his father's profession as a hairdresser, opening a shop on Clive Street. By the time of his death in 1924, he was a successful and prosperous businessman with an estate worth over a million pounds today.

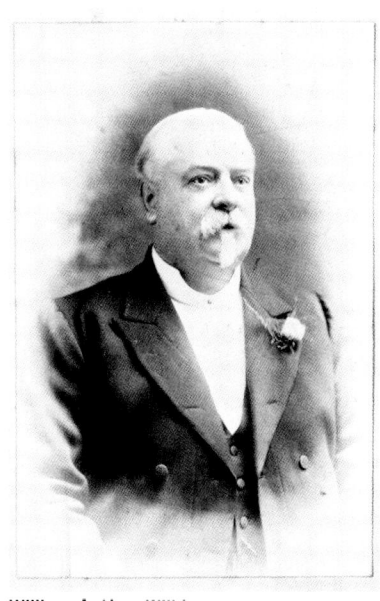

W. A. Wilkinson of King Street had become a respected and highly successful concern, supplying mineral waters, beers, spirits and wines to local hotels, pubs, corner shops and restaurants. They had their own retail shops for the general public and even carted drinks down to Tynemouth's beaches to quench the holiday thirst. A depot in Choppington was opened to make deliveries beyond North Shields more efficient. The company's temperance drinks, "Smila" and "Pineola" were especially popular. It was the "Smila" brand whose labels would litter the pavements after the bombing in 1941.

William Arthur Wilkinson.

William Arthur was the epitome of the Victorian entrepreneur of popular imagination.

He was the very paterfamilias. His marriage to Emma Turnbull in 1872, resulted in 13 children. All 3 of his sons worked in the business and Alfred Ernest (1884–1939) would go on to manage the company. Alfred Ernest's son, "Young Ernie", would be the manager when the business was all but destroyed by the Luftwaffe.

William Arthur was born in Gateshead on 20th May 1848, one of seven children to William and Elizabeth Wilkinson.

Moving to North Shields, William Arthur put down the scissors and moved into pop. He branched out into soda water manufacturing at Elder's Quay in 1875 and then traded as an Ales and Porter Merchant and Mineral Water Manufacturer from premises in Coach Lane in 1879. The growth of this business allowed him to move to larger premises in the East End of town. In 1886, Wilkinson purchased the old Mathews' Hall, also known as King Street Hall, at the corner of King Street and George Street. The family moved in across the road to No 27 King Street, Phoenix House.

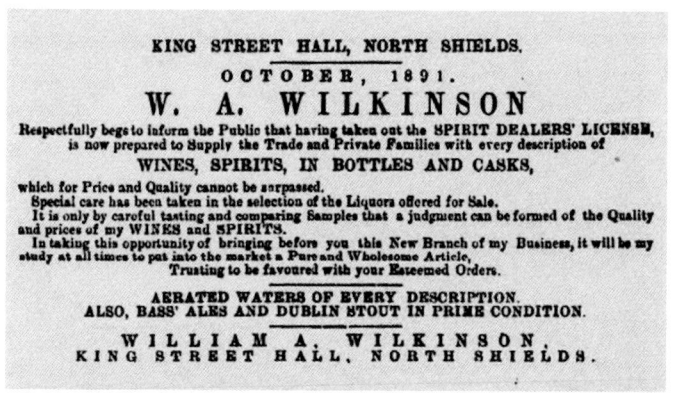

> **KING STREET HALL, NORTH SHIELDS.**
>
> **OCTOBER, 1891.**
>
> **W. A. WILKINSON**
>
> Respectfully begs to inform the Public that having taken out the SPIRIT DEALERS' LICENSE, is now prepared to Supply the Trade and Private Families with every description of
>
> **WINES, SPIRITS, IN BOTTLES AND CASKS,**
>
> which for Price and Quality cannot be surpassed.
>
> Special care has been taken in the selection of the Liquors offered for Sale. It is only by careful tasting and comparing Samples that a judgment can be formed of the Quality and prices of my WINES and SPIRITS.
>
> In taking this opportunity of bringing before you this New Branch of my Business, it will be my study at all times to put into the market a Pure and Wholesome Article,
>
> Trusting to be favoured with your Esteemed Orders.
>
> **AERATED WATERS OF EVERY DESCRIPTION.**
> **ALSO, BASS' ALES AND DUBLIN STOUT IN PRIME CONDITION.**
>
> **WILLIAM A. WILKINSON,**
> **KING STREET HALL, NORTH SHIELDS.**

W. A. Wilkinson trade advertisement, 1891.

Later, William Arthur's younger brother Joseph, would open a similar mineral water business in Gateshead. Both businesses would support each other with materials and staff. It is not known the extent to which W. A. was involved in Joseph's company.

The success of the business (and some enthusiastic marketing very much of the period) can be seen in the various and increasingly elaborate

Orders Executed on Shortest Notice — and Delivered Free of Charge.

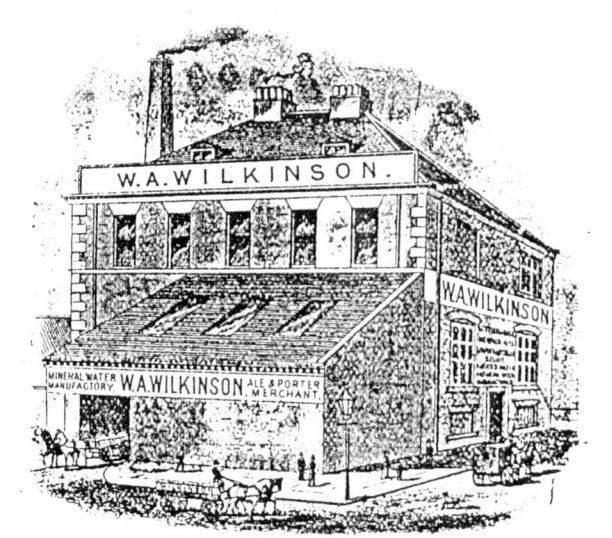

W. A. WILKINSON,

Wholesale and Family

Ale, Porter, Wine, and Spirit Merchant.

Agent for

Messrs. Bass and Co.'s Burton Ales,
Guinness' Dublin Stout, and
Findlater & Co.'s Nourishing Stout.

―o―

The Trade and Shipping Supplied in Casks and Bottles.

―o―

Manufacturer of

ALL KINDS OF ÆRATED WATERS

Of Purest Quality and always in Sparkling Condition.

CELLARS AND OFFICES—

KING STREET AND GEORGE STREET, NORTH SHIELDS.

A LARGE STOCK OF CIGARS ALWAYS ON HAND.

Also large assortment of Glasses of every description. Samples and Prices sent on application.

W. A. Wilkinson trade advertisement, 1901.

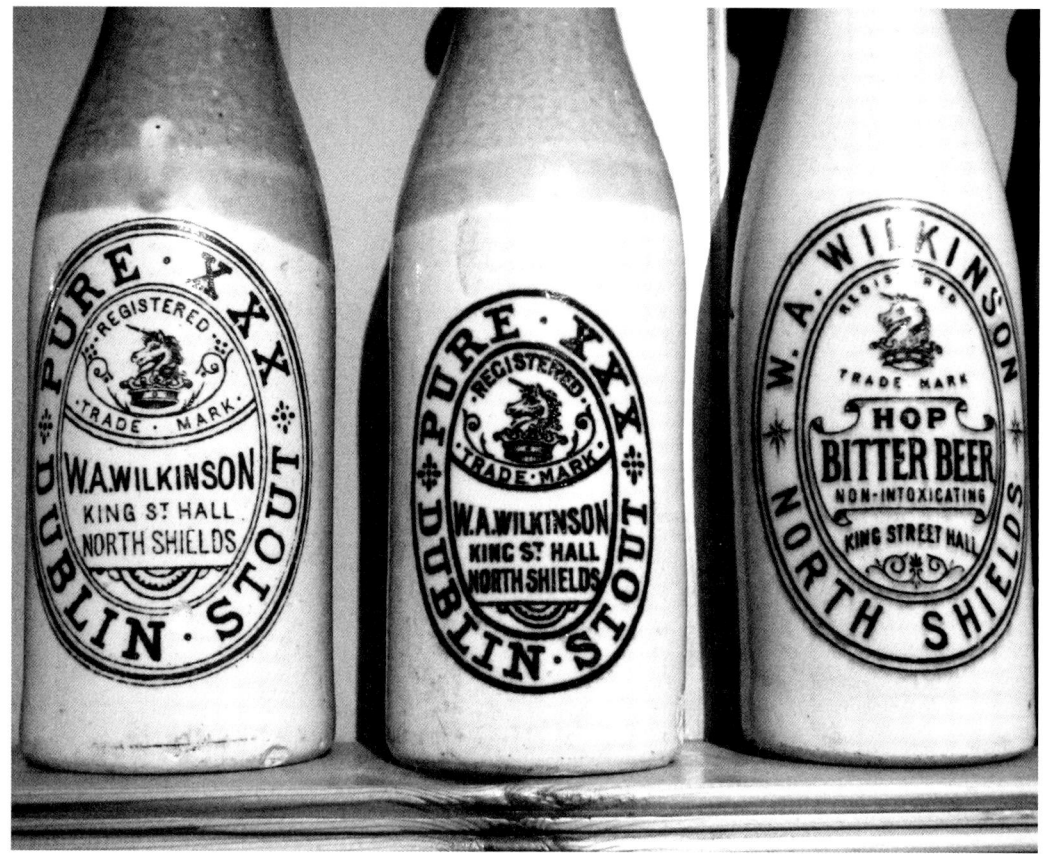

Two stout beer bottles and one hop beer bottle with unicorn trade mark. Courtesy of Jim Rickard.

adverts appearing in the local trade directories. In 1901, Wilkinson's offered a wide range of ales, porters, wines and spirits as well as "all kinds of aerated waters of the purest quality and always in sparkling condition". They were agents for Guinness and Bass' Burton Ales. A large stock of cigars was "always on hand" and a "large assortment of glasses of every description" could be hired. They even made vinegar supplied in casks. A range of earlier adverts announced that the business could supply bottles and glasses with name, trademark and any kind of lettering required. This side line was an astute move as bottle recycling and glass sandblasting allowed the company to mitigate against the rising costs and regular shortages of glass bottles.

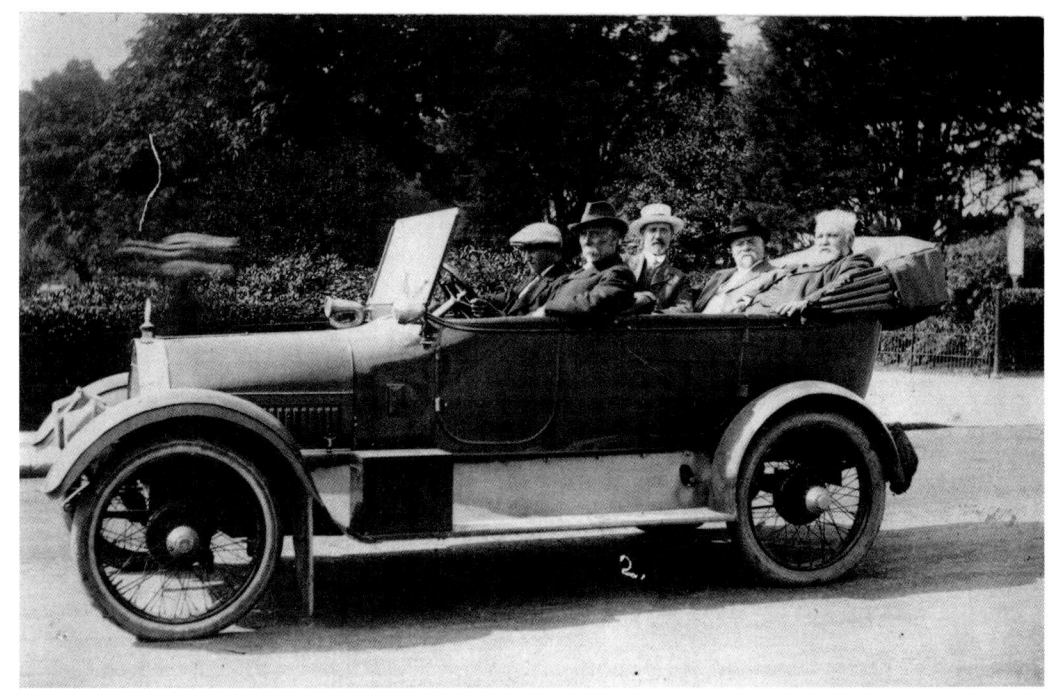

W. A. Wilkinson, seated middle on the back seat, in about 1921. The portly gentleman to his right is Henry Thompson, a long-standing friend. The location would appear to be outside Northumberland Park on King Edward Road, North Shields. Thanks to Mike Coates for the photo and identifications.

In 1909 Wilkinson's adopted new technology and added Tel. 173 to their advertising.

At the outbreak of war in 1914, Wilkinson diversified into the Groceries business, opening up a shop at 94½ Prudhoe Street. It is thought this business was managed by his second son, George Richard (1882–c1952).

Wilkinson enjoyed the fruits of his labour. He was a frequent visitor to London with his long-standing friend Henry Thompson. He was also reputedly one of the first owners of a motor car in North Shields. Latterly, he would enjoy trips out in his Humber driven by the company chauffeur Dave Moffitt.

There were family tragedies too. The deaths in infancy of several of his children were a sadness. In 1900, William Arthur Jr was injured by an explosion at the factory which shattered glass bottles. As a result, he lost

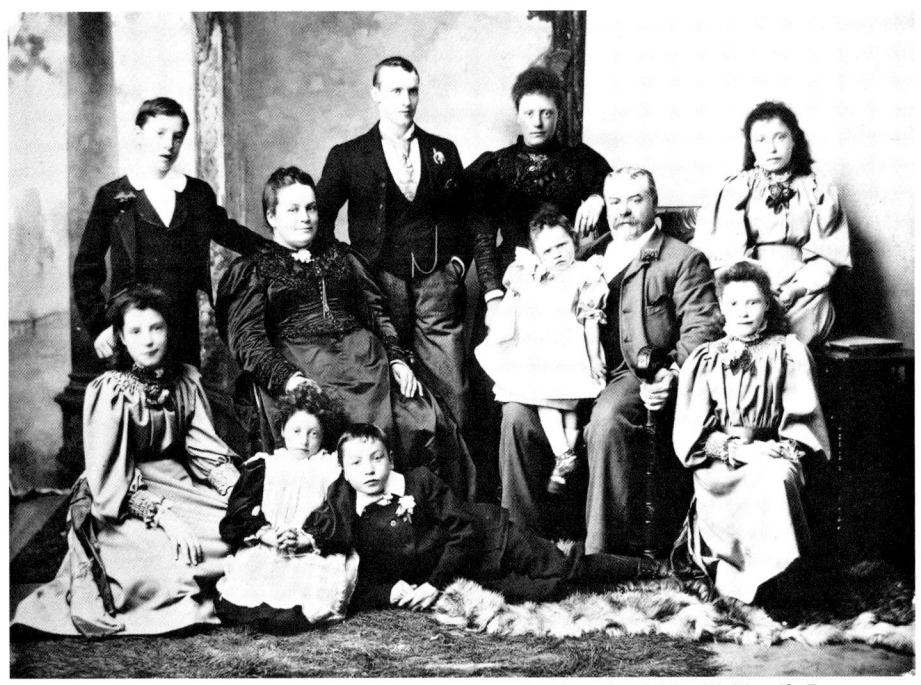

The Wilkinsons: William Arthur Wilkinson (Senior) is seated, holding the child, with his wife Emma seated on his left. Eldest son William Arthur (Junior) is standing with his hand in his pocket. George Richard is standing on the left. Arthur Ernest is lying down in the front row.

an eye as well as being badly cut around the face and neck. The injury did not however prevent him serving with the RAF during World War One. In later years William Arthur Jr became totally blind. In 1904, William Arthur's wife Emma died, aged 54.

Wilkinson proved to be a benevolent business owner, closing the factory for one day each year for a workers' excursion. The *Shields Daily News* reported enthusiastically in August 1905 on the employee's picnic trip to Morpeth.

> *The employees . . . held their annual pic nic to Morpeth on Wednesday last, leaving King Street in brakes at 7.30 going via Gosforth Park and Stannington. Morpeth was reached at 12.30 after a beautiful drive. Games of football, running, skipping etc were thoroughly enjoyed, for which prizes were given. At 5pm the company repaired to Mrs Dunn's refreshment rooms where a splendid repast was done full justice to. The party, after an*

enjoyable time, left Morpeth at 8pm, arriving at Shields at 11.15pm, all fully appreciating the treat provided by their employer.

William Arthur survived his wife by nearly 20 years, dying on 18th January 1924, aged 74 years.

> **WILKINSON** William Arthur of Phoenix House 27 King-street North Shields died 18 January 1924 Probate **Newcastle-upon-Tyne** 28 March to James Wightman auctioneer George Richard Wilkinson provision merchant Alfred Ernest Wilkinson mineral water manufacturer Robert Doubleday Forster assistant relieving officer and James Storey secretary. Effects £28830 9s. 8d.

The probate document showed he had left £28,830 9s 8d. According to the National Archives' currency converter, that would have been worth £1.2m in 2017.

The will makes for interesting reading:

- Gertrude Moffitt, daughter – was left all his linen and soft goods for her to share with her siblings.
- Alfred Ernest – half the shares in the company with the remainder divided equally among all his children
- Servant, Mary Tubby, if still employed by him at his death, to receive £50
- The Salem United Methodist Free Church on Linskill Street to receive £100

Everything else was be sold by his Trustees to fund his funeral and other expenses with the residue shared amongst his children. William Arthur also left Gertrude a variety of furniture and items at Phoenix House and gave her permission to live there for one year following his death, after which the house and contents were to be disposed of by his Trustees.

Wilkinson's prized Humber car was auctioned off, 3 months after his death. Phoenix House was sold and became an CIU club.

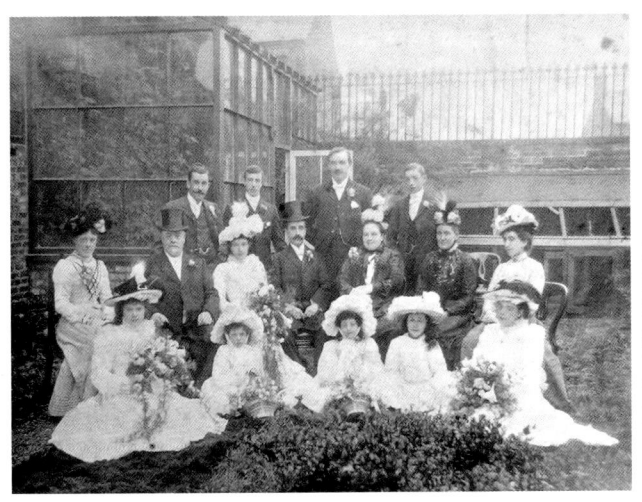

Daughter Emma married Robert Doubleday Forster (a clerk at Wilkinson's) in 1901. The wedding photo shows the gathering of Emma and Robert, taken at the rear of Phoenix House, opposite the factory in North Shields. It is the only known photo of this building.

Clearly a pragmatic man, Wilkinson the widower, thought it best to liquidate all assets other than the company itself, to ensure fair financial shares for all his children.

William Arthur is buried in a substantial family plot in Preston Cemetery, in the older, southern section just past the chapel.

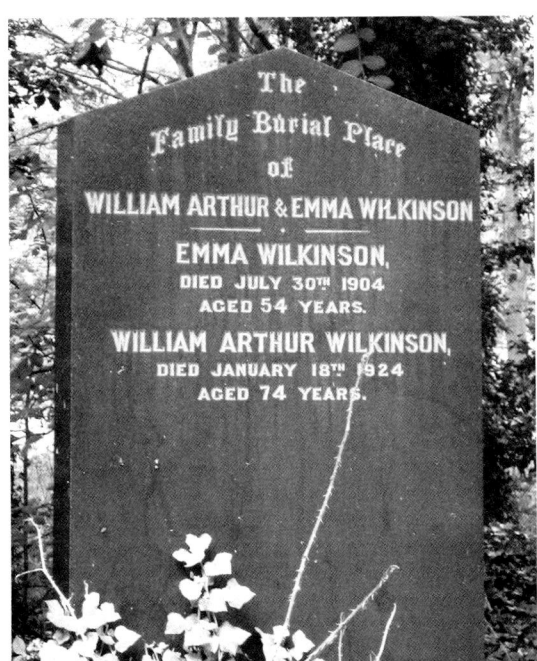

William Arthur and Emma Wilkinson's gravestone in Preston Cemetery, North Shields.

The death of William Arthur Sr. proved a damaging blow to the company's fortunes. He was the originating driving force and it was his business acumen which his successors found difficult to match. They had a hard act to follow. The Victorian and Edwardian heydays were a sunlit memory as the business coped as best it could in the 1920s and 1930s – decades of economic downturn, mass unemployment and the shadows of looming conflict.

Control of the company passed to his son Alfred Ernest (1884–1939).

In this period the business opened new retail premises at 39 Savile Street, North Shields and at 23 Percy Park Road, Tynemouth.

W. A. Wilkinson became a limited company in 1926. This fact helps in dating the company's bottles, which are often dug up at old tips or found in sheds. Anything marked W. A. Wilkinson Ltd is 1926 or later.

Alfred Ernest ran the company until his own death in 1939.

He was succeeded by his son, also Alfred Ernest (1908–1962) but known as "Young Ernie".

Young Ernie was the manager at the time of the bombing.

It is reported that David Moffitt, the company's motor driver, who had married Gertrude (W. A.'s daughter) in 1919, helped rescue people from the factory debris. He never spoke of the bombing subsequently.

Within weeks following the disaster, Young Ernie and Dave Moffitt had organised affairs so that the company could start trading again, albeit in much reduced form, from the company's stabling yard further

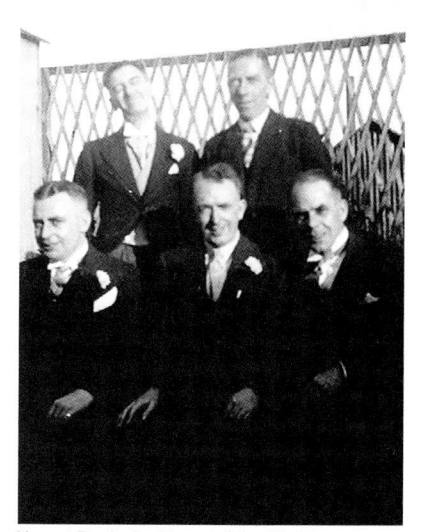

Young Ernie (bottom left) with his brothers-in-law.

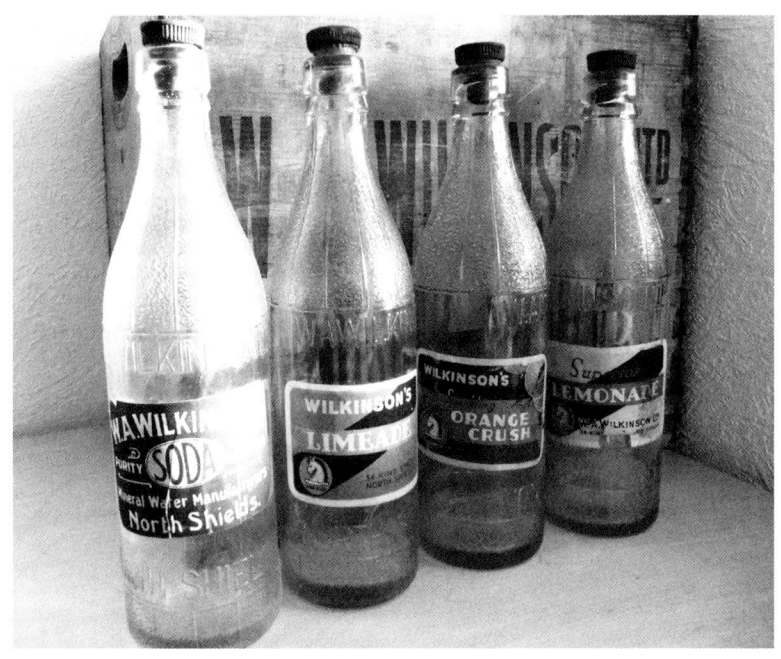

Wilkinson pop bottles, about 1940. Courtesy of Philip Tallent.

up and on the opposite side of King Street. The business from then on focused entirely on soda drinks. The well-known, company logo featuring the unicorn head might have been changed to that of a phoenix, risen from the ashes.

It was short-lived. Wilkinson's had had its day.

In 1954, W. A. Wilkinson Sr's younger brother, Joseph, sold his mineral water factory in Gateshead and bottles to Margaret Pearson of Sunderland.

The North Shields business was sold in 1964. In 1900, Wilkinson's was a big fish in the small pond of North

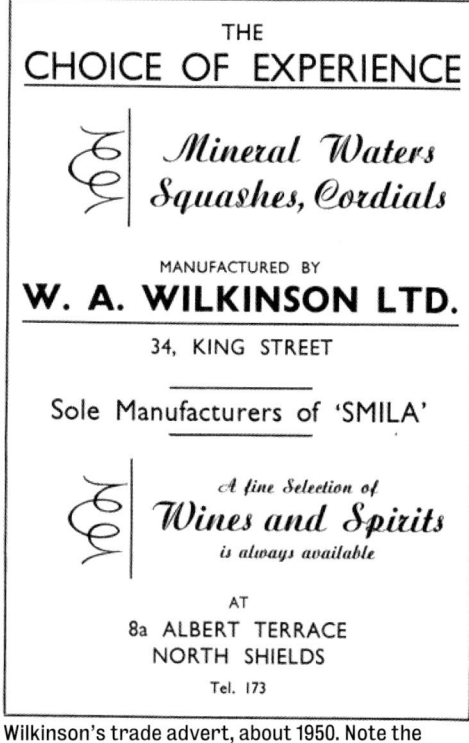

THE
CHOICE OF EXPERIENCE

*Mineral Waters
Squashes, Cordials*

MANUFACTURED BY
W. A. WILKINSON LTD.
34, KING STREET

Sole Manufacturers of 'SMILA'

*A fine Selection of
Wines and Spirits
is always available*

AT
8a ALBERT TERRACE
NORTH SHIELDS
Tel. 173

Wilkinson's trade advert, about 1950. Note the address change.

Shields, but by the 1960s they just couldn't compete with the larger national companies that dominated the market. Had it not been for that awful night in May 1941, Wilkinson's would be an ever-fading memory of a once successful business.

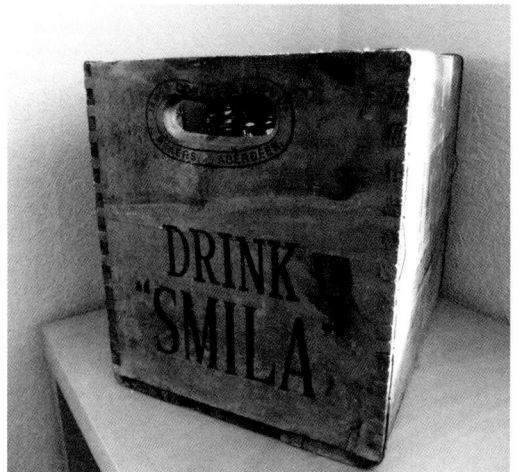

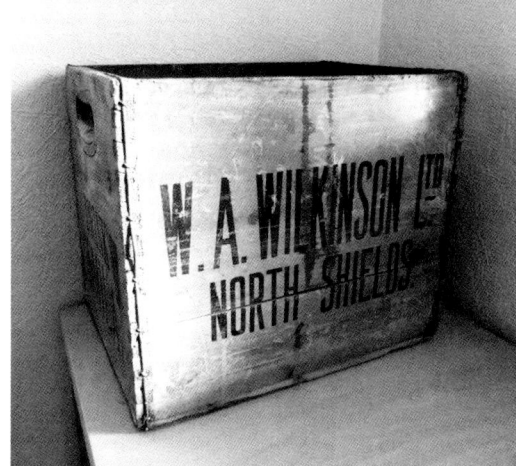

Very rare Wilkinson's wooden crate, post-1926. Courtesy of Philip Tallent.

Briefing

What did the buildings look like?

Sadly, there are no known photos of the full building.

The evidence we do have tells us that Wilkinson's factory was previously a large private dwelling built in about 1800 and known as Mathews' Hall. The original, extensive gardens of the Hall had been divided by the new railway line into Tynemouth in 1845 and further sold off and built upon. The original building, following the deaths of the owners, had been converted by the 1860s into tenements and then into a tea warehouse for John Reid.

William Arthur Wilkinson purchased the building in c1886. His trade adverts from the 1890s and into the early 20th Century boast line drawings of a substantial and impressive Georgian building. We see a three-storey structure, with a large industrial chimney and horse and cart delivery access onto George Street. There appears to be a shop entrance on the King Street/George Street corner. The building is referred to as King Street Hall in many of the company's adverts. It is uncertain if William Arthur was responsible for the name change. Any modifications to the building made by Wilkinson are unknown.

There are only 3 known photos which show Wilkinson's. One is an aerial photo taken in 1927 which can be zoomed to show a large but indistinct building on the corner plot. This image is on the Britain From The Air website.

With the likelihood of any official photos of the factory being destroyed in the bombing along with the rest of the company records and archives, I am left hoping for private photos turning up. The wonderfully evocative photo of snowbound George Street was supplied via a

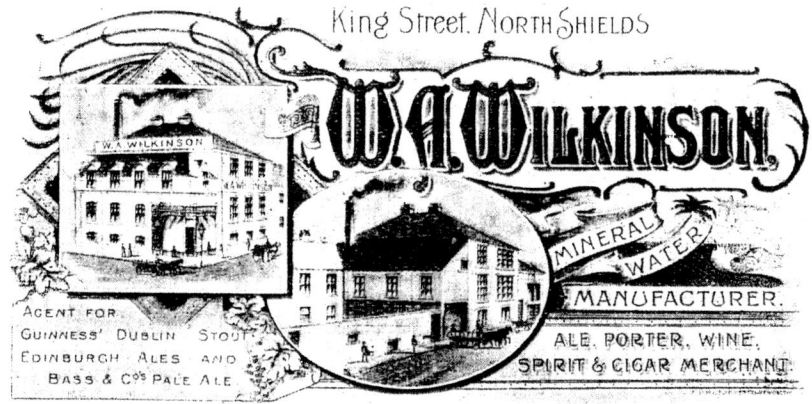

Wilkinson's trade advert showing front and side view of the main factory c1910.

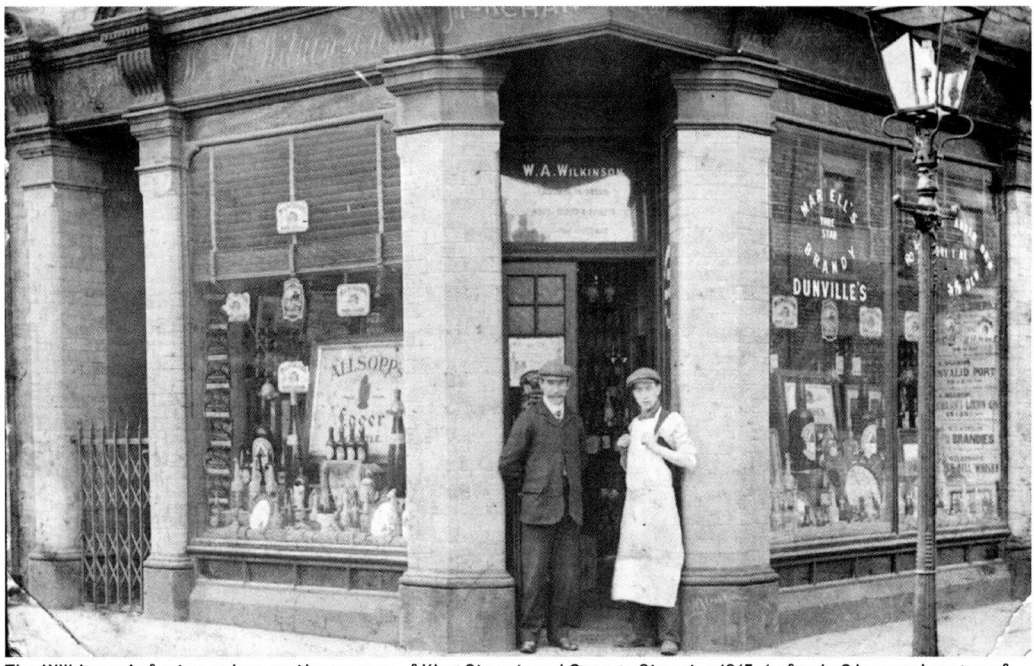

The Wilkinson's factory shop on the corner of King Street and George Street, c1915. 1 of only 2 known images of Wilkinson's. Courtesy of Philip Tallent.

Facebook conversation in 2019. There must be other images out there. Please check your old photo albums!

Oral testimony of how the building looked is scant and, where given, describes the shop. The descriptive focus has been on the air raid shelter.

There is also a written account, from the 1890s, of the origins of the building. This makes fascinating reading, not just with Wilkinson's in mind but in showing in microcosm the development of the East End of the town, from the large private dwellings of gentlefolk to the mix of light industry, commerce and terraced housing prevalent in the area in the 20th century.

Mathews' Hall, occupied by Wilkinson's from 1886 until its destruction in 1941, was built c1800 by Mr John Mathews, a solicitor from Whitby. Mr Mathews had married Miss Ann Wright, daughter of Mr Stephen Wright, ship owner, of 42 Dockwray Square.

When the Hall was built, there was a large garden to the rear which extended all the way to Tynemouth Road. In the garden there was an extensive conservatory and on the west side of the grounds facing in to Queen Street were some cottages belonging to the house. In front of the house was a small garden, and opposite to the house in George Street was a piece of ornamental ground upon which the Pine Apple Inn and other buildings now stand. When built, the site must have been a very pleasant one.

In 1845 the branch railway line to Tynemouth was made, and a portion of the garden cut off. Old John Nicholson who kept the Duke of York

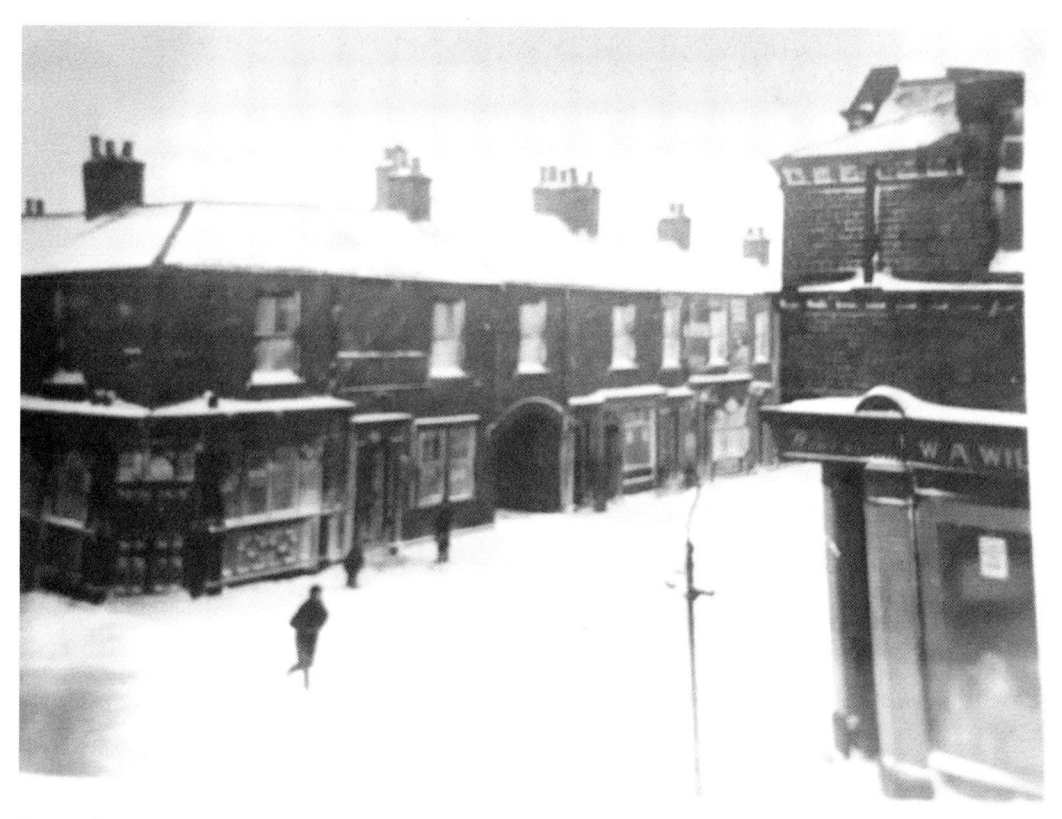

George Street/King Street junction c1930 showing Pine Apple Inn and, on the right, the Wilkinson's building with shop and partial signage. 1 of only 2 known images of the building. Courtesy of Heather Dunkley.

Inn on the east side of King Street and who was greatly celebrated for his good ale and London porter, which were dispensed in silver tankards, bought the severed land so that he could prevent anyone building upon it, and might always have from his house, a view of the trees at Tynemouth Lodge.

Mr Mathews died at the Hall in 1833 aged 87 years. His widow resided at the Hall until her death on the 5th of March 1848 aged 89 years. Two of her daughters, Miss Anna Mathews and Miss Sarah Mathews resided with her. The latter, for several years, conducted a Sunday School in the rooms in King Street which had formerly been her father's offices. Miss Mathews left the town shortly after her mother's death. Before she left the scholars gave her a farewell tea. She died in 1861 and was buried at Hornsey. Her memory is dear to many of her old scholars.

After the death of Mrs Mathews and the removal of her daughters to London, the Hall remained unoccupied for some time and then it was let into tenements. It was subsequently purchased by Mr John Reid, tea dealer, for a warehouse and after other mutations it was purchased by Mr Wilkinson who now carries on business in it.

The [Mathews] family like many more of the old families has entirely disappeared from our midst.

(from "Old Landmarks" by Horatio A. Adamson, *Shields Daily News* c1890)

11 Wilkinson's Voices

Even back in 2000 it was probably too late to entertain hopes of finding and interviewing former Wilkinson employees. The destruction of the factory in 1941 caused the total loss of the business' archives, including staff records. The various branches of the Wilkinson family have no remnants for us to examine. Despite a newspaper appeal at that time, nobody came forward.

Happily, we do have a 1990 interview with Billy Craig, a lifelong Wilkinson's employee who started in 1918, experienced some of the "golden age" of the business up to the death of its founder in 1924 and saw its slow decline in the face of competition and changing public consumption. He was still working for the company after the bombing when they moved over the road and operated a "pop" only concern from their former stabling yard. And Colin Sarin, presumed to be the last living employee (1961-1963), tells us Billy was still there driving a wagon, when he left just before the business finally closed in 1964. Hats off then, to Jim Rickard who discovered Billy living nearby and who had the foresight to interview him.

We also have interesting details from Mabel Moffitt, granddaughter of W. A. Wilkinson and daughter of Dave Moffitt who was a driver for the company for many years. She recalls her visits to the factory and the factory yard. Her father never spoke of the disaster. Her memories result from a recent interview with Terry Wilkinson, himself the great grandson of the founder. Terry adds his father's recall of the factory just as the War had started, as he sought to join the armed forces to "do his bit".

And we have an all too brief note about Mary Gargett, kindly supplied by her daughter, Edwina Thewliss. Mary worked for Wilkinson's in the thirties and up until the bombing.

It's a pity we don't have more records of the women who worked there. No doubt it was hard, tough work and their contribution was important. We know little of the day to day work experience of these local women. Perhaps more stories will come to light.

Billy Craig – Wilkinson's employee

In 1990, Dr Jim Rickard, one of the region's leading breweriana experts, interviewed Billy Craig, one the last employees of W. A. Wilkinson Ltd. Dr Rickard has given kind permission for me to republish the interview, edited, below. It first appeared in the *Northumberland & Durham Bottle Collectors Club Newsletter* (Number 107: p20-23). All copyrights belong to Jim Rickard.

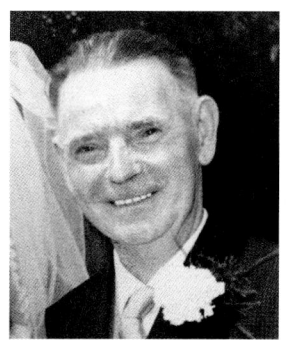

Billy Craig – Wilkinson's worker. Photo courtesy of Larrissa Lansdell.

We were exploring the old part of North Shields that was once home to William Arthur Wilkinson's thriving business. There was little evidence of his premises, the area had been redeveloped years before.

Still living nearby was one of Wilkinson's former employees, an elderly man called Billy. In his broad Shields accent he invited us into his small, terraced house to tell us his story. He took us into his front room and settled into his chair beside the gas fire. He talked about his years working for Wilkinson and showed tremendous affection for his old boss. His memory was sharp for a man in his eighties and we struggled to write even half of it down into our notebook.

Billy had lived all of his life in North Shields. He was born in 1904 and went to Eastern Board and then to Kettlewell School on George Street. At this time it was referred to as the "kipper college" because it was so close to the kipper factory. An

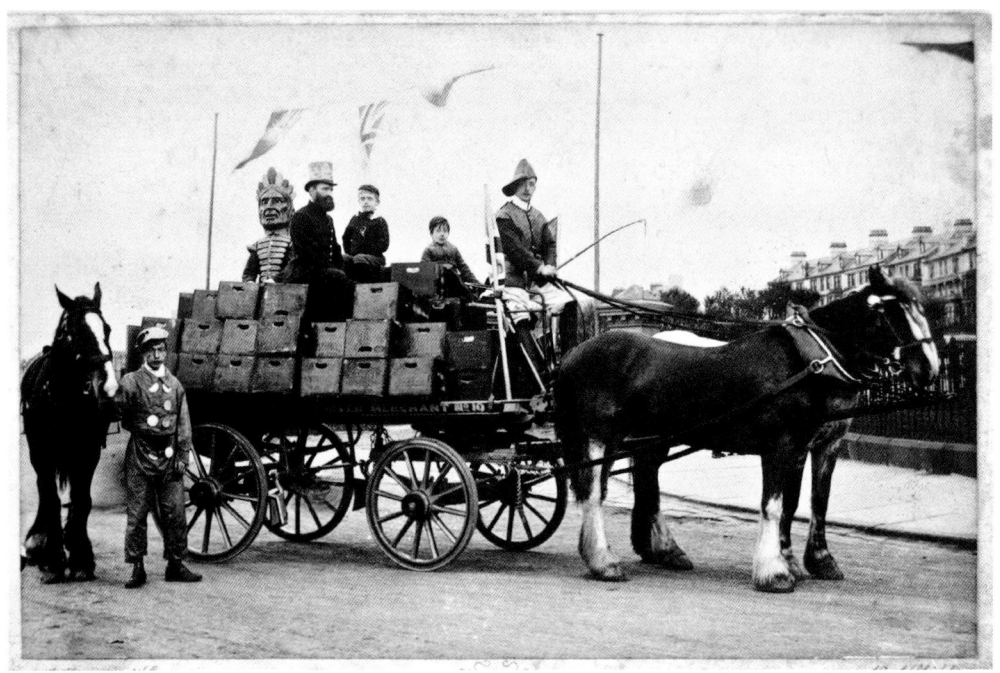

Wilkinson's delivery cart pictured outside Percy Gardens, Tynemouth, c1915. Empire Day/Trafalgar Day celebrations?

old school, it was founded in 1825 as a school for the Shields poor with a preference for orphans. During the First World War, soldiers were billeted at the school meaning that half the children had lessons in the morning and the rest had lessons in the afternoon. As was typical in those days, Billy left school at the age of 14 and went straight into work. His first job was as a delivery boy for Fred Hannah's bakery in North Shields.

Shortly afterwards, he saw that Wilkinson's were hiring delivery boys and he was hired just before the end of the First World War. On Armistice Day (11th November 1918), Wilkinson declared a day off, so Billy was able to enjoy the celebrations. To celebrate, he bought a packet of cigarettes, "5 Robins for tuppence. I was as sick as a dog, ever since then I've smoked Woodbines".

A day off was a rare treat for Wilkinson's employees as they had to work hard; often working from early in the morning until 8 o'clock at night (without being paid for overtime). They had to work Sundays and Bank Holidays and there were no trade unions to look after their interests.

William Arthur Wilkinson had 13 children, several of whom died in infancy, and all three of his sons worked in his business. His eldest son, also called William Arthur, worked at the factory. He lost an eye operating the Beavis bottling machine. His second son, George, worked in the firm's depot in Choppington. When Billy started, bottling wasn't carried out in Choppington. The filled bottles were transferred from North Shields and three draycarts, each pulled by two horses, were used for this purpose.

After the Choppington branch closed in 1918, George did selling and was in charge of deliveries. Wilkinson's youngest son, Ernest, was in charge of the factory itself. All the employees at the factory were women. Billy remembered an old woman who cleaned the bottles and women that pasted the labels onto the bottles by hand.

Billy himself used a smaller cart pulled by only one horse and usually did the round of Whitley Bay and area, 3 or 4 trips there and back each day. There were several other rounds although Billy would only do these when he was "on relief". He had occasionally done the round of New York and Murton villages and could recall delivering pop and cigarettes to the Rickard's general store in New York which was ran by my Dad Stew's uncle and grandfather. My Dad has fond childhood memories of drinking Wilkinson's delicious "Smila" brand lemonade, from pint screw top bottles. Aside from pop, Wilkinson sold Bass, Bulmer's cider, his own port wine (6 shilling a bottle) and Guinness. The Guinness had to be checked by a "traveller" to see that it wasn't too old. Wilkinson supplied many pubs including the famous Wooden Dolly in North Shields.

Delivery was central to the business and horses were essential, so they were well cared for. Horses were left with a filled feed bag overnight and were fed between 3:30 and 4:30 in the morning by a lamplighter, a part-time employee who did this after putting the street lights out.

Billy's first job was to muck the horses out and then clean and harness them. Every Sunday the leather harnesses and brasses also had to be cleaned. As Billy said, "This one Monday it had poured down and the harness was spoiled and everything was dull. As I was coming out of the gate, Wilkinson was standing there with his white hair and beard wearing a grey 3-piece suit and a gold Albert and shouted "Hey boy, stop that pony! Take that pony back into the stable, clean that harness and you'll do your deliveries when it's clean". All that work, and all for 8 bob a week."

Billy didn't like delivering the 6 oz codd bottles because not only were they heavy, he was also expected to haul them across the Long Sands beach at Tynemouth to supply the seaside kiosks. Aside from the hard work of delivery, it could also be dangerous. One day in 1920, Billy was making his usual Whitley Bay delivery. He left North Shields and as he ascended out of Spital Dene (which in those days would have been quite steep) his horse became unsettled and lurched away sharply. The jerk threw Billy to the ground and since the weight was all at the rear of the cart it tipped backwards spilling the delivery onto the road. Billy had to pick himself up quickly and run to catch the horse. It says a lot that Billy was more worried about turning up in the delivery yard with an injured horse and a spilt delivery than he was about his own injuries.

Unsurprisingly, we were keen to know what happened to the empties and as we might have known they were collected and re-used. If Wilkinson's ended up receiving another company's bottles they took them to South Shields bottle exchange and got paid a portion of the deposit on the bottles and also picked up any Wilkinson's bottles that had been handed in by other companies (but they had to pay the full deposit (a penny) on these so they ended up out of pocket overall). Billy especially remembered exchanging bottles from Evans and Reaveleys. Any broken bottles were collected by hawkers from Gateshead for "a few coppers". By the time Billy joined the company, stone bottles weren't used although they were still stored – sometimes Billy took them home to use as hot water bottles. The only stoneware bottles used were "gallon jars" in 1 & 2 gallon capacities for malt vinegar.

When other local mineral water manufacturers closed down, Wilkinson bought their bottles; Billy remembered half pint and pint glass bottles from Matthew Knott, Holliday & Co. (both North Shields) and Sam Vincent (Howdon) being stored in a garage in the yard (sadly emptied long ago).

In 1954, W. A. Wilkinson's brother, Joseph, sold his factory and bottles to Margaret Pearson of Sunderland. It wasn't long before W. A. Wilkinson met a similar fate; he sold up in 1964. In 1900, Wilkinson was a big fish in the small pond of North Shields, but by the sixties he just couldn't compete with the larger national companies that dominated the market.

When Wilkinson's factory closed, all of the old equipment and the bottles were taken away and dumped. Billy remembered making several trips to the municipal tip with a lorry full of old crates and boxes of bottles. It took Billy and the other workers about three days to complete, they must have tipped thousands of bottles. Anyone for digging 1960s dumps?

Mary Gargett – Wilkinson's Employee 1930s-1941

With many thanks to Edwina Thewliss who contacted the website regarding her mother Mary Gargett (1917–2014).

Mary was employed at Wilkinson's from the 1930s up until the bomb destroyed the factory in 1941. She worked on the bottling operation, washing returned bottles and crating up for deliveries. We do not know if she was in the shelter at the time of the raid. Unlikely, probably, as at that time she lived in Little Bedford Street. Mary died in 2014, aged 97.

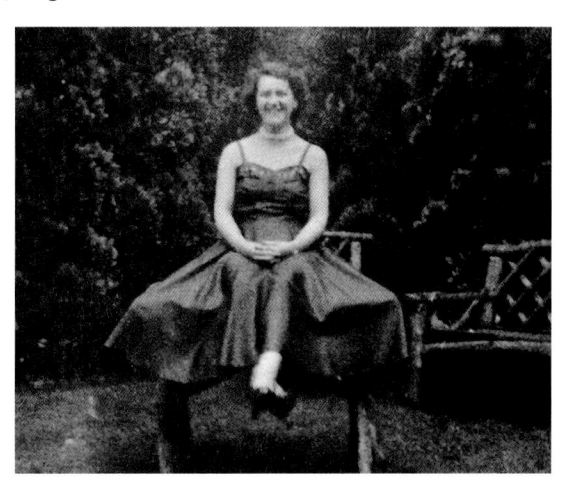

Colin Sarin – Wilkinson's last living employee?

Colin had left Linskill school and was 15 when he worked at Wilkinson's between 1961–1963.

At that time the business was being run from a yard just up from King St Club, close to the junction with Tynemouth Road.

Colin worked as a van lad for the 3 wagon drivers delivering Wilkinson's pop to businesses and homes across the town. He recalls the following old-timers: Charlie Cobb (drove a Comma van), Billy Craig (drove a bullnose Austin) and Gordon Madgin. He worked from 7.30 am-5.00 pm for £2.00 a week.

He remembers carrying 12 bottle crates of pop down to King Edward's Bay and along the Long Sands on hot summer days. In addition to deliveries, there were regular trips across to the Joseph Wilkinson factory in Gateshead.

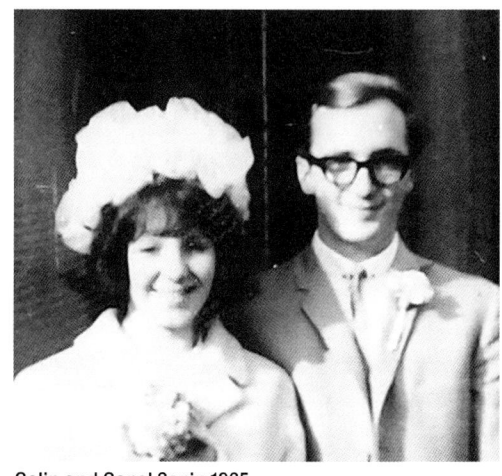

Colin and Carol Sarin 1965.

The manager in North Shields at that time (and here Colin's memory is less sharp) was an Albert or Alfred Towns?

There were also 3 women working in the factory washing bottles and re-filling them with varieties of pop. At that time Wilkinson's did not sell beer or alcoholic drinks.

Terry Wilkinson – great grandson of W. A. Wilkinson
Me and dad

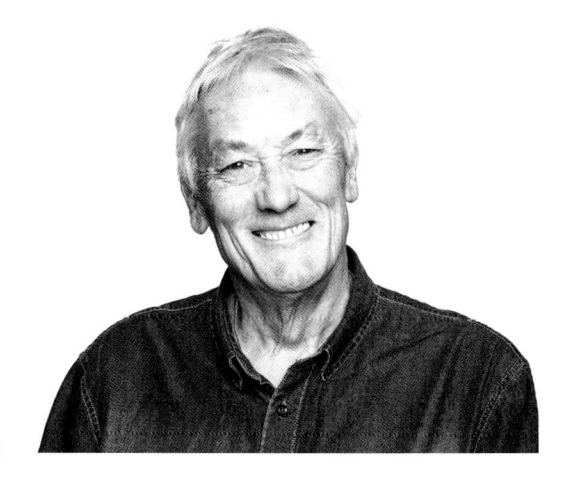

My first recollection of the tragedy that befell the North Shields factory was a mention from my dad, Les Wilkinson. I was probably in my mid 20s and, by then, married with two children and a mortgage. It clearly meant little to me at the time as I was more concerned with all of life's new travails. I knew little of my family's history and my only knowledge of North Shields was that it was on the other side of the river.

Now that I am writing this down, I have unearthed an earlier memory. My dad ran a small general dealership in Sunderland Road, South Shields in the 1960s. I was helping him to fill the shelves after we had closed. When it came to the lemonade, he told me that there was once a 'Wilkinsons Lemonade'. This was the early 1960s and I was a teenager – so if it wasn't sung by the Beatles, I didn't take much notice.

I think it was only about 10 years ago that I was talking to dad about family history. It was like turning on a tap. He showed me a family tree drawn up by my Auntie Connie. She was one of my dad's sisters. I will add at this point that both my great grandfather – the mineral water company founder – and his eldest son, my grandfather, and also a William Arthur, produced large families. Thirteen progeny each, I believe, so our extended family tree is labrynthine.

I think the behaviour of my grandfather – hereinafter called WAW Junior – so irked his father – hereinafter called WAW Senior – that he effectively evicted him. My only memory of WAW Junior is on Sunday afternoon visits to him and gran at their new bungalow in Prince Edward Road, South Shields. He was blinded in an accident at the North Shields factory in 1901 so never saw his grandchildren.

Auntie Connie was a few years younger than dad. The family tree was interesting and she was able to tell me a little about the factory and what happened on that tragic night in 1941.

So I consulted the God that is Google. And I found the website 'North Shields 173'. The rest, as they say, is history. In fact, it really was history. My history.

On talking to dad subsequent to that, I showed him the website and printed pages off for him. At that time, mam had succumbed to Alzheimers and was in permanent care. Dad visited every day.

Flashback to 1941

In early 1941, dad was desperate to join the RAF as a pilot. He had been in 324 Squadron ATC (Air Training Corps) in South Shields. He lived in the family home in Hawthorne Avenue, South Shields. There had been a break in the relationship with his father WAW Junior and he had packed his bags and moved across the Tyne.

Historical context to this:- the British Expeditionary Force had been pushed into the sea at Dunkirk in May 1940, leaving much of its ordnance scattered across the fields of northern France; the RAF had saved us from invasion in the summer of that year; the Nazi hordes were cutting a swathe across Europe, having invaded Czechoslovakia, Poland, Belgium, Holland, Norway and Denmark. France too fell. Austria had been 'Anschlussed' back in 1938 but that was hardly contentious. Hitler was Austrian anyway, wasn't he?

The War meant a lot to dad. Like most men of his age at the time, he wanted to do his bit. April 24th 1941 was his 17th birthday. He was working at Joe Wilkinson's factory in Askew Road, Gateshead. (Joe was WAW Senior's younger brother and also ran a lemonade factory. - two, in fact, as there was also one in Sunderland).

Without informing anyone, dad visited the RAF Recruitment Office in South Shields, wanting to join up. Halfway through the paperwork, the recruiting sergeant discovered that he had been registered by his employers ie his uncle Joe, as 'reserved occupation'. Dad was disappointed and not a little peeved. His dreams of fighting the Hun at the controls of a Spitfire, were dashed.

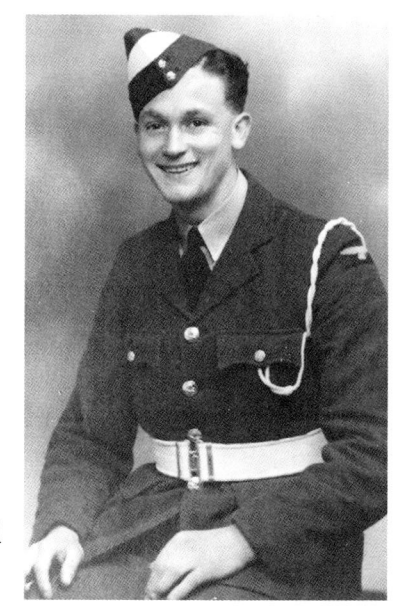

But the sergeant threw him a lifeline. Dad could rescind that 'reserved occupation' status. He did so at the stroke of a pen. Now he had to tell his family.

According to dad, Joe was none too happy. My father was then given all the menial, dirty jobs in the factory until such time as he was called up.

By the time he was serving in the RAF and had undergone early training, he was informed that they no longer needed pilots. The RAF had then been flooded by pilots from the Commonwealth, as well as Free French, Poles and Czechs.

So they suggested he retrain as a Navigator. Then, guess what – they had no further need of Navigators. Would he fly a glider? Dad wasn't keen about that – it wasn't exactly Biggles, was it? So he re-mustered in the Parachute Regiment. There, he became a Sergeant Instructor, training many of those who jumped at Operation Market Garden in September 1944.

At some point, after the War but before demobilisation, he was posted to the Isle of Wight where he met my mother and they married there in June 1947. I was born fully formed and ready for action, in December 1948.

Fast forward to 2009

Now fast forward to my chats with dad 10 years ago. At the time of the raid on the factory, he was working at Joe Wilkinson's Gateshead factory. This was possibly the time when he was biding his time waiting for his RAF call-up. He recalled hearing about it on the Monday ie 5th May. He doesn't recall any talk about the scale of the disaster or the death toll. He does have memories, though, during that week, of Dave Moffitt coming across with a horse-drawn dray to fill it with crates and bottles. The Tyneside version of Lend Lease.

Clearly, the North Shields site had been cleared but they needed bottles to continue trading in some way. Dad said he liked Dave. 'He was a good man'

Dad and I learned more when we visited Peter Bolger the following year. Sadly, after mam's death in December 2011, dad's own descent into Alzheimer's began. It was slow, sure and painful. He passed away in August 2016.

Mabel Moffitt

In October 2018, Terry Wilkinson (great grandson of W. A. Wilkinson, interviewed Mabel Moffitt. Mabel is the daughter of Dave and Gertrude Moffitt. Dave was a company driver for W. A. Wilkinson Mineral Water Manufacturers. Gertrude was the third daughter of company founder, William Arthur Wilkinson. Mabel is now in her nineties and lives in Cullercoats.

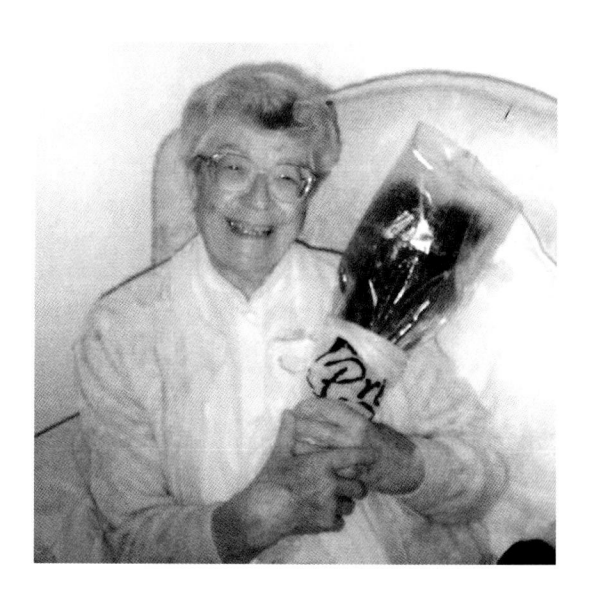

I asked Mabel what she remembers of the factory from any visits she made. She was doing teacher training at Durham when the raid took place on 3-4 May 1941.

So, you used to go in the shop. That's the one on the corner where they used to sell wines & spirits, tobacco . . .

>Yes, that's right. It was in front of the factory . . .

. . . on the corner of King Street and George Street?

>Yes . . . Mrs Tubby. I don't know how old she was. She just seemed to go on forever.

Was she the manageress of the shop?

>Well, yes, I would imagine so . . . and she always wore black.

I wonder if she was a widow . . .

> I don't know anything about her except that she was in charge of the shop. And whether there were living premises behind, I don't know. There was a curtain across the doorway that went to the back.
>
> [Mrs Tubby was William Arthur's domestic servant. She is mentioned in his will in 1924. She was to receive £50.00. It is likely that she was retained by the family and worked in the shop following his death]

I guess the shop would have needed some storage area. The square footage on the ground floor would have been quite big, I would have thought?

> Yes . . . and the horses.

Yes. Tell me about the horses . . .

> The horses were kept in the stables next to the house. Phoenix House.

And that's on the other side of King Street to the factory?

> Yes. Upstairs. And there were two lads who looked after them – Johnny and . . . I think it was Billy. I'm not sure. But they looked after the carthorses and if they were on holiday, my father would go to feed the horses and sometimes he would take us with him (i.e. Mabel and her younger sister, Dorothy). And we stayed downstairs, outside, because as soon as the horses were set free, they came thundering down the ramp . . .

So, they were upstairs . . . on the first floor?

> They were on the first floor.

How many horses were there?

> Just two. I would imagine that the carts were underneath. When my father freed them to muck out the stables, they came thundering down and galloped like mad things round and round the stable yard. And we used to jump up onto the water tank (laughs) in case we got mown down.

Darkie and Ginger they were called. One black and one ginger.

And my grandfather (ie William Arthur Wilkinson Senior. He died in 1924) I think was the first one to have a motor car. I think there were two who had motor cars in North Shields.

I've seen the photographs . . .

That's right – with one of his friends.

It looked as if he had a chauffeur as well?

I think one of the lads drove. He didn't drive. He sat in state in the back.

Going back to the horses. They were working horses so obviously got a lot of exercise, but they weren't free – they were in the shafts. So being let free for 15 minutes or whatever, would be . . .

They loved it. And they were huge!

Were they shire horses?

No idea but possibly. And of course, they would do quite long journeys during the day.

Talking of your grandfather – my great grandfather - you were born in 1921 and he died in 1924, just three years later. So you wouldn't have much of a memory of him, if any, do you?

I remember that when he was ill, he was in the front bedroom and the curtains were drawn. I wasn't allowed to go in.

Was this in his last days?

I think it must have been. I don't really remember much about him.

What memories do you have of other family members at that time? As we said, your grandfather died in 1924. He held the reins of the business which were then transferred to Alfred Ernest (Ernie) but he died in 1939. And then it was young Ernie.

Yes.

Did you ever meet young Ernie?

Oh yes, we used to go and see them in Park Avenue where they lived next to Northumberland Park. Auntie Frances, uncle Ernie - and Gertie and Winnie, their daughters.

Gertie disappeared from the landscape. She was the . . . erm, the adventurous one. I don't know what happened to her. Winnie married and went to live in Hexham. Her husband was the manager of that big store in Hexham. I've forgotten what it's called.

Robbs?

Robbs! Yes.

I think that's still there.

One of the departments he used to manage. That's right. Winnie – she was lovely. Very, very bonny girl.

What about their dad? What sort of a man was he? Do you remember him at all?

He was just uncle Ernie and that was it.

I know you were doing your teacher training in Durham when the bomb hit the factory. What year was it when you came back?

I started teaching in 1941.

So you were back in Shields not that long after the raid?

Yes, but my father never spoke about it.

Your dad was heavily involved in it, wasn't he? Helping with the rescue etc.

He was on fire-watch duty that night.

Do you know where he was on fire-watch duty?

Just down by the factory, I think. We went to Salem Church which was just two streets away and we lost quite a few of our Sunday School children.

Because they were in the shelter?

Yes.

What street was Salem Church in?

Linskill Street.

Not still there, I suppose?

No, that part of the town was all redeveloped.

Talking of the factory, the only pictures that I've seen, of course, are the ones of it on the morning after. It's not nice to look at but it gives you a fair idea of what the streets looked like at the time. You can see the houses in the background.

The machinery was on the first floor . . . not on the ground floor.

So what was on the ground floor? We know that the shop was there, on the corner . . .

And I would think that was either where Mrs Tubby lived or . . . storage places. I don't know. I never was in that part. There was upstairs where the lorries were loaded and the carts . . . from there. Because they were more or less level.

So you've got the ground floor, you've got the first floor which is more or less the loading area where the bottles and crates would come down . .

And the machinery.

And that, of course, is what caused all the damage when the bomb hit.

A-ha.

So you've got the basement, ground floor, the first floor. And what was there above that?

I don't know what was above that . . . if anything.

I sort of imagined in my head – because I've only seen drawings of the factory from adverts, of what the factory looked like . . . in most factories, the bosses, all the paperwork, the secretaries, the filing etc . . . would be on the top floor. Away from the actual work.

>I never heard of any secretaries.
>(At this point, I told Mabel that that my father – Leslie Alwin Wilkinson, the same generation as Mabel – remembered, vaguely, his dad (William Arthur Wilkinson Junior) taking him into an office which he told me was on the top floor. \

Is he the one (ie WAW Junior) who lost an eye?

>Yes. He used to come and visit us, you know . . . periodically.

What sort of a man was he, then? I only met him as a little tot.

>Oh, he was a canny man. Very independent. We would offer to go to walk him to the station to see that he was safe, really. But 'no, no', he would go himself. Very independent. Silver-haired.

Did you ever meet any of the other staff at the factory – apart from Mrs Tubby, Johnny, Billy?

>No.

It already sounds the cast from a sitcom, doesn't it?

>(laughs) Yes.

Was there a Mr Tubby?

>I think she must have been a widow. Probably that's why she wore the black. Except that, of course, it might have been more acceptable in those days to wear black behind the counter - to show dignity. She always used to come to us on Boxing Day and my mother would give her a Christmas dinner.

So, she'd be a work colleague of your dad's, really? Both employees of the WAW company.

Yes.

Where were you living at the time?

We lived in Windsor Gardens. My mother was the last one of the family at home and so when they were married, they just lived with my grandfather – to look after him.

And there was a lot of room in that big house.

Yes. I remember there was a big window halfway up the staircase. It was quite dark. There was a garden. I don't remember it having many flowers.

I remember seeing wedding photos taken in the garden. It looked like bushes and shrubs against the brick wall at the back.

And did they employ staff . . . in the house?

Now that I couldn't say. I would imagine so, but I really don't know.

Maybe when your mum (ie Gertrude Moffitt, one of WAW Senior's many daughters. She married Dave Moffitt, the company driver) was the last one left in the house – the last of the children, maybe they didn't have staff then. When there had been a house full of children, that would have been a different matter and perhaps that was when they had staff?

Yes, maybe.

Did you ever go onto the floor of the factory itself – where they did the bottling and all that kind of thing?

Yes, but I can't say I took much notice.

Was it very noisy?

I should think so.

Was it mainly lasses who did that sort of thing? During the War it would have been, obviously, as a lot of the men will have been called up. Do you remember a lot of lasses working there?

I don't remember. I think I was only once there. They slid the crates out onto the lorries and carts.

And they were all horse-drawn in those days, weren't they?

Yes they were until they got the lorry. My father drove it.

(We discuss what colour it was – she seems to remember it was red.)

That was where we got our first dog.

Was it?

Well, my father used to go on what he called his country runs on a Tuesday and a Thursday. He went round the villages. Cramlington . . . not too far afield. I can't remember where he was but wherever it was, he did two or three shops in this village and the dog followed him from one to another and then jumped in the cab. He thought it must be lost so he brought it home. We called it Pincher.

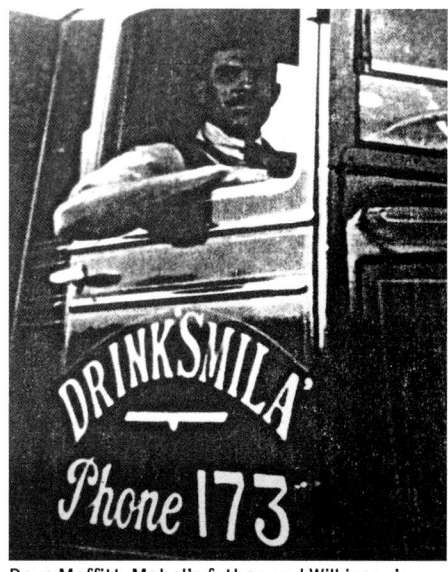

Dave Moffitt, Mabel's father and Wilkinson's lorry driver.

Pincher?

Yes, 'cos he pinched it! (laughs) And that dog was his shadow. It went with him every day. It went out with him to work in the mornings and if it was a day when he came in for his dinner, it would come in and have its dinner and then go out with him again. It just was his shadow.

And it was killed on a Sunday morning. We were out for a walk. I remember my sister Dorothy was in the pram so I would be only maybe five or six?

When the lads went out delivering, did they go on their own or in pairs, maybe?

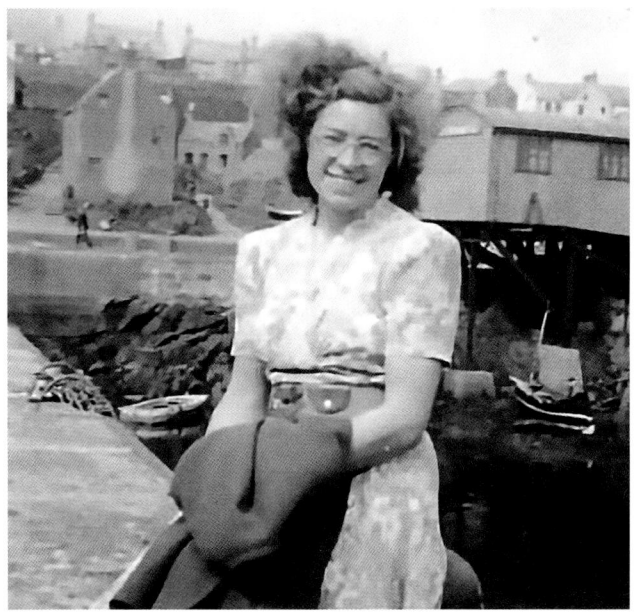

Mabel Moffitt. Courtesy of Mabel Moffitt/Alan Bainbridge

They went on their own. They each drove a cart. They were strong you know – lifting those crates with all the full bottles in.

Your dad must have been strong lad!

Particularly in the summer when he worked till nearly 10 o'clock. On the beach, there were stalls in those days and he would supply the stalls with pop. So it was up and down the banks, with steps to get onto the beach.

So it wasn't just parking outside a shop and delivering?

No.

When it was very hot as well . . .

My mother never liked the sand. When we first used to go to the beach, there were tents that you could hire and the tents had floors in them – wooden floors and a bench at the bank, where you could sit. They had wooden runners underneath. They hitched the horse to the tent and pulled it to wherever you wanted on the beach.

So you didn't have to cart it along and put it up yourself?

No, no. And you could have it open . . . well, in any way you wanted.

And you never had to put your feet on the sand. What were they? Did they have a name?

I don't think so. They were just tents. Square ones.

We're talking pre-war, are we?

Yes. The ordinary ones just had the sand for the floor so my mother used to sit on the lower prom.

Which beach are we talking about?

Tynemouth. Ee, the beach used to be packed. We often went down at dinnertime. She would say "I'll just take the tea down to the beach." Come down and you'll know where to find me. Near the bathing pool.

Briefing

After the raid

Following the disaster, the site was cleared.

The debris and rubble were used to fill in the burn which ran down Red Burn View in North Shields. Kathleen Parkin, remembered "scrambling over the debris and finding lots of household items: knives, forks, spoons and also lipstick and rouge and millions of bottle labels."

And Austin Jacob Mellor, a Facebook contributor commented that

> rubble from the pop factory is buried in the gardens of our streets. If you dig anywhere in the gardens, we unearth bricks. My grandfather even found a wedding ring amongst the rubble. It's all buried underneath Etal Avenue, Wooler Avenue and Ford Avenue just next to Norham High School.

The site was partially built upon in 1946 with two council houses. These were among the first new houses built by Tynemouth Corporation after the War.

Wilkinson's plot extended to the lane on George Street, which separated it from a row of terraced houses which when demolished, made way for East End Youth Club. The lane allowed loading from the side of the Wilkinson's factory.

By 1978, the Weekly News reported that the house at 11 George Street had started subsiding despite having had 65 tons of concrete poured into the foundations. The houses had started to tilt with cracks appearing in the walls. A decision was taken to demolish both houses to prevent any injury to tenants.

The houses were rebuilt c1979 and can be seen on the corner of King Street and George Street.

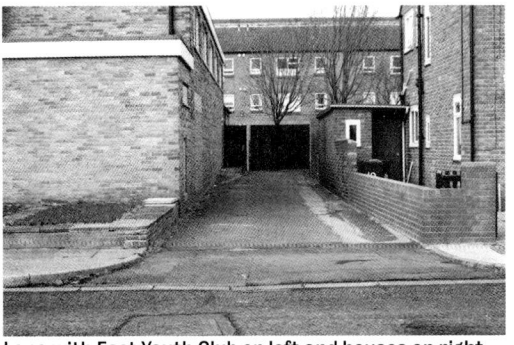

Lane with East Youth Club on left and houses on right. Taken from George Street.

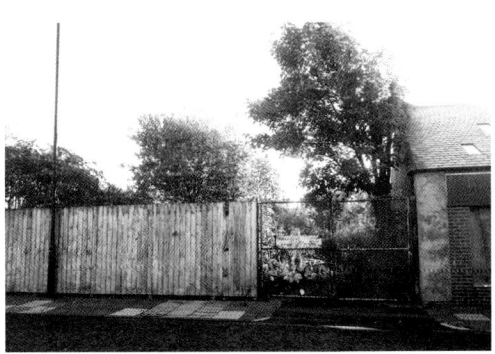

Wilkinson's Yard – photo taken in 2015.

Wilkinson's yard and stables were located over the road at the Tynemouth Road end of King Street. Following the bombing the business re-located to this location and operated from there until c1964. The land was sold and became a builder's yard. In 1983 the buildings and chimney were demolished and the rubble was sold and used as hard core for the Metro Centre in Gateshead. Photos of the yard and the demolition of the buildings can be found in John H Alexander's book, *Memory Lane, North Shields*.

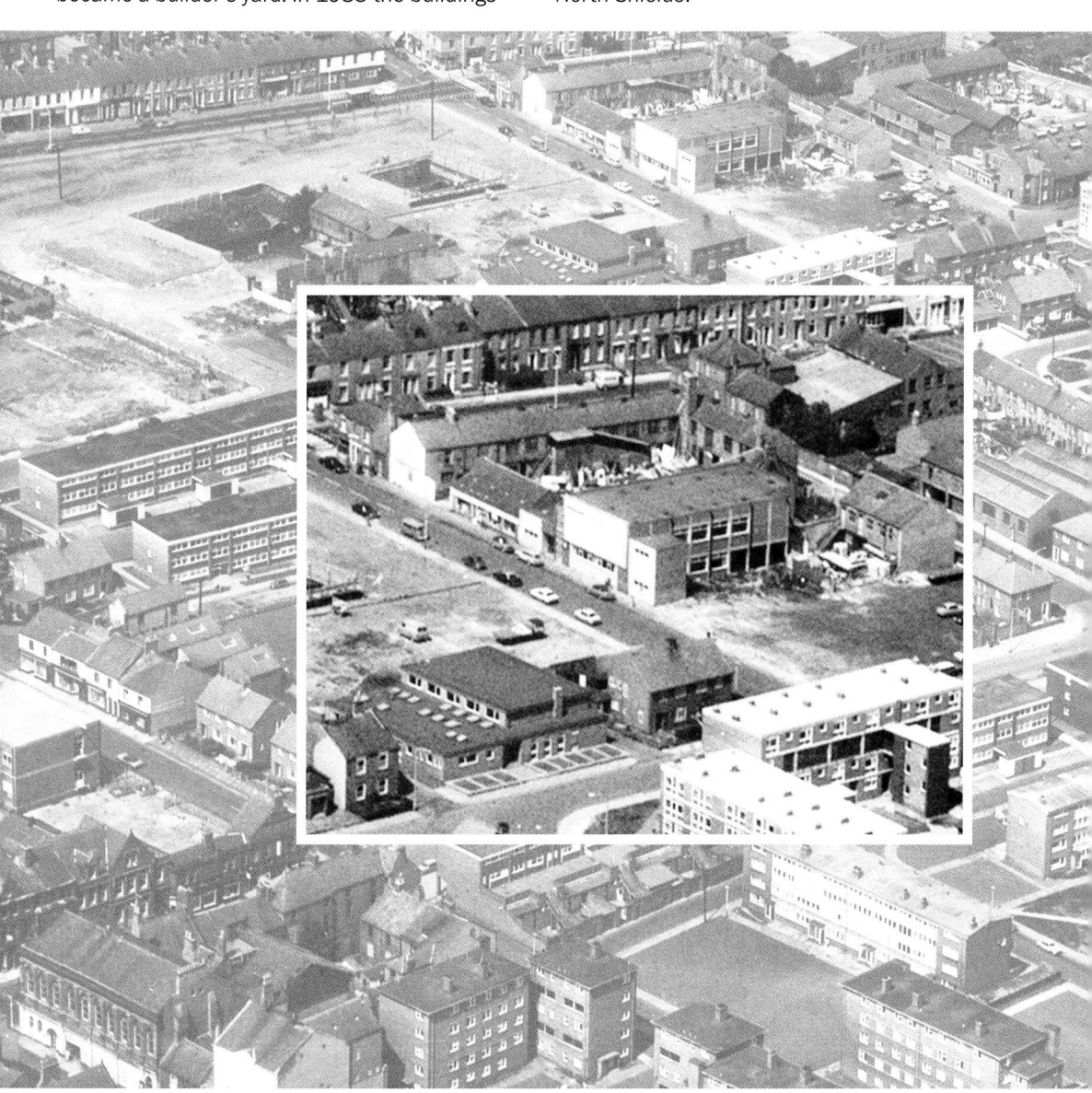

A 1973 aerial photo of North Shields showing the 2 houses on the corner plot. Above them is King Street Social Club and next is Wilkinson's Yard. You can still see the ramp from the first floor of the building which the horses would run down. [EAW259632] North Shields and environs, Tynemouth, 1973 © Historic England.

12 Bombing the Borough

It is useful to put the Wilkinson's incident into a wartime perspective, in terms of what was happening locally and nationally.

I am indebted to the late Brian Pears for permission to use his definitive "North East War Diary" (ne-diary.genuki.uk). The diary has detailed information about many of the bombing incidents in the Borough and readers are encouraged to consult it.

Tyneside was a major Luftwaffe target on account of its varied industrial activity including shipbuilding and repair and its armaments manufacture. Tyneside's role as an important military base should not be underestimated. Royal Navy ships caught in the river were a tempting target. The Tyne, as a strategic port, importing and exporting goods and material vital to the war effort, made it a target of significance. It was easily reached, too, from Luftwaffe bases in Belgium, Holland and Scandinavia.

German efforts to destroy and disrupt focused severally on minelaying activities along the East coast and at the mouth of the river, occasional multi-bomber raids and as the War progressed on different fronts, sporadic single "nuisance raiders" and "tip and run" attacks. North Shields' position at the river mouth also meant it became a dumping opportunity for enemy crews heading for home.

Local targets can be understood from German documents including the Stadtplan (a modified version of an OS map) and aerial photos which are marked with targets including the shipyards, docks, transport and public utilities infrastructure. Military targets, especially anti-aircraft gun batteries are also indicated. If there was any doubt about the nature of "total war", then the marking up of North Shields' hospitals is indicative.

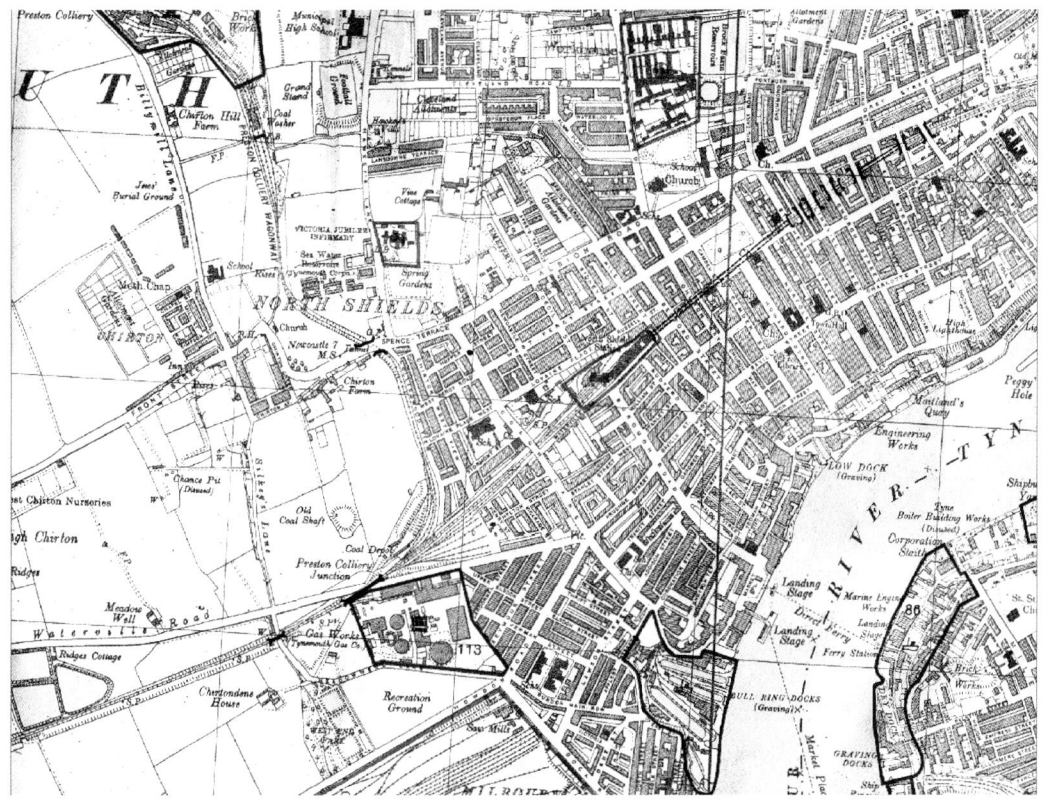

Stadtplan. At scale of 1:10,000. The Germans would have been able to buy OS maps without any problems in the years before 1939.

A heavy raid would result in detailed reports submitted by the Chief Constable/ARP Controller (Tom Blackburn) and the Town Clerk (Fred G Egner) to the Borough's Emergency Committee.

It is unfortunate that the Chief Constable's report on Wilkinson's is missing from Tyne and Wear Archives. An example of his reports can be found on the "North East War Diary" for the raid of Wednesday 9th April 1941, which lasted nearly 6 hours and cost 35 lives. The detail is fascinating, as is the picture it conveys of the concerted local response and the co-ordinated network of ARP services on hand to assist.

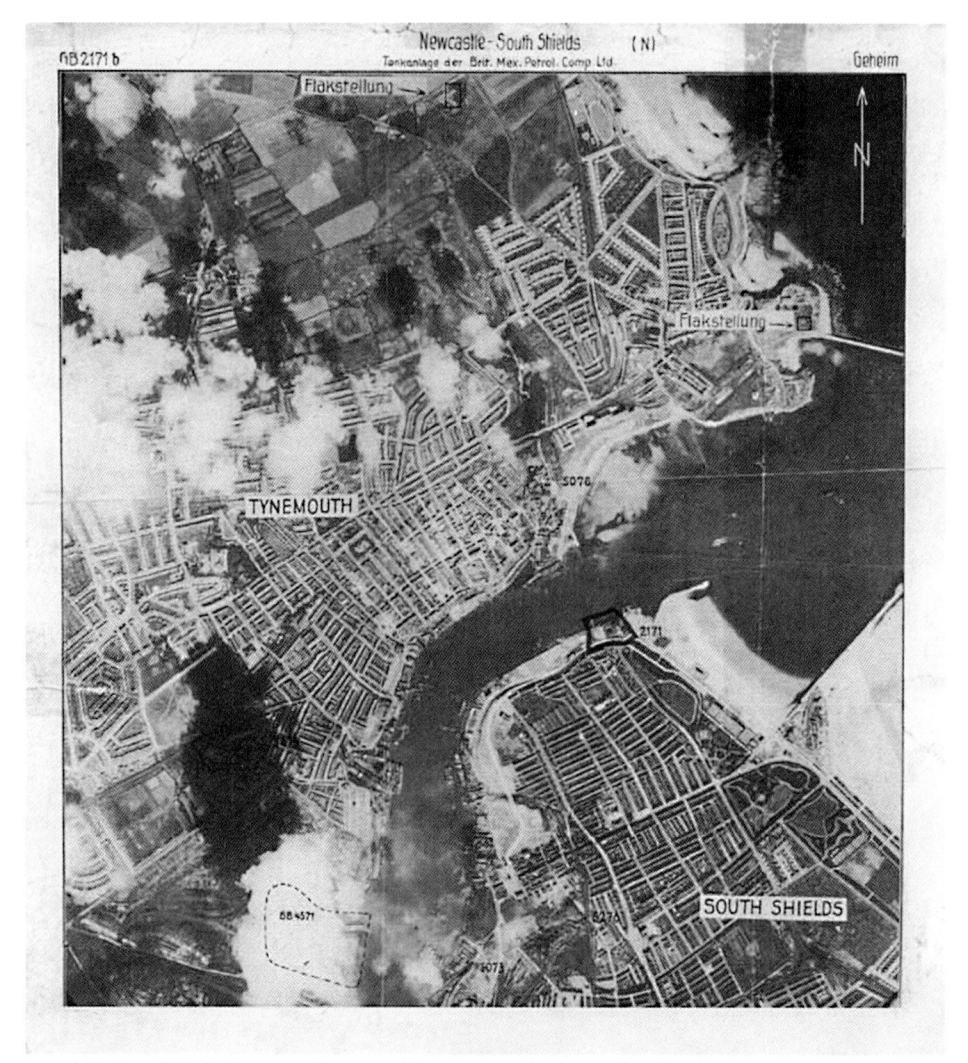

Aerial Photo, c1939. Anti-aircraft gun positions are marked as well as key targets.
Photo courtesy of Gary Carverhill.

The Town Clerk's report on Wilkinson's, less detailed and focused on the casualty information can be found on northshields173.org

The heaviest enemy raids in the Borough were experienced from April to October 1941. This "Blitz" period was characterised by heavy raids spread over a few days, followed by long spells of relative enemy inactivity.

The intensity of the raids brought severe damage to buildings and infrastructure and of course higher casualty figures. Fortunately, the

> **Report of the Town Clerk to the EMERGENCY COMMITTEE.**
>
> 14th May, 1941.
>
> **Air Raids in Tynemouth on 3/4th May and 5/6th May, 1941.**
>
> General Information Centre.
>
> Immediately after the "Raiders Passed" Signal sounded on the morning of the 4th May, 1941, the Town Clerk's Office was opened as a General Information Centre, and information was supplied to all enquirers.
>
> At 9 a.m. the Tasker Hall was taken over for this purpose, and kept open until 6 p.m. on each day until Thursday, the 8th May, 1941.
>
> The approximate number of enquiries dealt with during this period amounted to 600.
>
> Lists were prepared of persons requiring repairs to their properties, and these were forwarded to the Borough Surveyor for his attention. Similar lists in respect of furniture which required salving or removal were forwarded to the Salvage and Removal Officer.
>
> Casualty Information Bureau.
>
> The Casualty Information Bureau obtained the necessary particulars relating to injured and dead from hospitals and mortuaries, and lists were published outside the Town Clerk's Office, Tasker Hall and Police Station.
>
> Relatives of dead persons were traced and notified by post or messenger.
>
> The total number of casualties recorded, in respect of the raid on the 3/4th May, was as follows:—
>
> | | |
> |---|---|
> | Dead ... ... | 107 |
> | Admitted to Hospital ... | 36 |
> | Treated at First Aid Posts | 16 |
>
> The number of casualties in the raid on the 5/6th instant, was:—
>
> | | |
> |---|---|
> | Dead ... ... | 9 |
> | Admitted to Hospital ... | 2 |
> | Treated at First Aid Posts | 1 |
> | Outpatients at Hospitals.. | 4 |

The Town Clerk's report on air raids in Tynemouth, May 3rd–6th 1941.

periods of respite meant that ARP and Civil Defence services were never really overstretched. Public morale could be rebuilt, infrastructure repaired, ready for the next raid.

The ARP Control HQ at Cleveland Villa, Cleveland Road in North Shields, kept a detailed record of all bombing incidents in the Borough, marking each bomb dropped on a Borough Bomb Map. This can be consulted locally at North Shields Central Library.

The majority of bomb incidents were also photographed and filmed by Tynemouth Borough Police, presumably on behalf of Tynemouth Corporation and probably for War damage claims. The film footage, although of poor quality, is a moving record of what our townsfolk endured during the War. The film footage and various edits of it can be

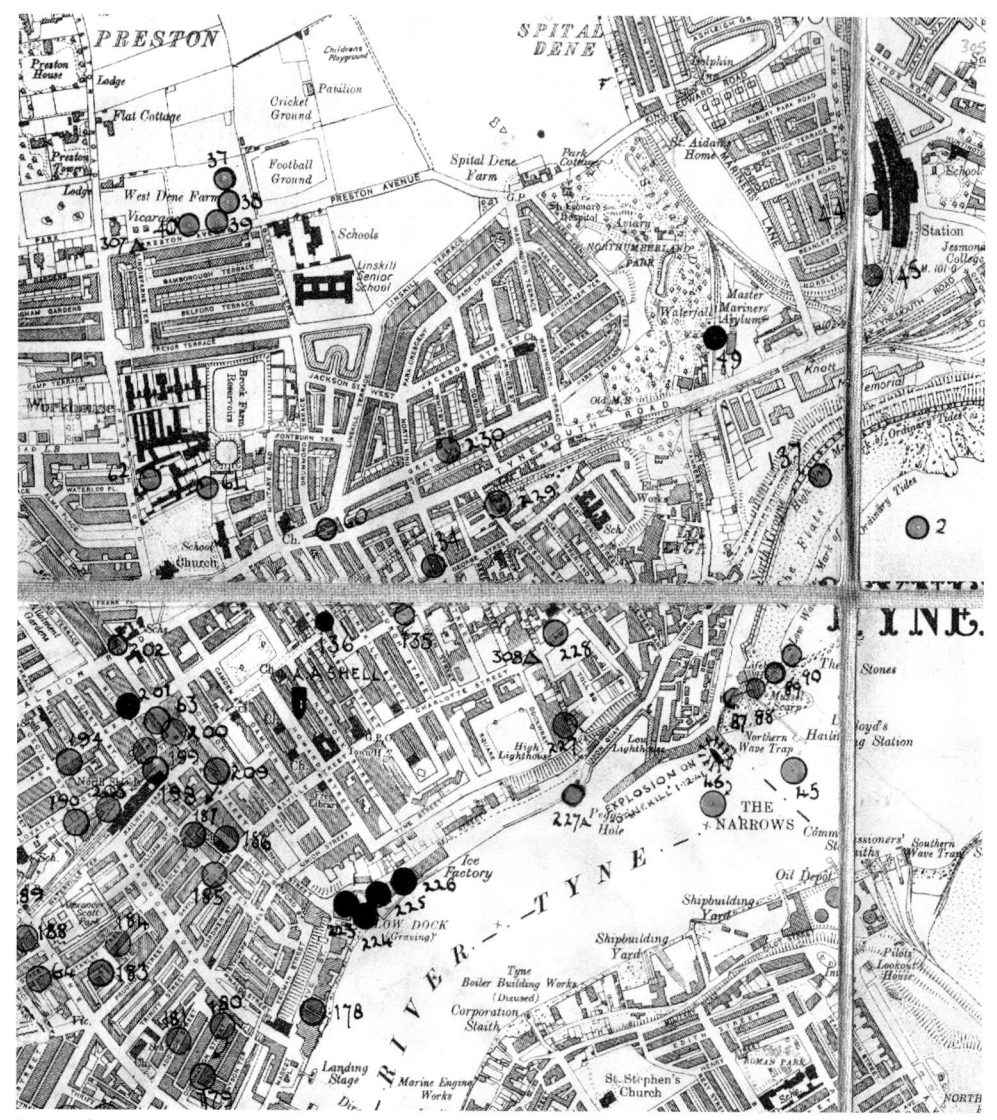

Detail of Borough bomb map showing the 4 HE bombs which fell on 3rd/4th May 1941.
Bomb No 134: Direct Hit on Wilkinson's Factory Shelter (107 people killed).
Bomb No 135: Direct Hit on house (2 killed). Bomb No 136: Unexploded bomb (0 casualties).
Bomb No 137: Exploded on beach (0 casualties).

found on northshields173.org and YouTube. The original footage is lost. Does anyone know of its whereabouts?

Inspector Harold White, Deputy A.R.P. Controller, gave the following summary report in October 1944 when the threat of further Luftwaffe attacks on the Borough was over.

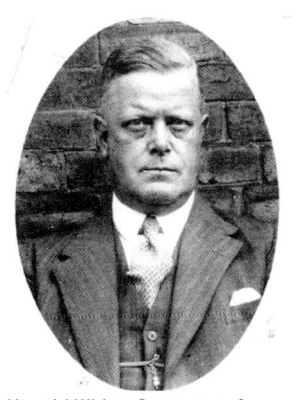

Harold White. Courtesy of Paul Sampson

During air raids on Tynemouth borough since June 22, 1940, 225 persons lost their lives, 150 were seriously injured and 325 slightly injured. A total of 310 high explosive bombs have been dropped in the town, 19 parachute mines and approximately 18,000 incendiary bombs. There have been 253 alerts and bombs have dropped on 31 occasions. The number of properties totally demolished was 166, while 281 were damaged beyond repair, 1303 seriously damaged and 9,928 slightly damaged. The number of shops, offices and public buildings damaged was 328.

Timeline

[HE = High Explosive / IB = Incendiary Bomb / PM = Parachute Mine]

1939

SEPTEMBER

Sunday 3rd (Day 1)
- War announced at 11.15am by Neville Chamberlain.
- Government ordered that gas masks were to be carried at all times.
- Closure of cinemas and theatres announced.
- National Service (Armed Forces) Act passed. All men between 18 and 41 were liable for conscription except those in reserved occupations.
- 44,000 Newcastle children had already been evacuated to locations in Northumberland, Cumbria and Yorkshire.
- National Census taken for mobilisation, rationing and registration. (29/9)

OCTOBER
- British men between 20-22 years of age now liable for conscription. (1/10)

1940

JANUARY
- Rationing begins - the allowances were: 4oz. of butter, 4oz. of bacon or ham and 12oz. of sugar, per head, per week. (8/1)
- Black Out speed limit reduced to 20mph to reduce road accidents. (23/1)
- Meat rationing began - the allowance was 1s 10d worth of meat for everyone over 6 years of age. (23/1)

MAY
- Germany invades Belgium, Luxembourg and Holland. (10/5)
- Chamberlain resigns. (10/5)
- Churchill forms National Government. (10/5)

Sunday 12th
- A stray barrage balloon damaged 17 houses at Tynemouth.

JUNE
- Churchill's "We shall fight them on the beaches" speech. (4/6)
- The last day to comply with the order to erect delivered Anderson shelters – they must be erected and covered with 15" of earth on top and 30" at the sides or they will be taken away and penalties imposed. (11/6)

Friday 21st/22nd
- Luftwaffe mine-laying operations along the east coast.
- High explosive (HE) bomb just off "The Flatts" and a second just south of the North Pier.

JULY – OCTOBER: THE BATTLE OF BRITAIN
- The Luftwaffe attempts to gain air superiority over the RAF. This was a decisive air campaign fought over southern England. By the end, the RAF had lost 1,542 aircrew killed and 1,744 aircraft destroyed. The Luftwaffe in comparison lost 2,585 aircrew killed and missing and 1,977 aircraft destroyed
- Luftwaffe targets coastal shipping. Minelaying activities were often the cause of a number of air raid warnings inland. (12/7)

AUGUST

Friday 9th/10th
- HE on the railway north of Cullercoats station.

- 3 bombs in fields west of Broadway. Some property damage. No casualties.

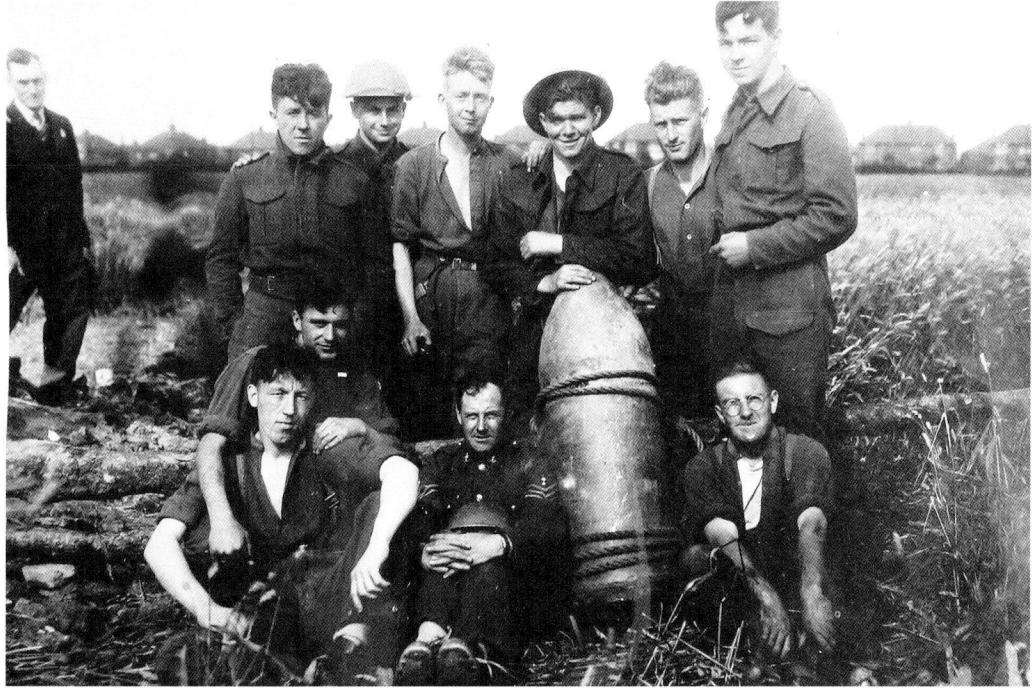

UXB removed at Marden Farm just off the Broadway, Cullercoats.

Thursday 15th
- Most intensive raid on the North East during the Battle of Britain with Luftflotte 5 Heinkel He111's and Junker Ju.88's attempting a flanking operation. Engaged out at sea, the Luftwaffe suffered heavy losses.
- 5 HE just below the Low Water Mark between Sharpness Point and the castle and 1 just south of the North Pier. Some damage reported.

Saturday 24th/25th
- 2 HEs dropped, 1 falling into the sea off the Long Sands, the other fell on the North End Foreshore.
- Galaland (later The Plaza) had a large number of windows broken and a few window frames damaged. No casualties.

Thursday 29th/30th
- 8 HEs were dropped in the New York and Murton Districts.
- Able Seaman Furse smothered IB which had penetrated roof of Moor Park Hospital preventing possible fire and fatalities.

SEPTEMBER – LONDON BLITZ BEGINS

Sunday 1st/2nd
- 1 HE dropped on the Long Sands at Tynemouth leaving a crater 8' in diameter. No damage was done to property or casualties reported.

Friday 6th/7th
- An enemy plane was observed dropping mines in the sea between the mouth of the Tyne and Cullercoats

Saturday 7th
- The London Blitz begins, lasting for 57 consecutive nights. Over a million homes were damaged or destroyed and more than 20,000 Londoners were killed

Saturday 21st/22nd
- 1 HE on the Short Sands and 3 HE just below low water mark. Property damage.

OCTOBER

Thursday 10th/11th
- 4 HEs in the market garden, Preston Road, 2 HEs in the river area near the harbour entrance and 4 delayed HE at High Flatworth Farm (2 exploded on the 11th)

Wednesday 23rd/24th
- A Parachute Mine (PM) on the bowling green in Tynemouth Park and another in a field at Kennersdene Farm near the LNER electric railway caused craters measuring 35 feet x 15 feet.
- Damage to Park Cafe, Bowling Club Pavilion, Beaconsfield House AFS Station, the Grand Parade First Aid Post and many other buildings including 280 houses. No injuries. Damage also to the Princes Theatre, Russell Street, North Shields.

Thursday 31st 1940
- The last daylight raid by the Luftwaffe. Generally considered to be the end of the Battle of Britain. Night time raids on a wide variety of targets continued through the Winter/Spring of 1940/1941 ending as the Luftwaffe focus attention on the Russian campaign.

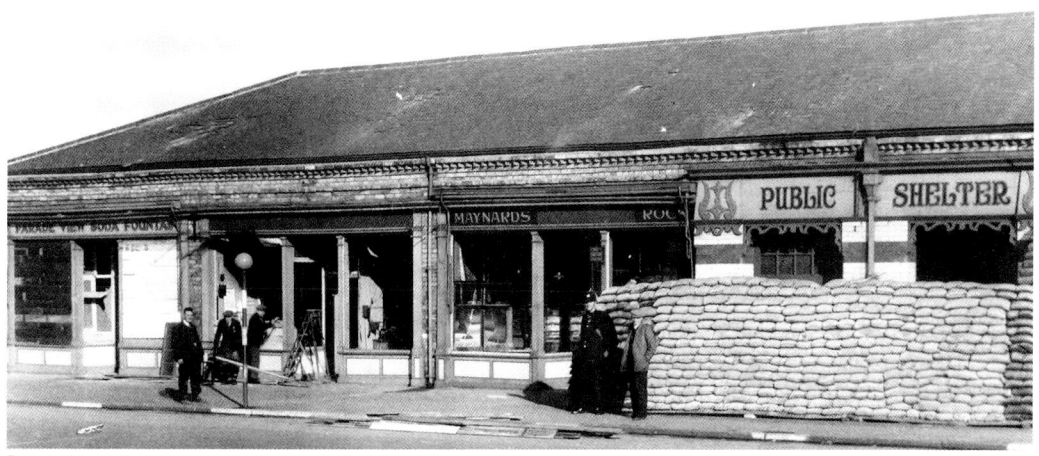

Bomb damage at First Aid Post on Grand Parade,

NOVEMBER
- Luftwaffe begins heavy bombing of British cities. Targets included Coventry, Southampton, Birmingham, Liverpool, Clydebank, Bristol, Swindon, Plymouth, Cardiff, Manchester, Sheffield, Swansea and Portsmouth.
- On November 14th, more than 4,000 homes in Coventry were destroyed. Approximately 600 people were killed and more than 1,000 were injured.

DECEMBER
- Heavy bombing raids on Sheffield, Liverpool and Manchester.

1941

JANUARY – MARCH
- Cardiff, Swansea, Clydebank and Plymouth bombed.
- Compulsory fire watching introduced. All men and women from 16 to 60 must register for part-time Civil Defence service. (20/1)

FEBRUARY

Sunday 16th/17th
- 1 HE in Northumberland Park and a second just west of Northumberland Terrace above Swaddles Hole.

MARCH
Monday 3rd/ 4th
- 22 enemy bombers of Luftflotte 2 attacked armament and industrial plant, dockyards and dock installations at the mouth of the Tyne and at Newcastle. They dropped 94 HE, 2,988 IBs and 56 Parachute Flares between 20.08 and 21.05. The Concentration Point was on the banks of the Tyne at Newcastle. Fires and damage were reported. Tyne AA guns in action. Minelaying carried out between Tyne and Tees.

APRIL
- Belfast and Plymouth sustained heavy bombing

Monday 7th/8th
- 9 small HEs were dropped in fields at Close's Farm, North Road, Preston, North Shields.
- Later an enemy aircraft was heard overhead and heavy anti-aircraft was experienced. Two parachutes were seen at sea SE of Cullercoats, gunfire and tracer bullets were also seen out at sea.

Wednesday 9th/10th
- Lifeboat Station near the Fish Quay hit.
- Preston Institute hit – X-ray Department demolished.
- 2 patients and 3 male attendants were killed.
- A police box was destroyed, a first aid and wardens' post damaged, two members of the police reserve, a female ambulance driver and a naval rating lost their lives. An ambulance received a direct hit proceeding from Whitley Bay and trains in sidings at Monkseaton were set on fire.
- 33 dead included five children of under 16. 15 people suffered serious injuries and 86 were slightly injured.
- Tyne AA guns were in action, firing 3,133 rounds

Tuesday 15th/16th]
- Some 100 enemy aircraft were in operation over the NE coastal areas.
- Tynemouth was attacked three times in the early morning. Chirton

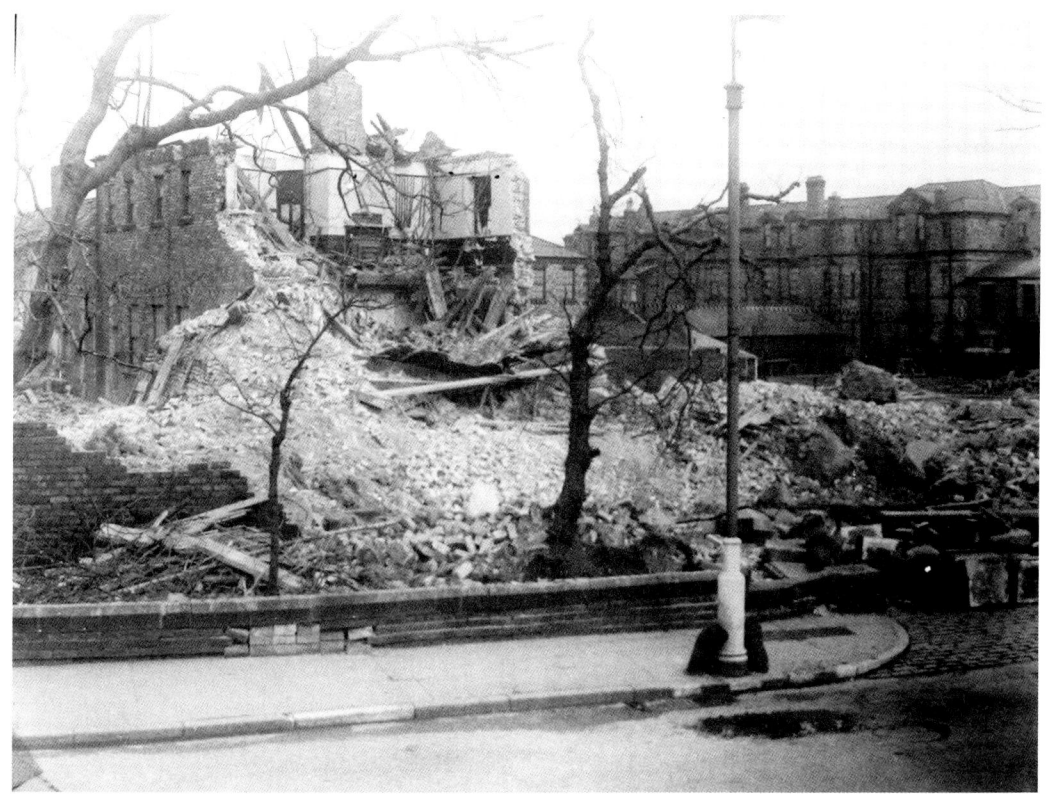

Preston Hospital/Holmlands damaged in raid of 9th/10th April

council school and a nearby Warden's post at the Rex Cinema were demolished by a mine, further mines were dropped in the town. An air raid warden and a firewatcher were killed at their post in Billy Mill Lane and a woman died in Balkwell Avenue.
- 6 HEs fell in fields in the Preston district. No damage or casualties were caused.
- At approximately 03.55 a PM dropped within 100 yards of a reservoir at the junction of Moor House Road and Rake Lane, causing damage to houses in Rake Lane, Moor House Road and Brookland Terrace, New York. Two people were slightly injured.
- At approximately 03.55 a PM was dropped in a field near White House Farm, Preston, North Shields. No damage was reported.
- A PM fell in the moat of Tynemouth Castle hitting a store, a second PM fell in King Edward Bay at Tynemouth. Much damage was done to

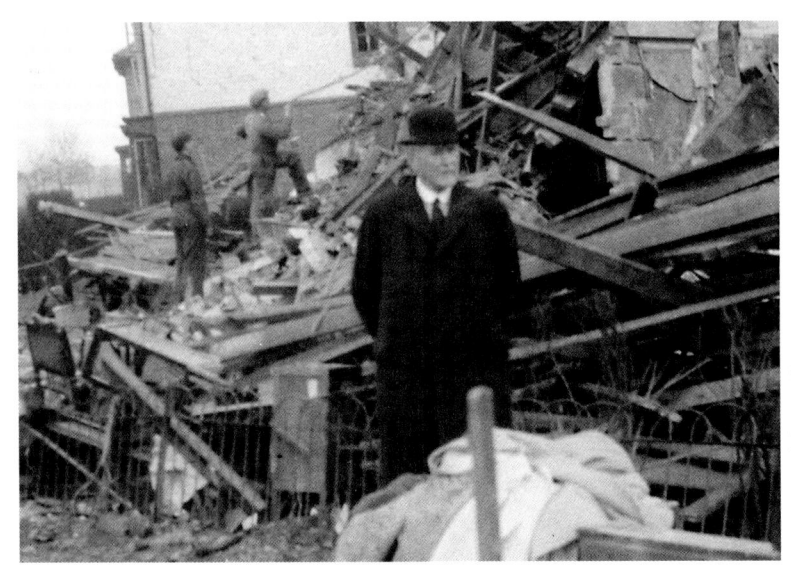

Chief Constable Tom Blackburn at Balkwell Avenue. ARP Demolition workers in background.

houses and shops in Front Street, Percy Gardens and nearby districts. The Catholic Church at Tynemouth was also damaged by blast. Hundreds of shops and houses in Tynemouth and Balkwell areas had windows broken.

- Hundreds of people were made homeless, three emergency Rest and Feeding Centres were opened and a total of 218 persons passed through. Many of the homeless made their own arrangements for billeting. The Information Bureau in the Tasker Hall, Howard Street was opened and representatives from the Billeting Officer, Food Office, Citizens' Advice Bureau and Assistance Board were available as well as the Town Clerk's staff. Additional assistance was given by the Librarian and a member of his staff. Information was supplied relating to missing relatives, repairs to property, removal and salvage of furniture, funeral arrangements and other, general advice. The Centre remained open each day from 09.15 to 18.00 on the Wednesday, Thursday, Friday, Saturday and Monday following the raid, and was closed at 18.00 on the 21st.
- The approximate number of enquiries dealt with, amounted to 1,500. Lists were prepared of persons requiring repairs to their property - these were forwarded to the Borough Surveyor for his attention,

similar lists in respect of furniture which required salving or removal were forwarded to the Salvage and Removal Officer. The total number of cases where property was removed from damaged buildings was 120. Of this number, 43 were placed in storage by the Corporation at Collingwood School which was taken over for this purpose.

Friday 25th/26th
- Shortly after the Alert was sounded, numerous flares lit up the whole of this and surrounding districts. 11 HEs (2 large and 9 medium) fell in a field adjacent to that occupied by the AA battery off Broadway, Tynemouth. 2 PMs fell on the Golf Course, King Edward Road, Tynemouth. 2 PMs fell in fields on the west side of the North Road, Preston Grange Farm. 2 PMs fell on the rocks near Bathing Pool, Sea Front, Tynemouth. An HE fell in a field off Norham Road, near the Knitwear Factory, Percy Main. 2 PMs fell on the rocks off Marconi Point, Cullercoats.
- Although many IBs were dropped in the Borough, the Fire Service was not required. IBs also fell on the Tyne Improvement Commissioner's property, some of them fell on Nos 4 & 5 Staiths, Whitehill Point, they were soon extinguished. An IB fell on board 'SS Rioazul' causing slight damage in the thwartship bunker which was extinguished by the ship's crew.
- A UXB fell on the railway embankment between the Park Hotel and Beaconsfield House, Tynemouth, damaging the track between Tynemouth and Cullercoats. The hole was about 3 ft. 6ins. in diameter and the UXB penetrated to a depth of between 30 ft. and 40 ft, railway traffic was suspended between Tynemouth and Cullercoats , this lasted for about a week.

MAY
- Winston Churchill gives 'Blood, Toil, Tears, and Sweat' speech.
- Merseyside suffered one of the last big raids on Britain before the German invasion of Russia. It involved 681 bombers which dropped about 870 tonnes of high explosive bombs and over 112,000 incendiaries causing extensive damage to the city centre and the docks.

Saturday 3rd/4th (N609)

Bombs fell at Newcastle, Tynemouth, Throckley, Catcleugh, Morpeth, Lynemouth, Gosforth, Clifton and Stannington in Northumberland, Sunderland, West Hartlepool, Gateshead, Tees Bridge Roundabout at Billingham, Lambton Park, Castletown, Ryhope and South Shields in Co Durham and York and Hull in Yorkshire.

Enemy activity at:

00.30 Newcastle
01.05 Newcastle
23.30 Northumberland
23.45 Northumberland
00.10 Northumberland – Lynemouth
00:00 North Shields – Tyneside's worst incident of the War occurred when HEs fell on North Shields; one scored a direct hit on Wilkinson's Lemonade Factory at the corner of George Street and King Street, North Shields

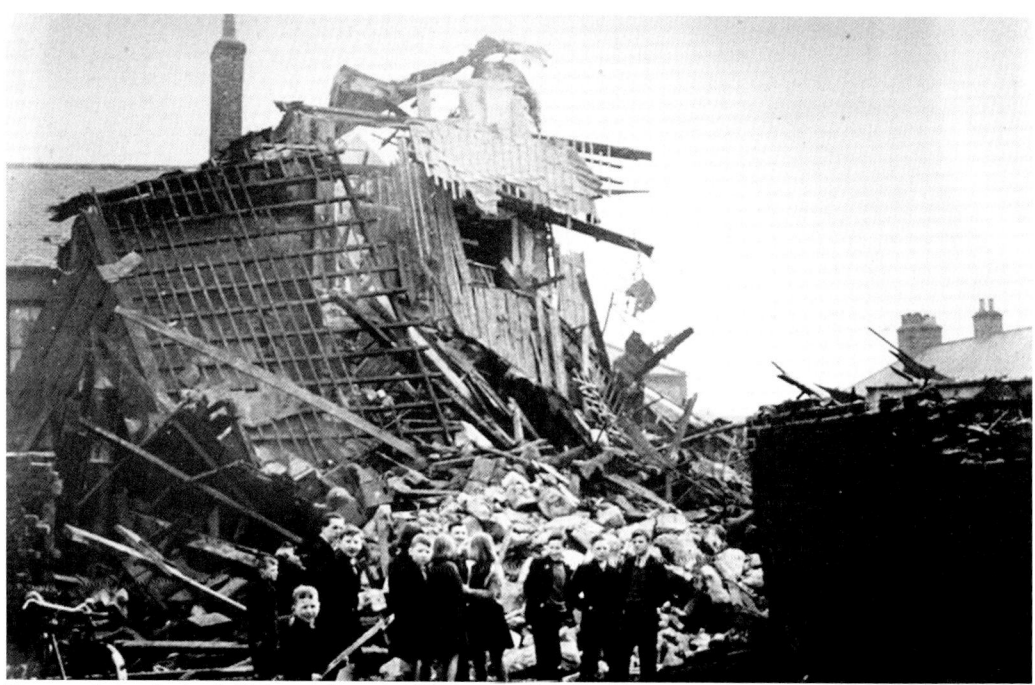

Famous photo of school children gathered at Wilkinson's. Note the bike propped up bottom left.

00:00 A single HE dropped on George Street, between Church Street and Queen Street

00:00 A single HE fell on the railway embankment near to Stephenson Street

00:00 A single HE fell at the high water mark on The Flatts. There was major property damage.

00:00 Gateshead

23.03-03.13 South Shields

Shortly before the siren sounded, approximately 600 incendiary bombs were dropped between the Stadium, Westoe and the Horsley Hill Estate. The few small fires which resulted were put out by the Street Firefighting Parties. No HE bombs were dropped in this raid.

Monday 5th/6th
- Some 386 enemy planes passed over the area in waves of about thirty every seven minutes or so, en-route to Clydeside. At Newcastle, enemy aircraft were overhead for most of the alert period.
- Bombs fell at Newcastle, North Shields and Cullercoats in Northumberland
- Six people were killed in Heaton Terrace, North Shields and three in Garden Square, Cullercoats.

Tuesday 6th/7th
- 2 HEs fell at Heaton Terrace, Billy Mill, between the junctions at Verne Road and Langley Road. There were 6 fatalities. 2 HEs fell in the vicinity of Front Street, Cullercoats. 2 HEs fell on the foreshore at Cullercoats Bay. 2 HEs fell adjacent to Birtley Avenue, Tynemouth, 1 beside Tynemouth railway station and the other on the railway at the southern end of the Avenue.

Wednesday 7th/8th
- Two HEs fell in open country between Preston Grange and Rake House. There was damage to property.

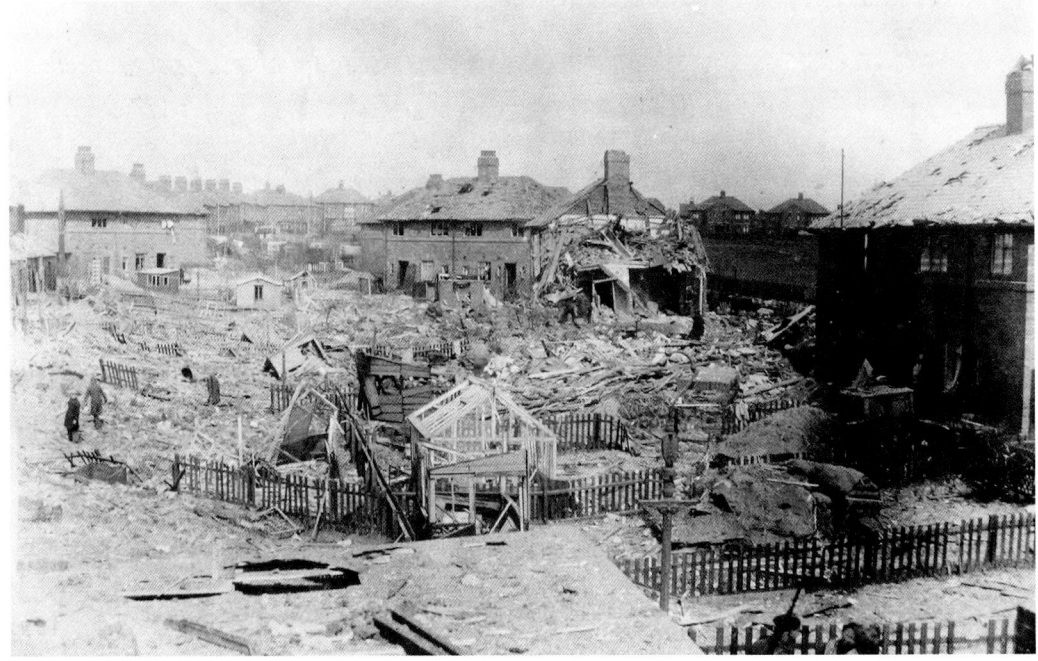

Devastation at Heaton Terrace after raid 6th/7th May

JUNE

Monday 2nd/3rd
- A Junkers Ju.88 A was shot down by a Hurricane, into the sea four miles notrth-east of Tynemouth at 22.29. Two of the crew were killed and two were taken prisoner.

Wednesday 18th
- King George and Queen Elizabeth toured Tyneside and visited shipyards and armament factories.

SEPTEMBER

Monday 1st/2nd
- Two HEs fell, one near the junction of Silkey's Lane and Waterville Road about 60 yards N of the LNER track, and the other on the tennis court in Smith's Recreation Park.
- Casualties were two fatal and eight injured, all the latter having been sent home after treatment. The bodies were received at the ARP Mortuary. Board.

Tuesday 30th/1st

- A major raid causing sixty-one deaths and widespread damage. 38 HEs dropped over residential areas in the eastern half of North Shields causing major damage to property including North Shields Railway Station. A single HE fell at Whitehill Point Ferry Landing. 7 HEs fell at Albert Edward Dock and the railway lines serving the docks. 4 HEs fell at Percy Main affecting Rothbury Terrace, Morpeth Terrace, Wallsend Road and Waterville Road and a single HE between Regent Terrace and Queen Alexandra Road.
- In North Shields: Bedford Street, Saville Street, and Coach Lane were among the streets hit. The buildings damaged included the Wesleyan Hall, which was set on fire, Prince's Theatre, Chirton Co-operative Store, and Queen Victoria Council School – the school was badly damaged, five classrooms were found to be unusable, pupils were transferred to the Western Board School
- The minesweeping trawlers 'Eileen Duncan' and 'Star of Deveron'

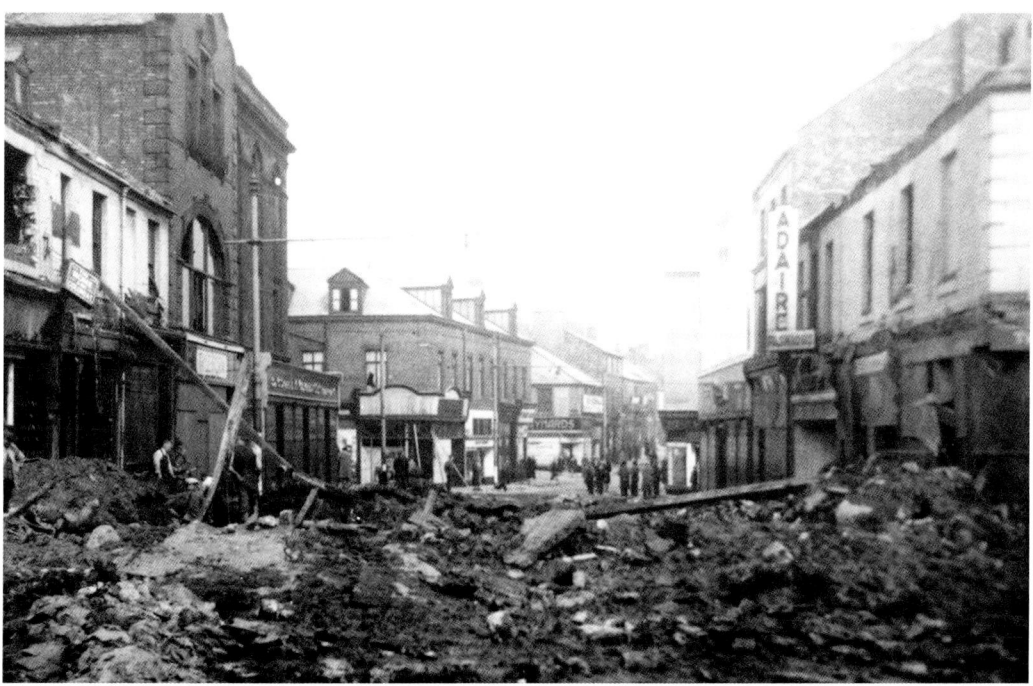

Major property damage across North Shields. Huge crater on Saville Street from raid on 30th September 1941.

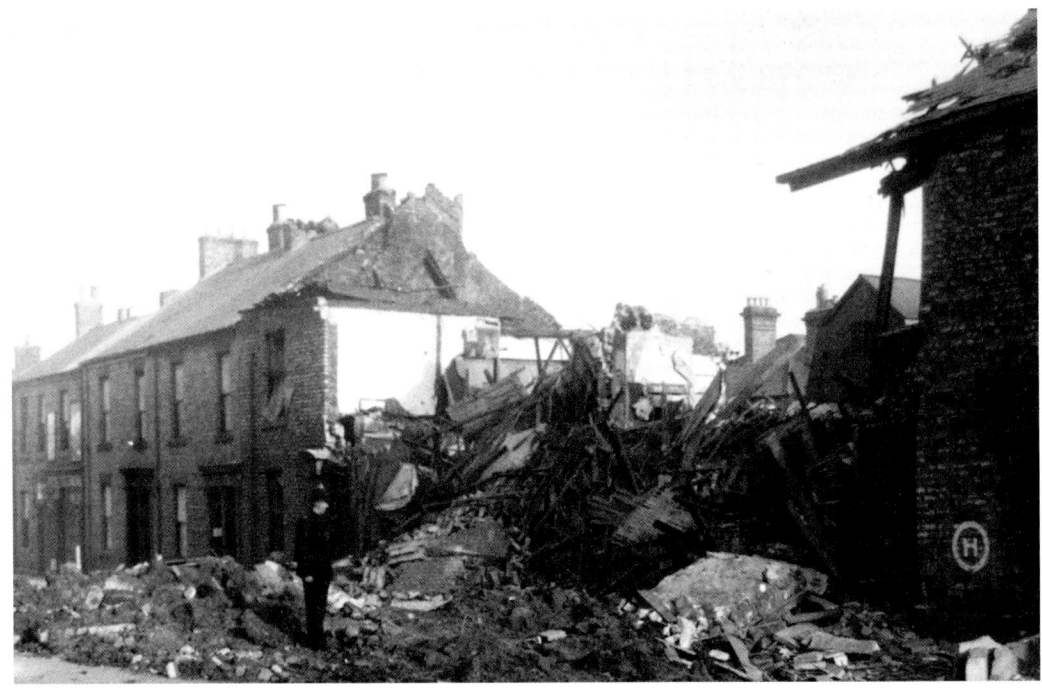

Grey Street, North Shields, 2nd October 1941.

were attacked and sunk, probably during this same air raid. Three bombs fell on Prince Albert Edward Dock. In South Shields, all of the E side of the Market Place was devastated including the Shields Evening News and Gazette building
- Preston Colliery – Homes damaged, a shelter hit and two people killed.

OCTOBER

Thursday 2nd/3rd
- 28 HEs fell, scattered over the Borough. 2 people were killed by an HE at Beacon Street shelter and another by an HE on the railway at Hudson Street near the junction with Tynemouth Road. There was much damage to property, the gasworks was hit and supplies affected.

DECEMBER

Monday 8th/9th
- A single HE fell at Flatworth Pit. 2 HEs fell in Prior's Park, Tynemouth.

1942

AUGUST

Saturday 8th

- In a hit and run, just after 20.00, St John's Methodist Church, Cullercoats was demolished and a thirteen year old boy was killed while practising the organ. A single HE fell on Marden Avenue, Cullercoats. A single HE fell beside the LNER main line near Beaconsfield House and a single HE beside Kennersdene Farm, Tynemouth near the LNER main line. Property and hospital damage in the Borough.

OCTOBER

Sunday 11th/12th

- At Cullercoats 7 houses were demolished, 10 severely damaged, 6 people killed and 17 seriously injured.

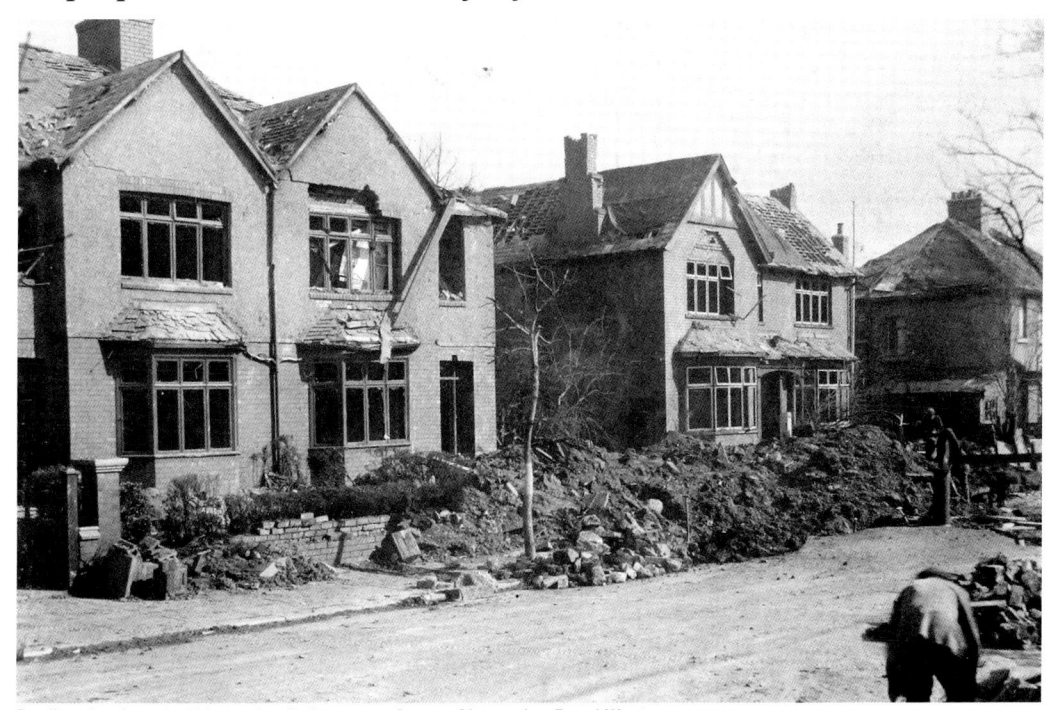

Perilously close to this author's home on Queen Alexandra Road West.

- 4 HEs fell on residential property between Cullercoats railway station and Newton Avenue. 4 HEs fell in a line between Dock Road and the Commissioners Staiths.

DECEMBER

Monday 14th/15th
- 6 HEs and 3 IBs fell on or beside The Broadway between Kennersdene Farm, Tynemouth and the northern boundary of the Borough at Cullercoats.

1943

MARCH

Friday 12th/13th
- IBs of various types fell around North Shields Gasworks and Tynemouth Cemetery and across a wide area of open ground along the northern extremity of the Borough.

Monday 22nd/23rd March
- 7 HEs and 5 IBs fell on fields north of Rake House, Rake Lane, 1 HE fell on the beach at Cullercoats and a single HE fell on the rocks beside the South Pier, Cullercoats.

Wednesday 24th/25th (N1299)
- Two HEs fell on Queen Alexandra Road West, close to the junction with Hawkey's Lane. These were the final bombs dropped on the Borough during the War.

1944

JUNE

Tuesday 6th
- D-Day

Tuesday 13th
- First V1 Flying Bomb Attack on London

SEPTEMBER

Friday 8th
- First V2 rocket attack on London. More than 2,500 Londoners were killed by this weapon. In total, 9,000 V-2s were launched against England. V-1 attacks continued to target London, Southampton,

Briefing

Which plane?

Despite enquiries over the years, I have been unable to shed much light on the plane, crew and mission of the bomber which attacked North Shields that night to such horrendous effect. This is the part of the Wilkinson's story which needs further specialist research.

As to what type of plane it was, the choice is really one of two. Either it was a Heinkel He-111 or a Junkers Ju.88.

Special Inspector Joseph Stuart, one of the first at the scene, identified the aircraft as a Junkers by the sound of its engines. World War Two historian and aviation expert, Bill Norman, author of *Luftwaffe Over The North*, agreed that it was more than likely to have been a Junkers Ju. 88 based on payload and the nature of the raid.

The Heinkel was used most commonly over Britain in 1940, but because of high losses due to its relatively light armament and slow speed it was withdrawn from daylight bombing. It was used in night bombing missions over London until the end of the War.

The Junkers Ju.88, a fast twin-engined, multi-role, medium range bomber, was used throughout 1940-1945.

Developed in 1936, it joined the Heinkel He-111 and Dornier Do 17 ('The Flying Pencil') as a mainstay of Luftwaffe bomber fleets during World War Two.

The Ju.88 had a crew of 4: pilot, bombardier/nose gunner, radio operator/rear gunner and navigator/ventral gunner.

The plane with variant designs proved to have impressive versatility and was used by the Luftwaffe for massed bombing raids, dive-bombing, mine-laying, reconnaissance and as a night fighter.

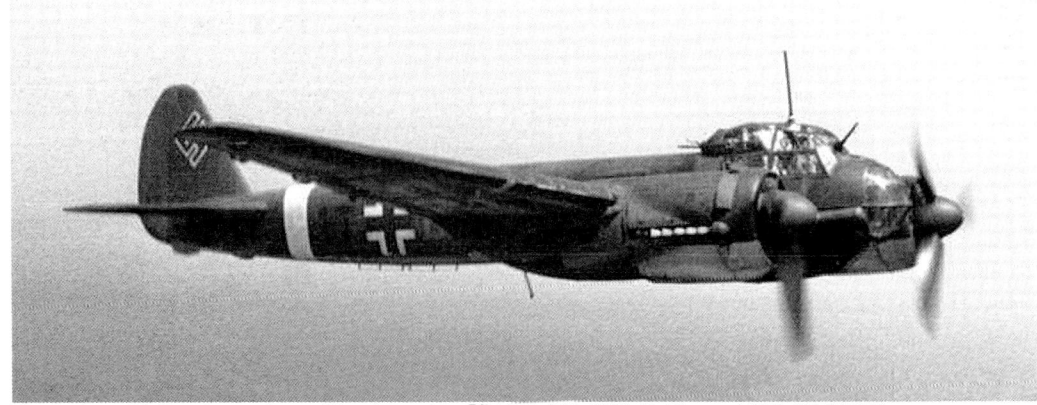

The Junkers 88. [Image courtesy of Bundesarchiv, Bild 101I-363-2258-11 / Rompel / CC-BY-SA 3.0]a

The Ju.88 could carry a bombload of two 500kg or 250kg bombs under each wing and twenty-eight 50kg bombs stored internally. It had 6 MG81 7.9mm machine guns

At had a maximum speed of 286mph at 16,000 feet and a maximum range of 1,553 miles.

Despite being extremely vulnerable to the speed and manoeuvrability of the Spitfire and Hurricane, the Ju.88 had a better attrition rate than the He-111 and Do 117.

It was the most produced Luftwaffe bomber with over 15,000 built during World War Two.

It is commonly thought that the Wilkinson's bomber was 'dumping' his bomb load before returning to base. It is more likely that the pilot thought he was over his target and released the bombs deliberately.

Navigation was very poor, so it is often impossible to even guess at the specific target that night without reference to German records of the raid. To add to the confusion we had numerous decoy sites around the area designed to mimic specific high-risk sites – these included the well-known 'Starfish' sites at Cleadon and Wallsend. The overall result was that places attacked were very rarely the intended targets.

The sequence of bombs as listed on the Tynemouth 'bomb map' suggests that the bomber was actually heading inland. The first area to be hit that night – in fact minutes before the sirens sounded in the area – was South Shields which was showered by incendiary bombs. This could well have been target marking. However, if the incendiaries were marking a target, it was an unsuccessful exercise – not a single high-explosive bomb fell on South Shields during the night.

Bill Norman in correspondence with Mr Haydon Sharp, a Wilkinson's eye-witness, comments:

> **... the Luftwaffe's main target on the night of 3/4 May 1941 was Liverpool/ Birkenhead and that the Luftwaffe Air Fleet mainly responsible for the attack was Luftflotte 2 (based in eastern France and Belgium). However, it is most unlikely that the offending German bomber was a participant in that raid.**

A more likely explanation – given that apparently only one aircraft was involved – is that the attack was carried out by a 'nuisance' raider or by an aircraft on an unsuccessful anti-shipping patrol who decided to drop his bombs on a coastal target before going home. Ju. 88's of Kustenfliegergruppen (Naval co-operation units) often patrolled the north-east coast looking for ships to attack and if none appeared they would operate over the coastal fringe looking for a 'target of opportunity'.

It is also known that there was a deliberate attack on Hull by a single Ju.88 at 0115 hrs that night which dropped one 1000kg landmine onto George Dock. At the same time, single Ju. 88s attacked Great Yarmouth.

The involvement of a plane from Kampfgeschwader 30 (KG30), a Luftwaffe bomber wing operating since 1940 out of Amsterdam-Schipol cannot be ruled out. KG30 was equipped with Junkers Ju. 88's and was initially trained as an anti-shipping and maritime attack unit.

Where did that plane fly from? What was the target? Who was aboard that bomber that night? What were their stories?

Perhaps, it's not too late to find out.

13 Wilkinson's Shelter: Sodom & Gomorrah?

In 1996, at a Reminiscence Event hosted by North Tyneside Libraries, a group of survivors were read an extract from *Children of the Blitz* by Robert Westall.

The extract is a reference to the Wilkinson's Air Raid Shelter disaster as told by a 'Tyneside Boy aged 12' (presumably Westall himself). As to be expected from a 12 year old, it is irreverent, accusing, and to me, slightly tongue in cheek. Needless to say, those present took great exception at how Wilkinson's was portrayed and especially it's comparison to Sodom and Gomorrah.

> *1941 A Nasty One*
>
> *My father came off duty looking pale and sick, and said the Germans had scored a direct hit on Wilkinson's Lemonade Factory, and hundreds had been killed, and some were still trapped down there in the cellars. He said there should never have been a shelter down there. There'd been heavy bottling machinery on the ground floor, just standing on wooden boards, and when the bomb hit, it all just collapsed on the people below.*
>
> *Terrible rumours started going round. People so crushed they couldn't be recognized; people sitting down there without a mark on them, just dead. Mothers with babies still in their arms. A man still holding his accordion…*
>
> *Everybody was just stunned; couldn't cope. Why had God let it happen?*

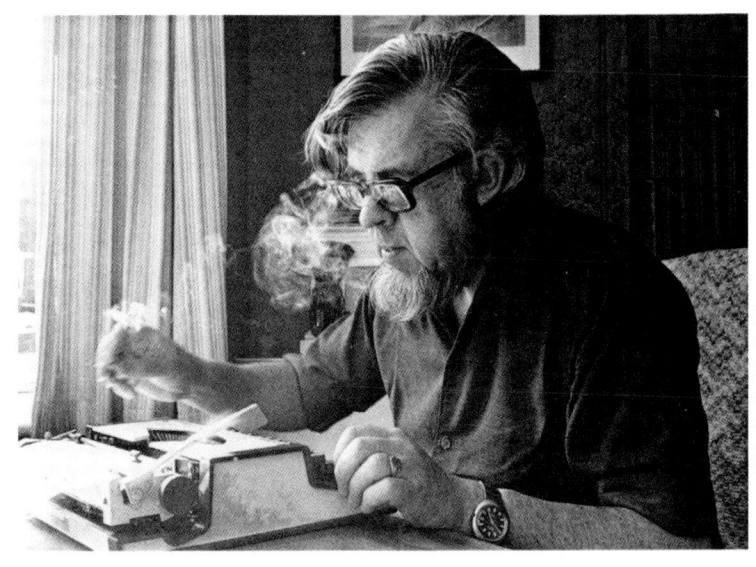

Robert Westall, award-winning North Shields author. Photo and quotation from Children of the Blitz by kind permission of the Robert Westall Estate.

Then the stories changed. Wicked things had gone on in that shelter. People had taken drink down there; held parties. Music and dancing every night. Immorality, and they didn't care who saw it...People went there even when there wasn't a raid going on. Gambling...

People said it was a Judgement. God is not mocked! It was like Sodom and Gomorrah.

Everybody felt much better after that.

Robert Westall – The Children of the Blitz (Viking 1985 p126)

Readers will recognise the authentic voice of an opinionated 12 year-old, living in the then green suburb of the Balkwell estate. We hear the disdain of a lad whose family had progressed up the ladder to a house with a garden and, of course, their own Anderson shelter. Of relatives living at Chirton West View, Westall would write in *The Making of Me*,

We were posher than my Aunt and much posher than her neighbours...they had no hope of greenhouses and central heating boilers and new radios and they lived in a terrace with backyards...Beyond the shops, all down to the river they got poorer and poorer. In the lower depths, they Drank."

Immorality and depravity in the "smoky jungle" of town, were convenient scapegoats for the inexplicable, for lives suddenly and violently snuffed out. It is the fear of a young boy that we read here.

The reality was that in the East End as elsewhere, adults had lives to lead, as best they could, despite the War and the air raids. Time spent in air raid shelters was boring, uncomfortable and unproductive. Rather than cowering underground, folk wanted to make the best of it. It was far from Sodom and Gomorrah.

Miss Grace Colman, the prospective Labour Party candidate for Tynemouth, writing in the *Shields Evening News*, 4th January 1941, criticised shelter provision in Tynemouth. "It is not enough," she said "for a shelter to protect against bombs; if people are to spend long hours in it, even all night, it must be dry, sanitary, not overcrowded, and reasonably comfortable"

Wilkinson's was, by all accounts, reasonably comfortable. It had bunk beds, benches, toilets and lighting. It may not have been too warm. However, Mrs Lee, the shelter warden, will have been attuned to what was needed to keep folk happy during the long hours of an enemy raid. It was not just about safety.

The shelter was in a tough, working-class part of town. It had opened in the summer of 1940. Locals had been divided as to its safety but there was a consensus that it was a lively place to be when the alert sounded. Millie Matthews, a shelter user, commented that it was an entertaining place with sing-alongs, card games, bingo and smoking. Robert Sutherst remembered a friendly place with sandwiches passed around. Jessie Dial's mother however, refused to go as she found the accordion player too noisy. Nora Sturrock also refused to go because of her dislike of the drinking and general atmosphere. And we're told by survivor Albert Lee, that it was a fairly quiet evening up until the bomb hit, with just a bit of singing and a hubbub of conversation.

More than anything, Wilkinson's was a community shelter. Everybody knew everybody else. Strangers were rare. The fear of the air raids was lessened people felt, by the shared experience of being together with friends, relations and neighbours in *their* shelter. 192 local residents packed the shelter that night undaunted by any bad reputation the shelter may have had.

Smoking was prohibited in public air raid shelters from late 1940. This was a tough restriction in an age when smoking was an almost universal habit. Smokers attracted further criticism by congregating at shelter entrances/exits causing obstruction. Wilkinson's informally designated smokers' area would appear to have been a pragmatic, local appeasement.

Of more interest perhaps, is the accusation of gambling in the shelter. A month after the disaster, 3 people were prosecuted for gambling in a Tynemouth public air raid shelter. Their defence was that "there was nothing else to do". Card games would similarly have just been one, common enough way of passing the time in the shelter. As Millie Cook (survivor) wryly commented, there was little or no money for gambling where they lived.

It was also an offence to be intoxicated in a public air shelter. There are accounts of people aiming for the shelter after a night in the pubs. Pubs were of course a key social resource. The number of pubs in North Shields at the time is mind boggling. In the mid-1930s, there were about 20 pubs, all within a short walking distance of Wilkinson's. By the early 1940s several had closed, including the Pine Apple Inn opposite the lemonade factory. Alcohol was more expensive during the War. Beer was about 3.5% ABV and would be described as low alcohol by today's standards (roughly 5% ABV). Spirits were generally unobtainable. Taxation, strength and availability acted as a triple whammy to influence public behaviour. It is easy to imagine individuals and perhaps small groups of people flouting this regulation at Wilkinson's. Less easy, to imagine mass drunkenness, given the shelter's attraction for families and children.

It is worth noting that there are no reports of drunkenness inside the shelter by any survivor or eye-witness. Nor have any reports been found of vandalism at Wilkinson's when such activity together with petty thefts were nationwide problems reported frequently in the press. The residents seemed to have valued their shelter. The only black mark I have discovered against Wilkinson's is contained in a Chief Constable's report on people sleeping in shelters when there was no raid on. Somebody was found to be doing so on one occasion. Again, hardly Sodom and Gomorrah.

This furore aside, Robert Westall is a superb writer. He grew up in North Shields during the War and his father was an ARP warden down in the docks. He was on duty at the time of the Wilkinson's bombing.

Although written for children, adults will enjoy his books, certainly those set in the fictional 'Garmouth', which is an amalgam of North Shields and Tynemouth.

He is best remembered for *The Machine Gunners* – a classic tale of children in wartime. The discovery and removal of a machine gun from a crashed enemy bomber gives the subversive Chas McGill and his gang, the chance to do their bit, clashing against adults and "authority" having befriended and protected, a downed German airman. Both the book and the later BBC TV series are fondly remembered by many.

The Kingdom by the Sea is a beautiful evocation of Tynemouth and the Northumberland coast, again set in a wartime of air raids and family loss. Essential reading though, is *The Making of Me*, a collection of autobiographical fragments, edited by Lindy McKinnel, which has fascinating descriptions of North Shields in the 1930s and 1940s.

In the news again

After the War, King Street hit the news again as the location of a particularly savage, jealousy murder.

In January 1950, Mary Victoria Longhurst, aged 23, and her young daughter Patricia moved into a bedsit at 26 King Street. Number 26 was next door to the CIU Club, previously the home of W. A. Wilkinson and now the site of the King Street Club.

Mary's boyfriend, George Finlay Brown, moved in, however the relationship did not go well and she asked him to leave after only a few weeks.

Mary quickly found a new boyfriend. Despite this, Brown began to pester her, demanding they get back together. Mary became so alarmed by his approaches that she complained to the police on Friday March 10th.

Later that evening, Brown let himself into Mary's flat and waited for her to return from visiting a friend. Mary's ground floor neighbour, Benjamin Hedley, heard an increasingly violent argument between the two, culminating in furniture being thrown and hysterical crying.

Hedley was so concerned he went to the Police Station. He returned to King Street just after midnight with Constable John Atkinson. Atkinson rang for assistance to get into the room. Within minutes Detective Constable Thomas Baikie arrived by car and forced entry into the room. He found Patricia hiding under the bedding. Her mother, Mary, had been assaulted and strangled and was lying dead on the bed.

By 01.00 the police had found Brown asleep at his mother's house and had taken him into custody. He was charged with Mary's murder. Brown denied any involvement.

After a two day trial in Newcastle opening on 30th May before Mr Justice Morris, the jury returned after only 30 minutes. Brown was found guilty of murder and was sentenced to death. His appeal in June was dismissed. Brown was executed by hanging at Durham Jail on 11th Tuesday July 1950. He was only 23. His executioner was Albert Pierrepoint.

A full account of this murder is given in *Murderous Tyneside* by John J. Eddleston.

It's impossible to think of another location in North Shields which has had a similar sad impact.

14 Afterword

I have no personal connection with Wilkinson's.

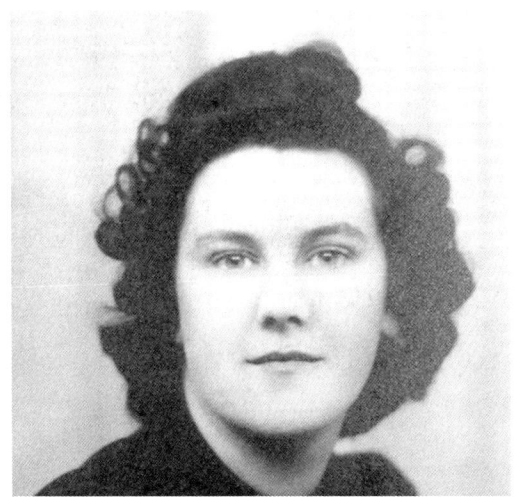

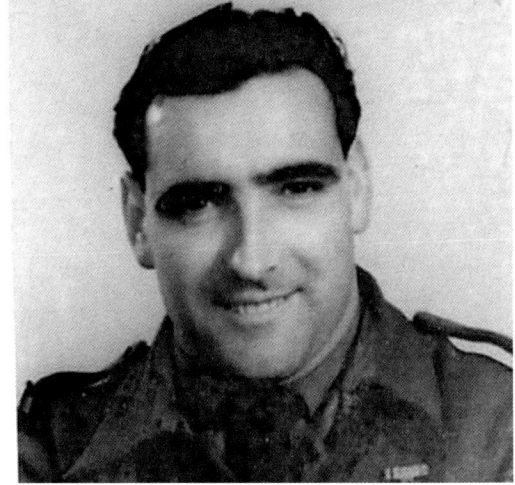

Monica.

Bobby.

Except that...when I was a bairn in the late 60s, aged about 7 or 8, my mam would occasionally say "Bobby, take our Peter out for a walk", which was code for, I want some peace and quiet for a few hours. Unfortunately for me, my Dad, ex-8th Army, liked a good route march. So, we'd end up on the Fish Quay, having walked from Billy Mill down to the River Tyne, along by the old wood yards and on towards the mouth of the River. Points of interest were explained. I think he was careful not to "explain" the various pubs we must have passed. Anyway, we'd go up the bank at the Low Lights, turn left at the top and walk along to King Street. We'd stop there and he'd say that a terrible thing had happened there during the War. And he'd talk about the poor people in the shelter, not having a chance. I don't think I took much in. I was too knackered after the walk! Turning right at Tynemouth Road meant it was the full march to Tobruk. Turning left, meant the No 11 bus home. "Monica…we're back", he'd say with some satisfaction. Job done.

Any factual errors in the text are entirely my own. Apologies.

Feel free to email me with questions, comments and corrections at

    info@northshields173.org

New stories about Wilkinson's emerge regularly. Photos are found in old albums. Bottles are dug up. Old wooden crates are discovered in garden sheds. Sadly, we are losing the people who were there. We need their stories before it is too late.

We need, too, to value Wilkinson's as an important part of our town's history. It tells us much about our community during the War – of fortitude and courage in the face of devastating loss.

It is an amazing story.

Thanks for reading the book.

That time-bending telephone call to North Shields 173 which I mentioned right at the start?

I know what I'd say now. I think I'd order a crate of Smila to be delivered by Billy and Ginger the Horse. Bet it tasted lush!

15 Thanks to...

I have been researching Wilkinson's since 1999. Back then, the idea was to create a project on the disaster for use in local schools. The idea was Peter Hepplewhite's and the original research, his. I was asked to develop the project website. I did…and I forgot to stop. So, twenty years later, **northshields173.org** is still there, recording and exploring the disaster, updated on a regular basis and acting as the information bank on the bombing. I view it very much as a "community website".

I've met and chatted with hundreds of people about Wilkinson's. They have kindly shared their stories and family photos. My thanks in particular to the survivors of the tragedy. There are still a handful with us. Their stories are particularly poignant. As are those of the townsfolk we lost. Their families have been very supportive in sharing their memories. For many of those involved, this happened yesterday not decades ago during the War. The emotion and sadness is tangible. Thank you all for talking with me. The best way to learn about history is to speak with those who lived through it.

Mick Sharp of Black Dog Design in Whitley Bay has steered the book production. The indefatigable Joyce Marti at North Shields Library has hunted snippets of information. Terry Wilkinson, great grandson of William Arthur opened the doors to the family side of things. And, Peter Hepplewhite, who started it all, asked the questions a proper historian would.

My thanks to:

Andy Wilkinson
Philip and Carol Tallent
Bill Atkinson
Dr Jim Rickard
Michael Coates
Mabel Moffitt
Colin Sarin
Brian Burdis
Patricia Lydon
George Darling Black
John Boothroyd
Judith and Peter More
Steve Hislop
Ken Robson
Alan Bainbridge
Stephen Harman
Heather Dunkley
Brian Chandler
Danny Lawrence
Chris Ord
Julie Simpson

I have, where possible, attributed copyright/ownership to photographs. If I have mistakenly credited the incorrect owner of any photograph, please contact me for rectification in the next edition of the book.

Cycle Rides South-West
Dartmoor

Robert Hesketh

Bossiney Books • Launceston

First published 2008 by
Bossiney Books Ltd, Langore, Launceston, Cornwall PL15 8LD
www.bossineybooks.com
© 2008 Robert Hesketh   All rights reserved
ISBN 978-1-906474-05-8

Acknowledgements
The cover design is by Heards Design Partnership
The maps are by Graham Hallowell
Printed in Great Britain by St Austell Printing Company Ltd

Introduction

Dartmoor offers a wonderful variety of cycle routes, set amidst the highest and wildest scenery in southern England. The moor's stark beauty and character – each rocky tor has its own peculiar profile – is complemented by attractive villages and small towns of granite and thatch. Many are included in this book, along with a range of historic buildings, from moorland inns and churches to castles, abbeys, prehistoric and industrial heritage sites.

I have assumed a reasonable level of rider competence, so the routes range from 11.5km (7 1/4 miles) to 38.5km (24 1/4 miles). They are arranged in approximate order of difficulty (rather than length), with the easiest first. If you're out of practice, it's best to work your way through the book and build your stamina. Many of the rides can be linked to make much longer routes.

All are designed to avoid noisome traffic by using Dartmoor's network of quiet lanes. Hardly made for speed, these winding lanes are ideal for exploration by bike. Some are lined with flower-rich hedgebanks, some with dry stone walls, whilst others stride over hills and down deep wooded combes. But do remember that while the narrowness makes them attractive, you may meet the odd car, tractor or van travelling without cyclists in mind. You may need to do their drivers' thinking for them.

Dartmoor also benefits from two extended near-level cycle tracks on former railway lines: Plym Valley (Ride 1) and the Granite Way (Ride 9). Four more routes in this book have traffic-free sections, all comfortably ridable on standard bikes. Please watch for pedestrians and remember they enjoy priority.

Whilst the routes give a full flavour of Dartmoor and a cross section of its scenery, along with visits to some of its most interesting places, they are also selected to avoid extremely long, harsh ascents. However, cycling Dartmoor inevitably demands uphill climbs – and some swift descents. Low gears are a terrific bonus and good brakes essential.

Apart from hills, you can expect some mud, loose gravel and surfaces less than perfect – this is not Hyde Park. It must also be admitted Dartmoor ponies and especially sheep have no road sense at all and are never likely to, whilst winding lanes hold bends that will remain forever blind. Keep alert and be prepared to dismount.

Dartmoor cycling requires nothing exceptional in the way of equipment, though safety counsels a helmet and reflective clothing. Changeable weather makes waterproofs a must. Leg covering is also advisable for the odd occasion when you may need to get off into the nettles to allow other vehicles to pass. The sketches in this book are a general guide; maps are essential – Ordnance Survey Landrangers are ideal as they give sufficient detail without being unwieldy. Numbers 191, 201 and 202 cover all the rides.

Please take plenty of drinking water – you can dehydrate fast on a bike – and a snack. Although Dartmoor has several cycle hire and repair shops, it's wise to carry a basic tool kit and spare inner tubes.

1 Plym Valley Cycle Way

The Plym Valley Cycle Track is a great route for novice cyclists and children. It can readily be shortened – Coypool and Plym Bridge car parks offer alternative starting points. Traffic-free except for one road crossing controlled by lights, it leads into well-wooded countryside with views onto Dartmoor. A special bonus is the chance to see nesting peregrine falcons through powerful telescopes provided by the National Trust at Cann Viaduct.

Chelson Meadow is signed from the eastern end of Laira Bridge, off the A379 Kingsbridge road. With your back to the river, turn left out of the car park, ALL ROUTES. Follow the road parallel to the river to join the PLYM VALLEY CYCLE WAY (ROUTE 27). Keep left 1 km ahead. Cycle ahead at the next path junction, PLYM VALLEY 27. Follow the path under the A38 flyover to the B3416. To avoid the heavy traffic on this road, do *not* turn right. Turn left CITY CENTRE and cross safely at the traffic lights immediately ahead. Pedal ahead LEIGHAM. Turn first right PLYM VALLEY CYCLE PATH. Turn left past Coypool car park. Continue ahead PLYM VALLEY CYCLE WAY 27.

Reaching a lane, divert left under the old railway bridge to see Plym Bridge. Return to the cycle track and continue for nearly 5 km to Shaugh Bridge Tunnel. Turn your lights on in the tunnel.

The final 2 km from Goodameavy to Clearbrook may be omitted. If done, it is best to leave the cycle track and take the lane left at Goodameavy. The short, steep climb is rewarded with terrific views of Dartmoor. Turn first right for refreshments at the Skylark. If you choose to use the cycle track to Clearbrook, follow the signs and be prepared for some very rough surfaces and a steep push.

The return route can be completed in half the time taken for the outward journey, because it is almost entirely downhill!

Start/finish: Chelson Meadow car park near Laira Bridge, Plymouth, SX 506545. Or Coypool car park (closed from 7 pm and on Sundays – check in advance for spaces on 01752 348179) or Plym Bridge car park

Distance: 26.5 km (16.5 miles). From Coypool 21.5 km, or Plym Bridge 17.5 km

Terrain: Easy. Mainly dedicated cycle path with slight gradient

Refreshments: Skylark Inn, Clearbrook. Saltram House (in season)

Public toilets: None   **Map:** Landranger 201

Peregrine Watch: Warden 01752 341377. www.plymperegrines.co.uk

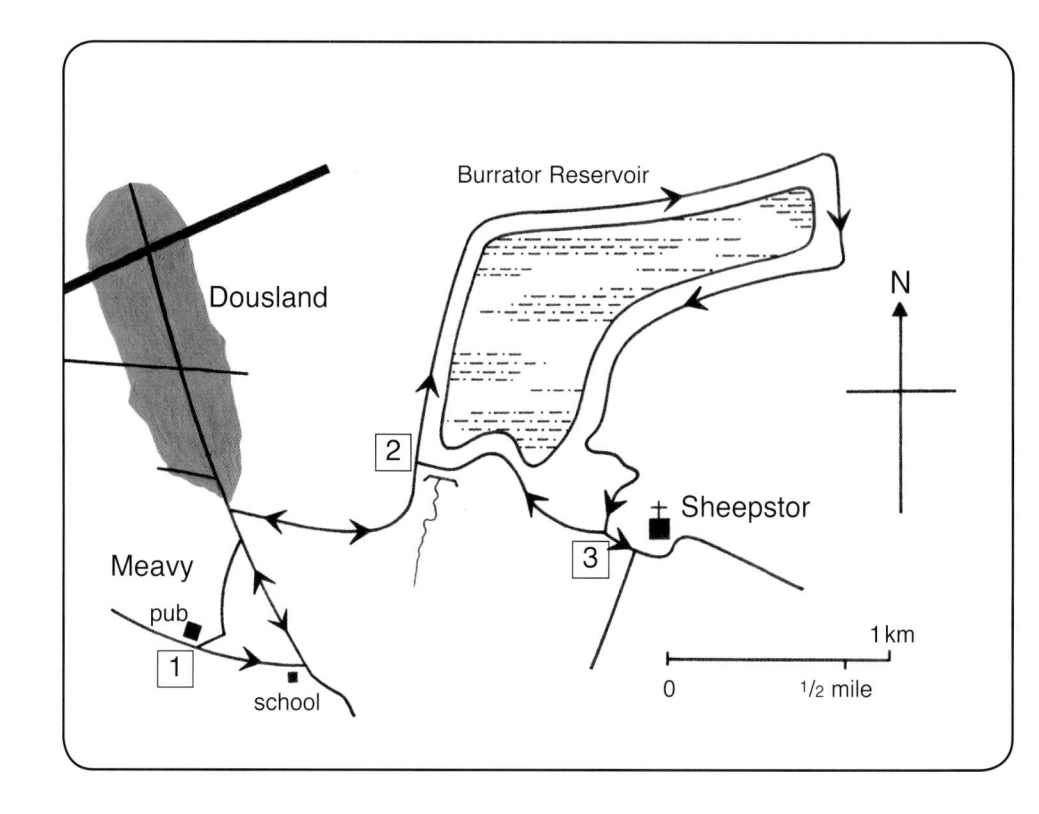

2 Meavy and Burrator

Burrator reservoir is the main feature of this route. Built in 1898, it melds beautifully into the Dartmoor scenery of rocky tors and huge skies. At only 7.5km, the quiet, easy circuit is the perfect short ride, a great introduction before the more demanding moorland circuits later in the book.

You can either park and start your ride from Burrator dam or, by adding another 4km and a steep uphill beginning to the ride, start at Meavy, one of Dartmoor's most interesting and attractive villages. Meavy's church, cross and inn are grouped around the village green, shaded by an ancient and massive oak tree. The Meavy Oak may not be the one mentioned in the 1086 Domesday Book – though this is debated – but all agree it is ancient.

Not surprisingly, the village pub is the Royal Oak. Like many Devon inns, it began as a church house. Built of stone and cob, the Royal Oak was used by monks travelling between Buckfast and Tavistock abbeys.

Inside are a cavernous log fire and a range of period and modern photographs showing village life. A sketch of 1810 portrays the inn as it was and a framed document of 1588/9 mentions it.

St Peter's, Meavy, was consecrated in 1122 but is largely 15th century. It has wagon roofs with carved and painted bosses. Built of granite, it is typical of Dartmoor churches.

Sheepstor's church is equally characteristic. It has a fine rood screen and carved bench ends – and a surprising connection with Sarawak in the East Indies. The tombs and memorials of the Brooke family cover a remarkable chapter in British imperial history, recorded in some detail inside the church. Sir James Brooke, who bought the Burrator Estate in 1858, was the first 'White Rajah of Sarawak', founding a dynasty that lasted until after the Second World War.

(1) Park carefully by Meavy village green. Start with the Royal Oak on your left and the village hall on your right and cycle ahead past the school. Turn left, DOUSLAND and follow the lane steeply uphill. Turn first right, SHEEPSTOR BURRATOR RESERVOIR.

Pedal ahead from the western end of Burrator (2), ARBORETUM CAR PARK – or park and start the route from here. Continue ahead at the next sign, NORSWORTHY BRIDGE and simply follow the lane around the reservoir.

Having circuited most of the reservoir, you will reach a T-junction (3). Turn left (no sign) and pedal on to Sheepstor church. Return to the junction and continue ahead, following the lane uphill and then across the dam. Turn left and return to Meavy.

Start/finish: Meavy village green (SX541672) or Burrator Dam (SX551680)

Distance: 11.5km (7 miles) including Meavy or 7.5km (4¾ miles) from Burrator Dam

Terrain: Steep climb from Meavy to Burrator, then near level around reservoir. All quiet lanes

Refreshments: Royal Oak, Meavy

Public toilets: Burrator Dam

Maps: Landrangers 201 and 202 (both needed) or Outdoor Leisure 28

Link: Can be added to all or part of Ride 1, the Plym Valley Cycle Way, by cycling the 3km between Meavy and Clearbrook

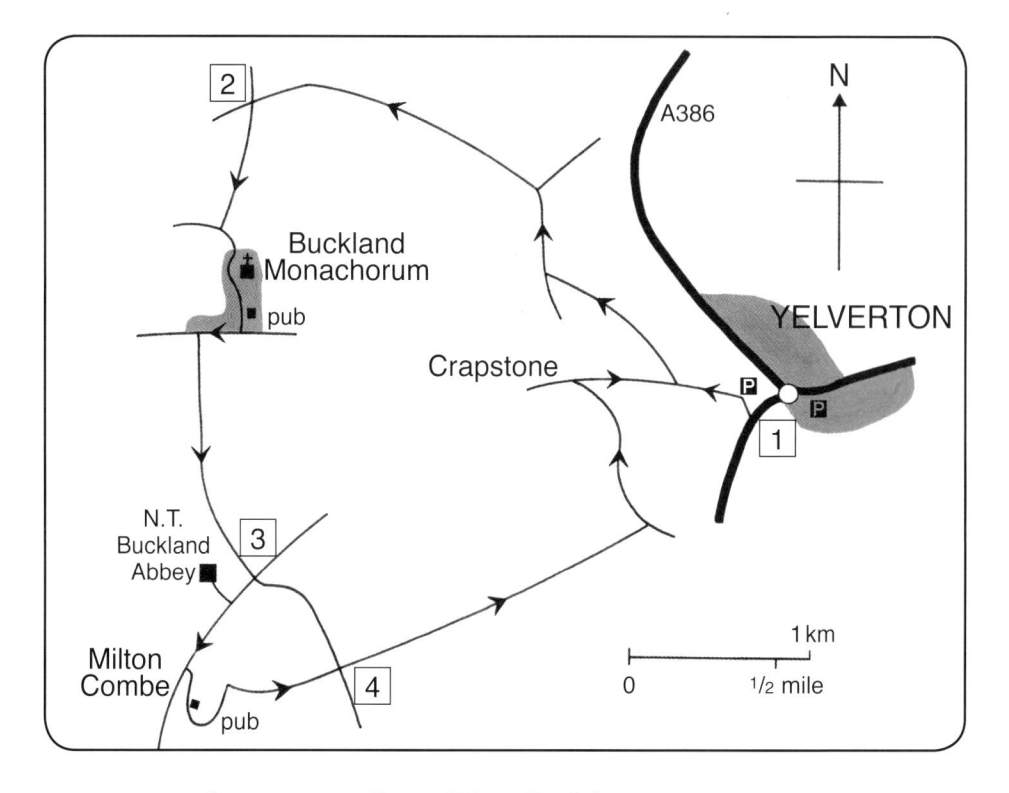

3 Yelverton and Buckland Abbey

The area immediately to the west of Yelverton was requisitioned in 1941 as the Harrowbeer airfield. It had been assumed in 1939 that Plymouth was out of range for the Luftwaffe – but the invasion of France changed that, so Harrowbeer's runways were constructed from the rubble of the Plymouth blitz. The strange layout of roads and the numerous car parks in the area are relics of the airfield, as are Yelverton's many single-storey buildings – their upper storeys were removed as a hazard to flying.

Buckland Abbey began as a Cistercian monastery and later became the home successively of two of Elizabethan England's most famous seamen, Sir Richard Grenville of *The Revenge* and Sir Francis Drake himself, explorer, naval general and, some would say, pirate. Open through the National Trust, it has an Elizabethan garden, craft workshops and a huge 14th century barn.

St Andrews, Buckland Monachorum, has an elegant tower and a beautiful nave roof, where sixteen carved angels each play a different instrument. Drake's most famous ship, the *Golden Hind*, is carved on a pew and the Drake coat-of-arms hangs in the Drake chapel.

The 16th century Drake Manor Inn at Buckland Monachorum has a beamed ceiling, a large fireplace with a bread oven and a collection of period photographs.

(1) Yelverton has several car parks and a rather confusing plan, so for simplicity the ride starts from the roundabout. Take the Plymouth road, A386 and after 100m turn right LEG O'MUTTON/ CRAPSTONE, then follow CRAPSTONE (ROUTE 27) over the cattle grid. Take the first right (ROUTE 27). At a crossroads turn right LONG ASH/HORRABRIDGE. Turn left LONG ASH (ROUTE 27).

At a staggered crossroads (2) turn left for BUCKLAND MONACHORUM. At a T-junction, turn left CRAPSTONE, then follow the CRAPSTONE sign into the centre of Buckland, past the church and the Drake Manor Inn, and up to a T-junction. Turn right, MILTON COMBE, then first left, MILTON COMBE/BUCKLAND ABBEY.

At Abbey Cross (3) you have choices. For a start, the entrance to Buckland Abbey is just 100m away on the right.

The short-cut from Abbey Cross (3) to Blowiscombe Cross (4) has a fairly steep descent and ascent, but these are as nothing compared to the very steep descent into the attractive hamlet of Milton Combe, with its pub, the Who'd Have Thought It Inn, and the seriously steep ascent back out.

For Milton Combe, turn right at Abbey Cross and take the first left, MILTON COMBE. Follow the lane steeply downhill, then turn sharp left at the pub and follow the lane up to Blowiscombe Cross (4). Pedal ahead, HORRABRIDGE/TAVISTOCK. Ignore side turnings.

At a T-junction turn left, CRAPSTONE. The road swings right, then takes a long curve to the left. Where it begins to straighten, turn sharp right, on an unsigned road which leads back to Yelverton.

Start/finish: Any of the Yelverton car parks
Distance: 13km (8 miles)
Terrain: Quiet country lanes. Some steep gradients, the toughest of them avoidable by using a short cut
Refreshments: Pubs in Yelverton, Buckland Monachorum and Milton Combe. Shops in Yelverton
Public toilets: Yelverton
Maps: Landranger 201 or Explorer 108
Buckland Abbey (National Trust): Seasonal opening, closed Thursdays (01822) 853607

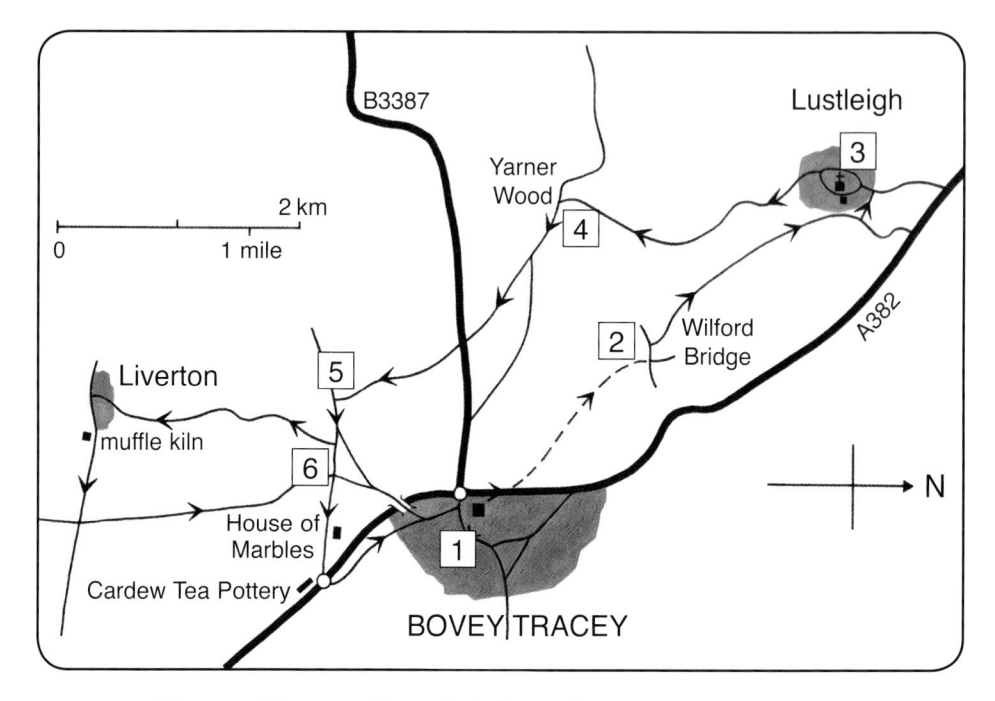

4 Bovey Tracey, Lustleigh and Liverton

This attractive ride amid the Dartmoor foothills offers wonderful scenery and a great deal of interest. Winding through woodland and small farms by quiet lanes and a section of railway trackbed, it is delightful throughout the year, not least in spring when the sheltered Bovey Valley is rich in wild flowers.

Lustleigh is an especially attractive cob, granite and thatch village, centred on its handsome medieval church and the 15th century Cleave Hotel. The splendid fireplace with its oak beam and bread oven was discovered in the 1950s. In the hall is a collection of period photographs, including Lustleigh Station and Lustleigh May Day.

The optional 5.4km (3 mile) loop from Brimley includes some characteristically Devonian cob and thatch cottages and a preserved muffle kiln at Liverton. This and the three muffle kilns at the House of Marbles, Bovey Tracey, are the only four extant kilns of their type in England.

(1) Turn left out of Bovey's lower car park. Follow Station Road to the roundabout. Take the third exit, LUSTLEIGH AND MORETONHAMPSTEAD.

Just before Hole Bridge, turn left through a wooden gate onto the permissive path. Follow this over the river by the old railway bridge. Continue for 2 km – watch out for pedestrians and tree roots.

Just before Wilford Bridge (the end of the path), bear right to join the lane at a wooden gate (2). Turn left, LUSTLEIGH, and only 50 m ahead, turn right before crossing the river.

Pedal ahead at the next junction, LUSTLEIGH. At a second junction, turn left towards the village, crossing the old railway line via a bridge next to the former station house.

At Lustleigh church (3) turn left, RUDGE. Only 100 m ahead, cross a small bridge and bear left. Pedal on past houses and a cemetery. Turn left at the next junction and pedal downhill to a T-junction. Turn right and cross the Bovey via a bridge with a 1684 datestone recording a repair. Pedal on. After 500 m the lane climbs steeply.

Turn left at Reddaford Water (4). Take the first turn right, HAYTOR with a street sign LOWER DOWN. At the Edgemoor Hotel cycle ahead along Chapple Road for BRIMLEY. The tramway is on your right at the foot of the hill. Turn left towards Bovey Tracey at the end of Chapple Road (5). Take the second turning right.

Decision time. Either pedal on to Thorns Cross (6) or add the Liverton loop to your ride, taking the first turning right at Brimley Cross onto a lane marked UNSUITABLE FOR LONG VEHICLES. Pedal on to Liverton, past cob and thatch cottages. Turn left, NEWTON ABBOT – the kiln is in Pottery Yard. Continue through the village to Cummings Cross. Turn left onto the blue cycle route for BOVEY TRACEY. Pedal on to Thorns Cross.

At Thorns Cross pedal ahead, NEWTON ABBOT if you took the short cut or turn right, NEWTON ABBOT if you took the Liverton loop. Continue past the House of Marbles. Take the second exit from the roundabout, signed CHURCHES AND SWIMMING POOL. Pedal back to Station Road. Turn right for the car park.

Start/finish: Lower car park, Bovey Tracey, SX 815784

Distance: 17.5 km (11 miles) or 12.5 km (7¾ miles) with short cut

Terrain: Fairly easy. Undulating, occasionally steep. Mainly quiet lanes. Section of gravelled railway bed

Refreshments: Pubs, cafés, restaurants and shops in Bovey Tracey; pub and tea room, Lustleigh

Public toilets: Bovey Tracey and Lustleigh

Maps: Landranger 191 or Explorer 110

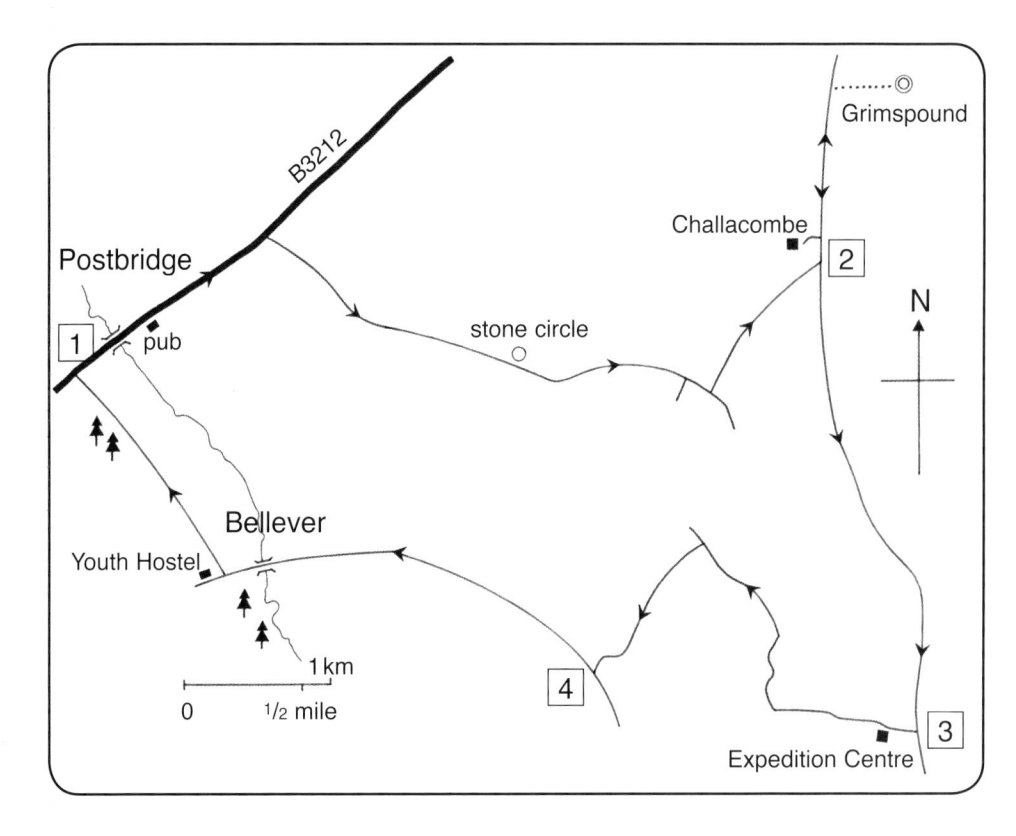

5 Postbridge

As well as splendid scenery, this classic circuit has a great deal of historic interest, including two clapper bridges and a stone circle with over twenty standing stones and a cist (stone coffin) in the centre. The diversion up Challacombe reveals a medieval field system and a Bronze Age pound containing the foundations of round-houses.

The route crosses the East Dart by the well-built 1790 stone bridge at Postbridge. This was constructed at the same time as the Moretonhampstead to Tavistock turnpike, part of the post road linking Exeter and Falmouth. (The tollhouse and turnpike stood near where the petrol pumps are today.) Beside it is the best preserved of Dartmoor's several medieval clapper bridges, a simple construction of two flat stone slabs resting on three piers. Before this was built the river was most probably forded at this point. There is a second clapper bridge later in the route at Bellever, though with one span missing.

The 1.5 km climb up Challacombe (also included in Ride 7) can be omitted, but it is well worth the effort. A deep and beautiful valley, Challacombe is flanked by two high ridges, Hamel Down and Challacombe Down. Clearly defined on Challacombe Down is a medieval field system. The characteristic terracing was created by erosion combined with ploughing.

These fields and the scars of later tin mining at Headland Warren are best seen by taking the short walk to Grimspound. One of the most impressive Bronze Age sites on Dartmoor, Grimspound contains 24 hut circles, some of them reconstructed by the Dartmoor Exploration Committee, which undertook a number of similar restorations in the late 19th century. The perimeter wall was probably built to impound domestic animals and protect them from wolves, rather than as a fortification.

(1) Turn left out of Postbridge car park. Cycle over the bridge and past the East Dart Hotel. Turn right, WIDECOMBE. Stop to view the stone circle on the left of the road at Soussons Down, just at the edge of the wood. Pedal downhill and take the next turning left.

Turn left again at the T-junction (2) to include the Challacombe diversion. Pedal 1.5km uphill and lock your bike by the parking area to visit Grimspound. Retrace your route to the T-junction and pedal on.

Take the second turning right (3), BROADAFORD CATOR. Cycle past the Dartmoor Expedition Centre. Follow the road when it curves 90° right. Cross the West Webburn and cycle on through a beech avenue. Follow the road sharp left (do not take the No Through Road). Continue uphill through the beech avenue to Cator Green (4).

Turn right BELLEVER. Cycle past Cator Court, over the Walla Brook and steeply downhill to Bellever Bridge. Pedal uphill and follow the road round right. The road continues uphill and down to Postbridge Cross. Turn right and almost immediately left to the car park.

Start/finish: Postbridge car park and Information Centre, SX 647789
Distance: 21km (13 miles) or 18km (11 miles) excluding Grimspound
Terrain: Moderate. One long, steady ascent to Grimspound. Quiet lanes, short section of B road
Refreshments: East Dart Hotel
Public toilets: Postbridge
Maps: Landranger 191 or Outdoor Leisure 28
Link: Can be linked with Ride 7, Widecombe, at points 2 and 3

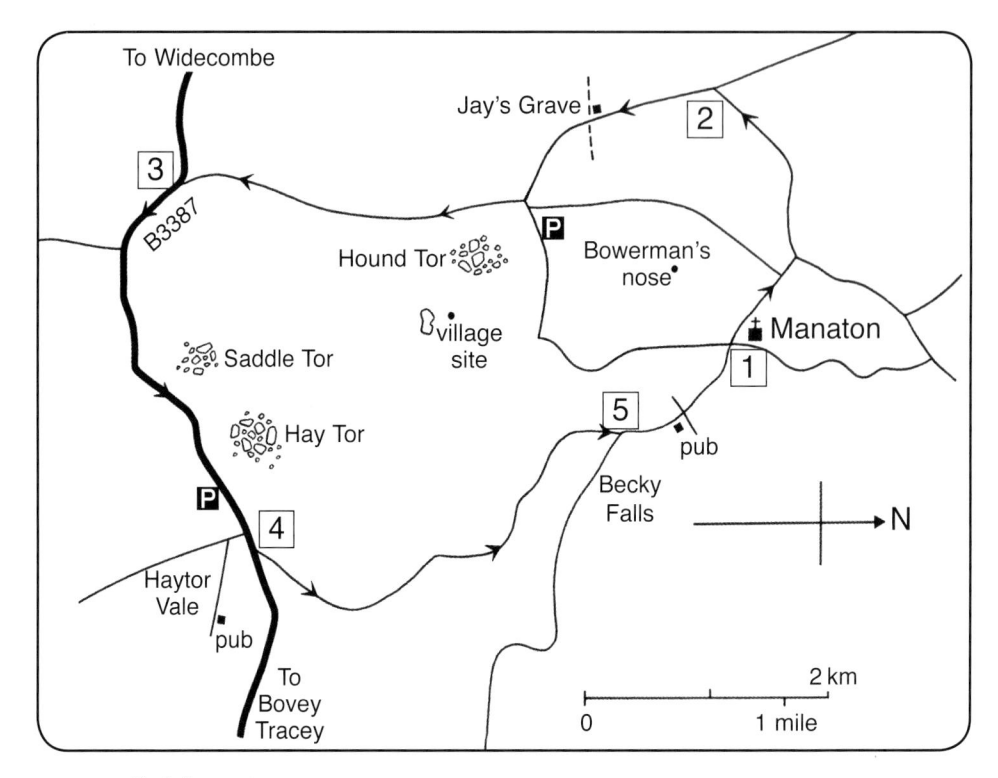

6 Manaton

This beautiful route encompasses some of eastern Dartmoor's most dramatic scenery, including Haytor Rocks, Hound Tor, Saddle Tor and Rippon Tor, in only 17 km. There are also superb distant views of many more tors and on to Haldon and the sea.

Manaton church is noted for its carved screen (circa 1500) and wagon roof. Bowerman's Nose, a distinctive granite pillar on Hayne Down, overlooks the first stage of the route. Legend has it that huntsman John Bowerman – who was buried at North Bovey in 1663 – was turned to stone for hunting on Sundays, whilst his pack of hounds were petrified as Hound Tor.

Jay's Grave, which you pass on the way to Hound Tor, bears a sad tale. According to Dartmoor writer Beatrice Chase, Mary Jay was born around 1790. Orphaned, she was brought up in Newton Abbot Workhouse and apprenticed to a local farmer at Ford Farm, Manaton. She was buried at this lonely spot because she committed suicide, probably after being jilted and left carrying the baby. Suicides were not permitted burial in churchyards before 1823 and were therefore interred in unconsecrated ground, such as this lonely wayside.

Hound Tor's impressive medieval hamlet is on the far side of the tor itself. A kilometre walk from the car park, it retains the foundations of longhouses, a farmstead and ancillary buildings and was abandoned around the time of the Black Death (1348-9).

After swooping down to Haytor Vale, the return begins with fresh views eastwards. At the beginning of a climb, the lane crosses Haytor's Granite Tramway. Built in 1820, it was Devon's first railway and served five quarries. With hand-cut granite rails and horse-drawn wagons, it took stone 12km to the canal at Teigngrace. Another steep descent brings you back to Manaton and the Kestor Inn.

(1) Turn right out of the car park HOUNDTOR WIDECOMBE MORETON-HAMPSTEAD. Bowerman's Nose stands on the skyline to your left. Ignore the turning for North Bovey. Pedal on to Heatree Cross (2).

Turn left HOUNDTOR HAYTOR WIDECOMBE and cycle uphill to Jay's Grave, which lies immediately on the right of the lane by a gate. Continue to Hound Tor. Do not turn left. Keep ahead, with Hound Tor on your left, to Harefoot Cross (3).

Turn left onto the B3387 HAYTOR BOVEY TRACEY. Ignore the right turn at Hemsworthy Gate. Cycle on with Saddle Tor and Haytor Rocks on your left. It's an exciting descent from Haytor Rocks, but watch out for ponies and pedestrians.

Turn left 100m beyond the red phone booth beside the Haytor Vale turning onto an unsigned lane (4). This crosses the tramway beside a granite pillar. Pedal on under the flank of Black Hill and make a steep descent to Leighon Cross (5).

A short diversion right leads to Becky Falls (seasonal opening, entrance fee). These waterfalls are best seen after heavy rain. Otherwise, turn left and return to the start via the Kestor Inn.

Start/finish: Manaton church car park, SX750813. Alternatively there are car parks at Hound Tor and at Haytor Rocks

Distance: 17km (10½ miles)

Terrain: Moderately demanding. Some steep gradients, the rest undulating. Country lanes and B road

Refreshments: Kestor Inn, Manaton; Rock Inn, Haytor Vale; snack/ice-cream vans at Hound Tor and Haytor car parks

Public toilets: Haytor car park

Maps: Landranger 191 or Outdoor Leisure 28

Link: Can be linked with Ride 7, Widecombe

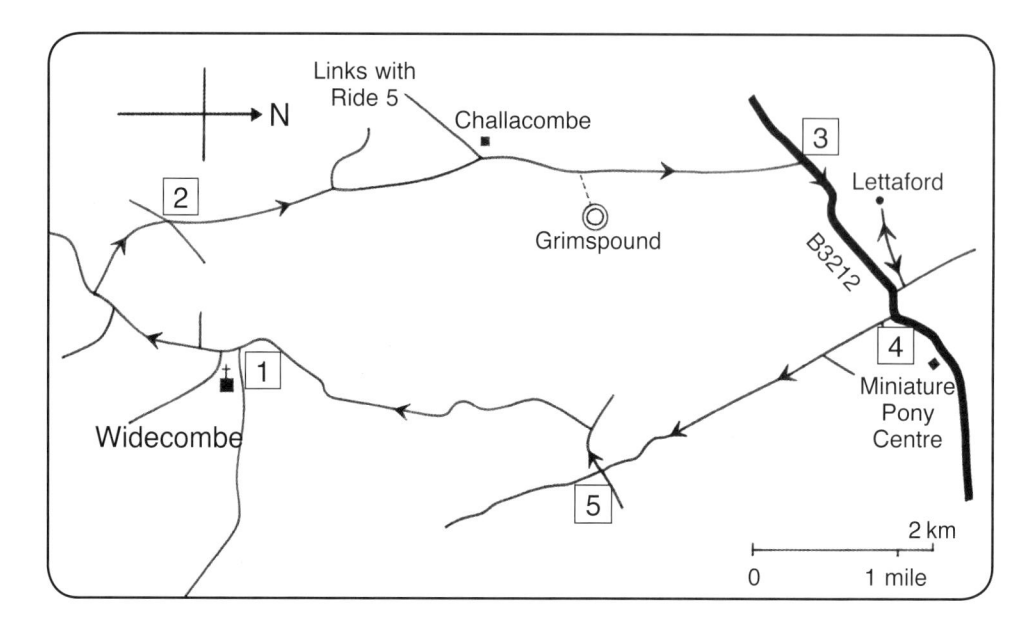

7 Widecombe

This characteristic Dartmoor route combines sweeping moorland views with several points of interest. It begins by the graceful granite ashlar tower of Widecombe Church. At 43.5m, it is a landmark for miles around and was originally financed by tinners in the 15th and 16th centuries. Look for their mark, the 'tinners' rabbits' (three hares joined by the ears) among the ceiling bosses inside.

The 16th century Church House, now a National Trust property, is noted for its granite piers and is the finest example of Devon's fifty or so extant church houses – the forerunners of village halls and the venues for 'church ales' in pre-Puritan England. The Sexton's Cottage next door is a shop and information centre with a good selection of Dartmoor books.

A short diversion takes in Hutholes, the excavated remains of a cluster of medieval farm buildings, including early longhouses. In a longhouse, the farmer and his family lived at the upper end of the building, separated from the animals at the lower end by a cross passage. This simple and very practical design, which is also found in other upland areas of Britain, is plainly shown by the Lettaford longhouses visited later in the route.

The ride continues up Challacombe, a deep and beautiful valley flanked by two high ridges, Hamel Down and Challacombe Down. Clearly defined on Challacombe Down are the terraces of a medieval field system and the scars of later tin mining at Headland Warren.

A short walk leads to Bronze Age Grimspound, which contains 24 hut circles. See page 11.

Lettaford was a typical medieval Dartmoor hamlet, which began as three longhouses.

(1) Turn right out of Widecombe car park and follow the road round left past the Old Inn, BUCKLAND DARTMEET POSTBRIDGE. Continue past Dunstone. Turn right at Easter Lane Cross, POSTBRIDGE PRINCETOWN MORETONHAMPSTEAD. Keep right when the lane forks.

At the next crossroads (2), take a short diversion to the left for 200m. A path through a wicket gate on the right leads to the Hutholes medieval longhouse settlement.

Pedal ahead at Blackaton Cross, MORETONHAMPSTEAD. The lane climbs steadily. (To visit Grimspound, lock your bike by the parking area at Firth Bridge and take the footpath right for 250m.) Cycle ahead to the main road across the moor, B3212 (3).

Turn right at Challacombe Cross, MORETONHAMPSTEAD B3212. Take the first turning left, LETTAFORD. Turn first left again, LETTAFORD. After visiting this fascinating hamlet, retrace your route to the B3212. Turn left. Take the first turn right (4).

Watching Place Cross has a worn granite cross, but is said to have gained its name from the gruesome practice of leaving gibbeted corpses on a crossroad gallows as a warning. Cycle ahead at the next crossroad MANATON.

Turn right at Heatree Cross (5) HEATHERCOMBE NATSWORTHY. The lane climbs steeply to a fork. Here stands a granite post inscribed with three fishes and 'Thine is the Power'. Keep left, NATSWORTHY WIDECOMBE. The lane provides an exciting downhill finish straight to Widecombe Green. Turn left there for the car park.

Start/finish: Widecombe car park, SX719769

Distance: 22km (13½ miles)

Terrain: Moderately demanding gradients. Mainly quiet lanes. Short B road section

Refreshments: Two pubs and tea rooms, Widecombe

Public toilets: Widecombe

Maps: Landranger 191 or Outdoor Leisure 28

Link: Can be linked with Ride 5, Postbridge, or with Ride 6, Manaton

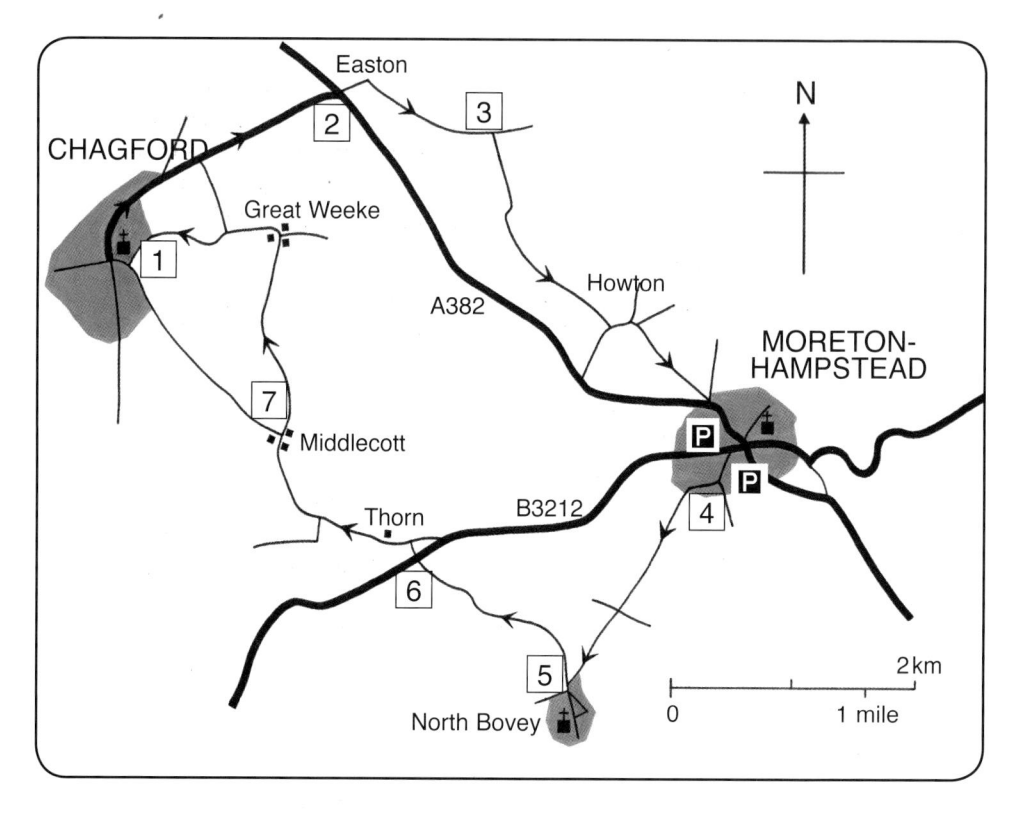

8 Chagford

As well as excellent views of Dartmoor, this circuit offers a great deal of interest. Chagford, Moretonhampstead and North Bovey each have a handsome selection of vernacular buildings, many of them granite and thatch.

Chagford's parish church is solid granite ashlar. It has medieval painted screens and many points of interest besides. Opposite is the Three Crowns. Granite and thatch, it was originally built as a manor house, incorporating parts of a 13th century monks' hospice. Later, it became a church house, then an inn, and witnessed two tragedies. In 1641, a jealous former lover shot Mary Whiddon on the day of her wedding as she returned from St Michael's Church, which is probably the origin of the famous scene in *Lorna Doone*, in which Lorna is shot at the altar on her wedding day by the villainous Carver Doone. Two years later, Sidney Godolphin, poet, MP and Royalist officer, died of his wounds at the Three Crowns following a skirmish with Parliamentarians. Godolphin's portrait has pride of place in the bar. His ghost and Mary Whiddon's are said to haunt the hotel.

A very short detour into North Bovey is rewarded with another beautiful granite church, typical of Dartmoor, with a carved 15th century screen and bench ends. Across the village green with its granite cross and iron pump, The Ring of Bells dates from the mid 13th century. With its thick granite walls, low ceilings and thatched roof, it has changed remarkably little.

(1) Turn left out of Chagford car park and right by the Globe Inn. The Three Crowns is on your left, the church on your right. Turn right at the Square with its 'pepperpot' market house, MORETONHAMPSTEAD OKEHAMPTON. Continue to the A382 at Easton Cross (2).

Cross over and pedal ahead, UPPACOTT. The lane descends steeply, then rises sharply. Look back for a wonderful view.

Turn right, HOWTON (3) and enjoy a downhill swoop. Don't take the next turning right, but pedal uphill past Great Howton and bear right at Howton Cross, MORETONHAMPSTEAD. Turn right then left onto the main road to Moretonhampstead. (To visit the church and almshouses, turn left into Cross Street opposite the White Hart.) Otherwise, turn right just past the Union Inn, POSTBRIDGE PRINCETOWN. Turn left into POUND STREET just beyond the White Horse.

Follow the lane right at the next junction NORTH BOVEY (4) and continue ahead at Hospit Cross. Detour left at Pound Rock (5) into North Bovey. Retrace your tracks as far as Pound Rock. Take the unsigned lane ahead – not the Moretonhampstead lane.

Cross the B3212 at Week Cross (6) onto a narrow lane. Turn left at the T-junction ahead ('The Old Barn, Thorn Cross'). At Singmoor Cross pedal ahead CHAGFORD. Continue ahead at Middlecott Cross GREAT WEEKE (7). At Great Weeke keep ahead CHAGFORD. A stiff but mercifully short climb leads to the start.

Start/finish: Chagford car park (SX 702875). Alternatively, car parks in Moretonhampstead or North Bovey

Distance: 17.5km (11 miles)

Terrain: Moderately demanding. Steep ascents and descents. Mainly quiet country lanes. Short section B road

Refreshments: Cafés, pubs, shops and restaurants in Chagford and Moretonhampstead, pub in North Bovey

Public toilets: Chagford and Moretonhampstead

Maps: Landranger 191 or Outdoor Leisure 28

Link: Can be linked with Ride 14, South Zeal

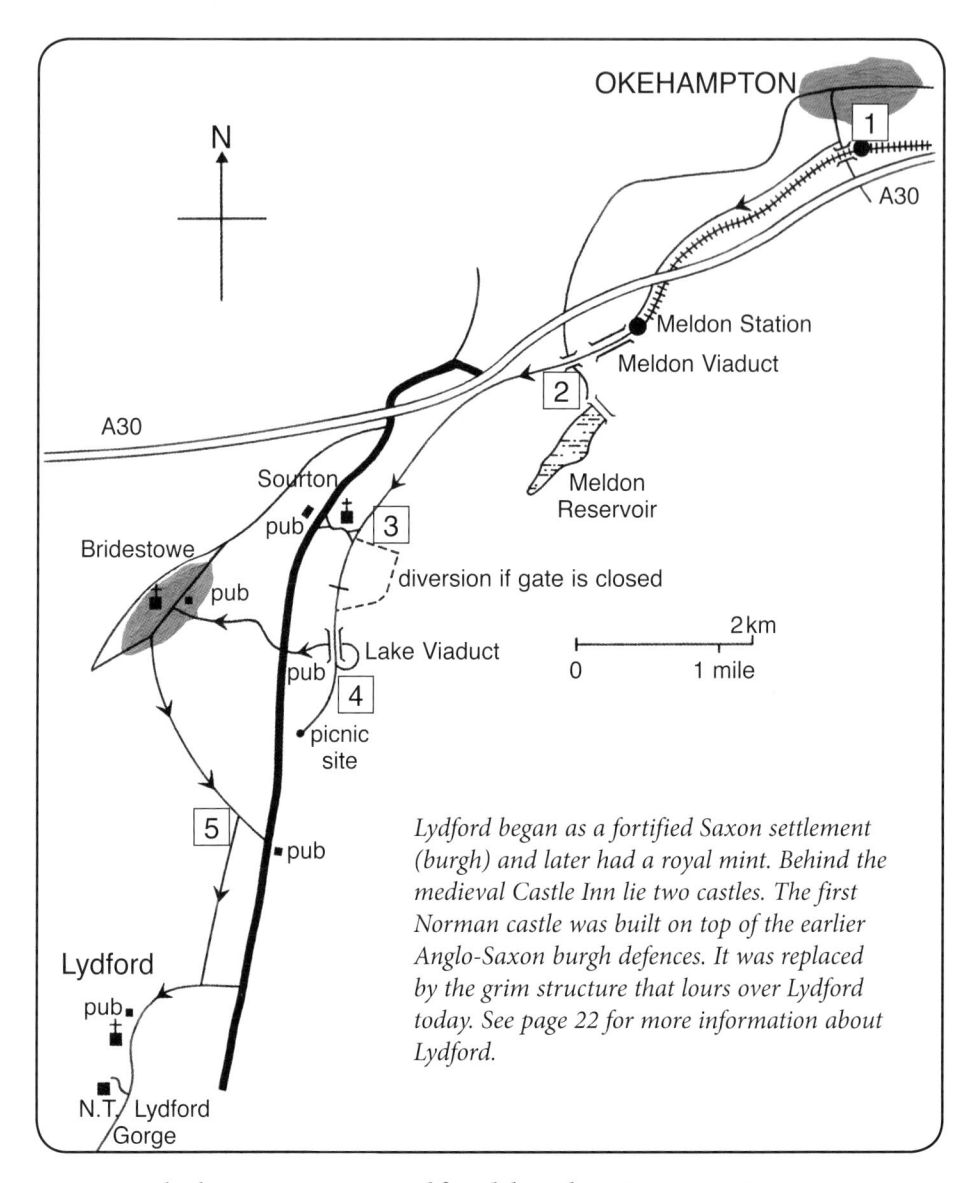

Lydford began as a fortified Saxon settlement (burgh) and later had a royal mint. Behind the medieval Castle Inn lie two castles. The first Norman castle was built on top of the earlier Anglo-Saxon burgh defences. It was replaced by the grim structure that lours over Lydford today. See page 22 for more information about Lydford.

9 Okehampton to Lydford by the Granite Way

From Okehampton station to Lake Viaduct, the Granite Way provides 10.5 km (6½ miles) each way of continuous traffic-free cycling. Using the former Southern Railway, the well-surfaced cycle path is level or near level throughout, making it ideal for families and beginners. I suggest using cycle route 27 to extend it by lanes as far as Lydford with its gorge and castle, plus small diversions to Meldon Dam and Sourton. This gives a full day's cycling, packed with interest.

The visitor centre at Meldon Quarry station provides information on the quarry, the railway and the viaduct.

(1) From Okehampton Station cycle down to Station Road. Cross over and take GRANITE WAY, CYCLE ROUTE 27. Continue past Meldon Visitor Centre and over Meldon Viaduct.

Turn left (2) off the cycle track, MELDON RESERVOIR. Pedal to the middle of the dam for superb views. Return to the cycle track.

Divert right SOURTON (3) to visit its unique Highwayman Inn, inscribed medieval cross and historic church. Just beyond the Sourton turn, the railway path is crossed by a metal gate. The next 230m is a right of way only during August and Bank Holidays. Otherwise, access is by kind permission of the landowner. If this section is closed cyclists must back-track to Sourton and take the bridleways parallel to the railway path as indicated on the map fixed to the gate.

From the far end of Lake Viaduct (4) turn left LYDFORD. Alternatively, pedal on along the railway path for 1.6km to the picnic site. Cross under the viaduct and follow the gravelled track to the A386 at the Bearslake Inn. Cross carefully and follow the blue cycle sign (Route 27). Turn left at the T-junction and coast down to Bridestowe. Turn left opposite the church on Route 27. Ignore the next turn right and pedal uphill to Station House.

Turn right at the Route 27 sign (5) to resume the railway track.

Follow the track to a lane. Turn right to visit Lydford Castle and church and Lydford Gorge.

Lydford Gorge (National Trust) is five minutes further by bike. Lock your machine to the rails. The spectacular gorge and waterfall make a delightful 5km walk, but make sure you have sufficient time and energy for the return cycle – 17.3km without any diversions.

Start/finish: Okehampton Station, SX592944. (Note closing time for gates.) Parking at the rear of the station; alternatively roadside parking in Station Road or Okehampton's long stay car parks

Distance: 38.5km (24 miles) including diversions

Terrain: Easy – 25km of the total on level or near level traffic-free cyclepath. The rest quiet lanes, with some steep but short ascents. One main road crossing

Refreshments: Pubs at Okehampton, Sourton, Lake, Bridestowe and Lydford. Buffets at Okehampton and Meldon stations. Tearoom at Lydford Gorge

Public toilets: Lydford   **Maps:** Outdoor Leisure 28 or Landranger 191

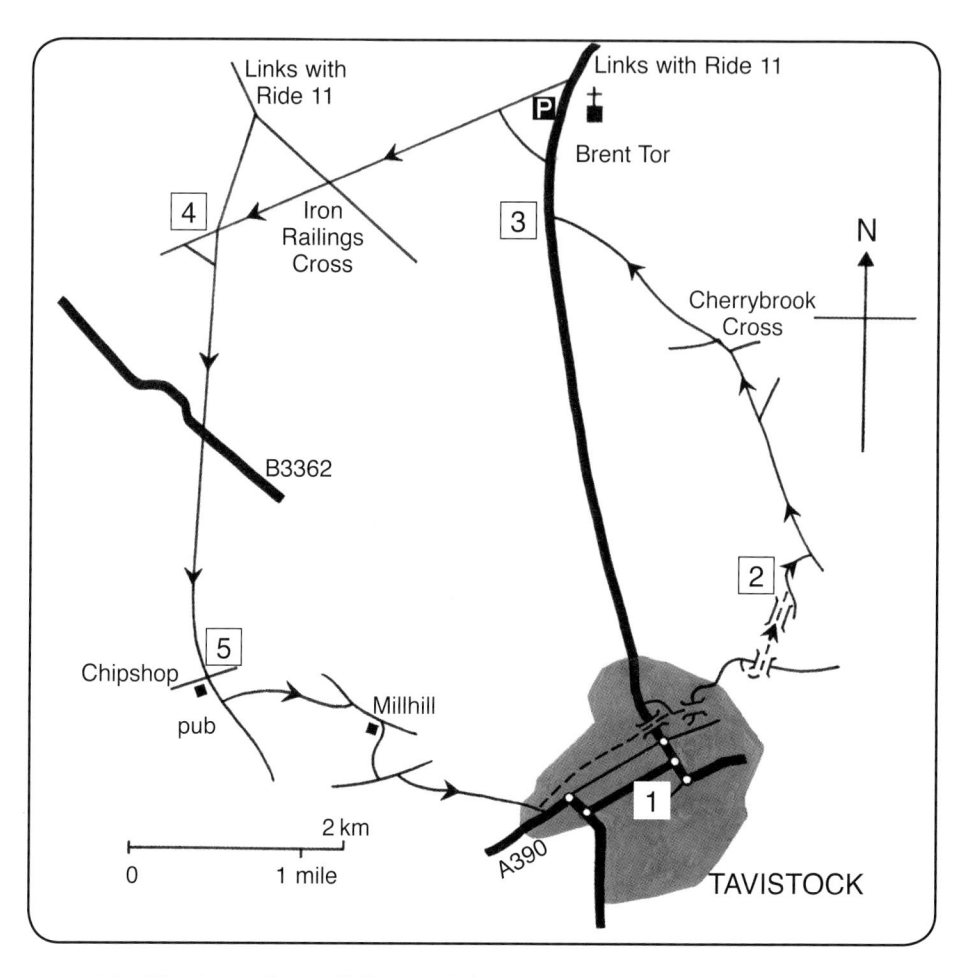

10 Tavistock and Brent Tor

The best route out of Tavistock follows Cycle Route 27. Using sections of converted railway and quiet lanes, the effort of climbing 200m is rewarded with a great vista of western Dartmoor and a classic view of Brent Tor. From Brent Tor, the cycling is much easier, with some fast downhill riding in the later stages via Chipshop.

Brent Tor (334m) is a landmark for a great distance around and well worth a short diversion on foot. (Remember to lock your bike!) Crowned with a tiny Norman church and the remains of an Iron Age hill fort, it was once an ocean floor volcano. It offers wonderful views, including a range of Dartmoor tors, the patchwork fields of the Tamar Valley and on to the heights of Bodmin Moor.

You will pass the curiously named Chipshop. It may be an Old English name, denoting a 'log built shed or workshop'. However, it was not recorded until 1765 – very late for an English place name. The 1841 Census showed all the men and boys of Chipshop employed as either blacksmiths or carpenters ('chippies'). An alternative explanation is offered for the Chipshop Inn – that local miners were paid in tokens or 'chips' only redeemable at company shops.

The return to Tavistock is by cycle track and the impressive viaduct of the London and South Western Railway. Built in 1889, it recalls Tavistock's days as a boom mining town, the centre of world copper production.

(1) Turn right out of the long stay car park and pedal ahead. Turn left at the mini roundabout by Bedford Square. Keep straight ahead at the following mini roundabout, WEST DEVON CYCLEWAY 27. The road climbs steeply under the 1889 viaduct. Turn right at the blue cycleway 27 sign and climb past the old railway station to join the cycle track proper. Turn right onto the lane ahead. Pedal uphill, then down to rejoin the cycleway at the next blue sign.

Turn left at the lane junction, ROUTE 27 (2). Turn left again (ROUTE 27). The lane climbs steadily and then begins to level. Cycle ahead at Cherrybrook Cross, ROUTE 27. Keep right at the fork.

At the T-junction (3), turn right BRENTOR. Just beyond the sign for the Brentor church car park, turn left MILTON ABBOT. Continue ahead at Iron Railings Cross and then onward to Long Cross (4). Turn left, LAMERTON TAVISTOCK. Pedal on at the next crossroads, CHIPSHOP. Continue ahead at the Chipshop Inn, GULWORTHY (5).

Turn next left by a converted chapel at the first of a series of brown cycle signs leading back to Tavistock. Bear right at the next junction and take the next turning right. Turn next left, TAVISTOCK. Turn left at the blue cycle sign on the outskirts of Tavistock to resume the old railway track. Cross the viaduct and turn right at the blue cycle sign. Turn left and left again under the viaduct. Retrace your route to the car park via Bedford Square.

Start/finish: Tavistock's long stay car park, SX 481742
Distance: 23km (14 miles)
Terrain: Moderately demanding. Cycle path and country lanes
Refreshments: Pubs, cafés, shops in Tavistock. Pub at Chipshop
Public toilets: Tavistock and Brent Tor
Maps: Landranger 201 or Outdoor Leisure 28
Link: Can be linked to Ride 11

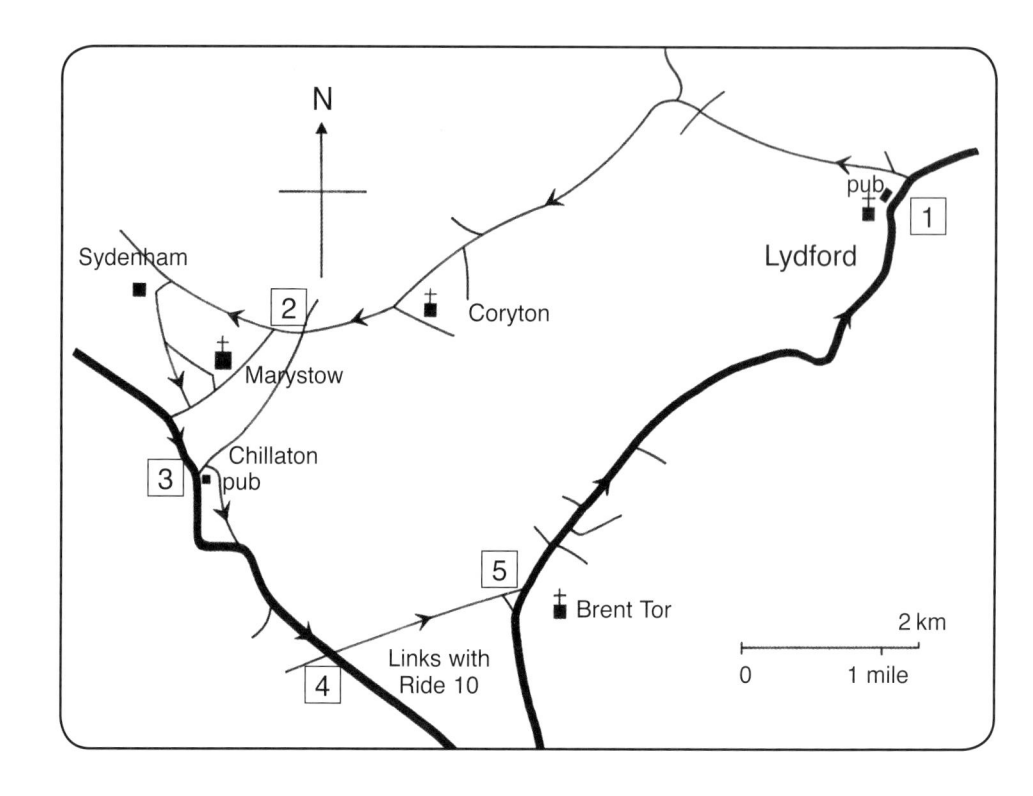

11 Lydford and Brent Tor

There is a great deal of interest in this pleasing and moderately demanding circuit. The route starts at Lydford car park, which has a helpful display board. Two castles and a Saxon royal mint were built here – Saxon coins can be seen in the Castle Inn. The first Norman castle was built on top of Lydford's earlier Saxon burgh defences. It was replaced by the impressive stone structure that still grimly dominates Lydford today. Employed as the notorious Devon stannary prison, it was used as a courthouse as late as the 18th century.

St Petrock's opposite is a characteristic Dartmoor granite church. It is noted for its carved screen and bench ends, as well as the 'Watchmaker's Tomb', with its witty epitaph: 'Integrity was the mainspring/And prudence the regulator/Of all the actions of his life…'

After a short climb from Lydford, you make a swift descent into the Lyd Valley. Turning south at Sydenham, an impressive 17th century house built by Sir Thomas Wise, Sheriff of Devon, you pedal on to Chillaton, where the Chichester Arms is well placed for midway refreshments. The route climbs again to Quither Common and Brent

Tor. Crowned with its 12th century church, Brent Tor is a marvellous viewpoint overlooking western Dartmoor, Plymouth Sound, the Tamar Valley and on to Bodmin Moor.

Like Brent Tor, Lydford Gorge must be explored on foot. (Remember your lock!) With its 30m high White Lady waterfall and remarkable ravine, the Gorge makes a first class 5km walk. The National Trust provides bike racks and reduced entry charges for cyclists.

(1) Turn right out of Lydford's village car park. Pedal through the village and turn left at the war memorial, CORYTON. Follow the CORYTON signs ahead and start the long, swift descent to Lowertown. (Were cycling always thus!) Ignore the signs left to Coryton church and continue to the crossroads (2).

Cycle ahead, SYDENHAM PORTGATE and the first of a series of helpful brown cycle signs. Turn left at Sydenham Cross, SYDENHAM MARYSTOW and follow the lane left past Sydenham. Cycle ahead at Stewardry Cross. At a T-junction, turn right CHILLATON, then at the next T-junction turn left CHILLATON.

In Chillaton (3) take the narrow lane slightly to the left of the Chichester Arms, bearing the brown cycle sign. The lane climbs steeply, swings right and continues climbing. After it levels out, bear left at the T-junction (no sign here at the time of writing).

Turn left at Iron Railings Cross (4). At the junction (5) opposite Brentor church (5) turn left again, LYDFORD – or divert right here to visit the tor. Follow the road straight on to Lydford via Lydford Gorge. Beware of the narrow lane and steep downhill gradients leading in to the village.

Start/finish: Free car park opposite Castle Inn, Lydford, SX 510848
Distance: 23.75km (14 3/4 miles)
Terrain: Moderately demanding. Some steep ascents. Quiet lanes and 'C' road
Refreshments: Pubs in Lydford and Chillaton. Tea room Lydford Gorge
Public toilets: Lydford
Map: Landranger 201
Lydford Gorge (National Trust): Seasonal opening (only the waterfall is open during winter)
Lydford Castle (English Heritage): Free entry at any reasonable time
Link: Can be linked to Ride 10 at Point 4

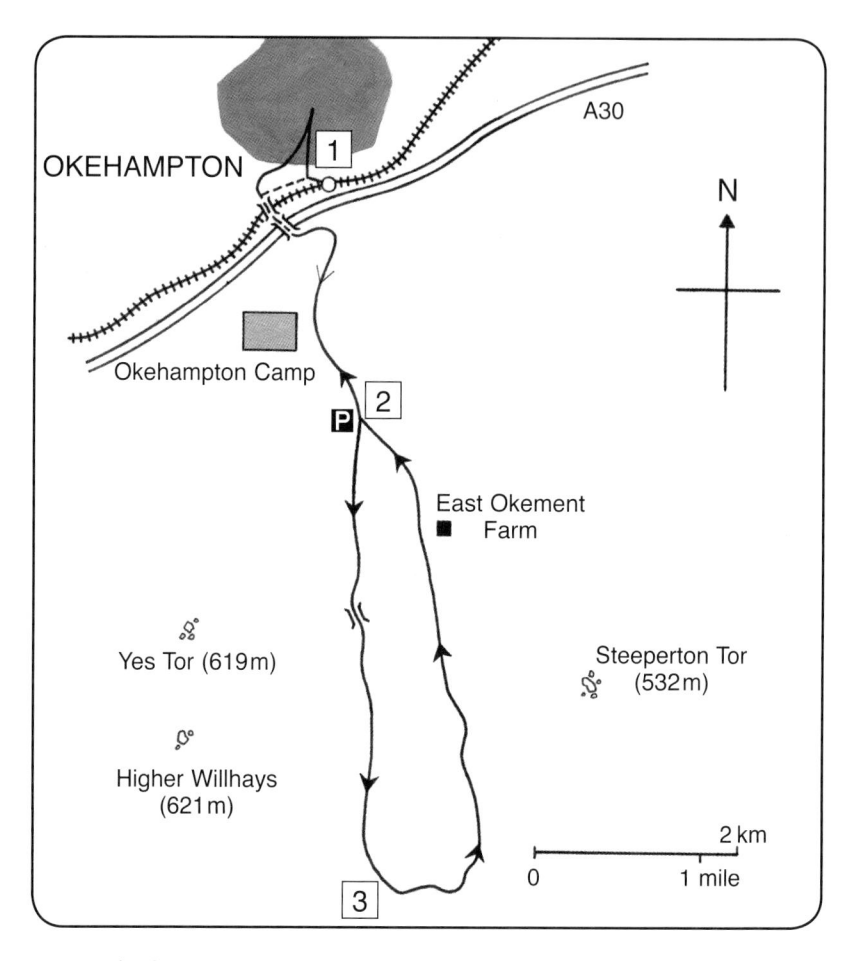

12 Okehampton to East Okement Head

This is a ride on the wild side, different in character from the others in this book. It will take you into the heart of Dartmoor, via military roads which are stony and potholed in places and which ford two brooks. The roads crisscross and are unsigned, so it is wise to take a compass to check your route.

Choose a clear day free of rain and strong winds – the views of the high moor and on over the patchwork fields to Mid Devon to Exmoor are splendid, but there is no shelter. The climate can be severe, even in summer, as I discovered riding this way in a July hailstorm.

The full route starts from Okehampton station, restored in the 1990s to period Southern Railway style and offering steam and diesel trains to Meldon and Sampford Courtenay. After a short section of cycle track it climbs very steeply over the railway and the A30. There is more, but less demanding, uphill work to reach the furthest point (3) at 564m above sea level. This adds up to 345m of ascent – the good news being that the second half of the ride is almost all downhill!

To reduce the ascent dramatically to 130m, start at Point 2.

(1) From Okehampton Station cycle down to STATION ROAD. Cross over and take GRANITE WAY, CYCLE ROUTE 27. After 500m, bear right off the Granite Way, following the road left and over the railway bridge. After climbing very steeply, the gradient slackens somewhat and levels towards Okehampton Camp. Turn left by the notice board, where the lane divides. Pedal over the cattle grid and bridge, past the house and wind turbine. Keep ahead on the tarmac, ignoring side turnings, to a fork in the road at Point 2. (There is ample roadside parking on the approach to Point 2.)

Keep right at the fork and head south, gaining height steadily. On the right are Yes Tor and High Willhays, the highest points on Dartmoor. At 619m and 621m, they just qualify as mountains.

At SX602878, follow the tarred road as it swings left by a military observation post. Follow the road steeply downhill to a ford – crossing it means wet feet after rain. Pedal on to a second ford. Bear left and uphill to Point 2.

Recover your car if you left it at Point 2. Otherwise, retrace your route to Okehampton Station.

Start/finish: Okehampton Station, SX592944. (Note closing time for gates.) Parking at the rear of the station; alternatively roadside parking in Station Road or Okehampton's long stay car parks

Shortened route: Roadside parking at Point 2, SX597922

Distance: 17.5km (10³/₄ miles) full route, 11.5km (7 miles) short version

Terrain: Very demanding and steep in parts. Military roads, rough and stony in places, minor road, and cycle track

Refreshments: Okehampton Station and choice of pubs, restaurants, cafés and shops in Okehampton

Public toilets: None   **Maps:** Landranger 191 or Outdoor Leisure 28

Special notes: Most of the route is within the Okehampton Firing Range. Check whether the range is closed for firing before you start on 0800 458 4868, www.dartmoor-ranges.co.uk, or Dartmoor National Park on 01626 832093, www.dartmoor-npa.gov.uk. Leave alone any strange objects you find in case they are unexploded shells and contact the police with a map reference

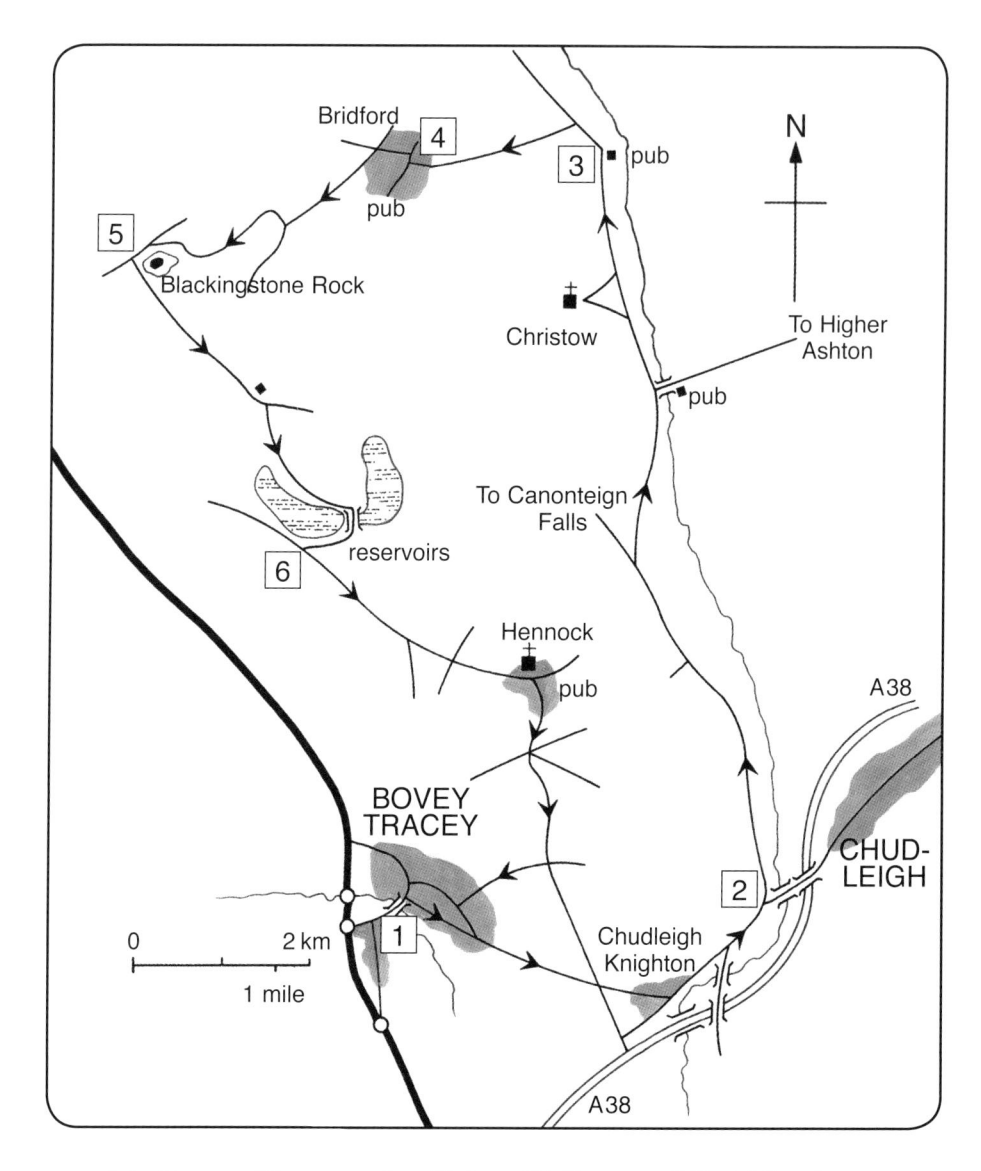

13 Bovey Tracey, the Teign Valley and Bridford

The Teign Valley road is a favourite with cyclists as it offers easy riding by the river. In spring it is lined with wild daffodils. A tough ascent to Bridford is rewarded with superb views of the valley below. The views from Blackingstone Rock – Dartmoor's most easterly granite tor – are even more impressive. From Blackingstone, the return route is largely level to the reservoirs, which have melded beautifully into the landscape.

Enjoy the easy coast home through Hennock. Few rides are better provided with attractive pubs. The Palk Arms at Hennock and the Bridford Inn are well placed. Both are historic buildings, with a range of interesting features, including stone fireplaces. Bridford, Hennock and Bovey Tracey also have exceptionally beautiful churches.

(1) Turn right out of the car park over the town bridge. Take the first right. Cycle on over Knighton Heath, a Devon Wildlife Trust nature reserve, to Chudleigh Knighton. At the T-junction just past the Claycutter's Arms turn left, CHUDLEIGH. Join B3193, CHUDLEIGH.

Just before reaching the A38 (2), turn left, TEIGN VALLEY DUNSFORD. Stay on this road for the next 10km. At Spara Bridge you could divert right for 200m towards Ashton for the Manor Inn.

Pedal on past the Teign House Inn (3) and take the next left, BRIDFORD. Arriving at the T-junction in Bridford (4), turn left, BRIDFORD INN, for the centre of the village, the church and inn.

Return to the T-junction and follow the lane around to the left. Turn left at the next crossroads, RESERVOIR BOVEY. Take the next right at Laployd Barton Cross, MORETONHAMPSTEAD. Cycle past the northern face of Blackingstone Rock to a junction. Turn left and almost immediately (5) left again, CHRISTOW AND HENNOCK.

To visit Blackingstone Rock, dismount at the footpath sign ahead on the left. Push your bike up the path (or lock it). Steps lead to the summit. Enjoy the view, then resume your route. Turn right just past Kennick Farm onto a lane, HENNOCK BOVEY TRACEY. Follow the lane ahead and then right past Trenchford reservoir to Bullaton Cross (6).

Turn left, HENNOCK. Cycle through the village (the church and the Palk Arms are together). Follow the BOVEY TRACEY signs to Little Helstonsbench Cross. Turn right, BOVEY TRACEY. At a T-junction, turn right. Pedal past the church and down the main street to the start.

Start/finish: Lower car park, Bovey Tracey, SX815784

Distance: 35km (21 3/4 miles)

Terrain: Moderate. Fairly level apart from steep 2km ascent to Bridford and a long descent into Bovey Tracey, plus a few short slopes. Part on B roads, part on lanes

Refreshments: Pubs in Chudleigh Knighton, Teign Valley, Bridford, Hennock, Bovey Tracey, plus shops and cafés in Bovey

Public toilets: At start

Maps: Landranger 191 or Explorer 110

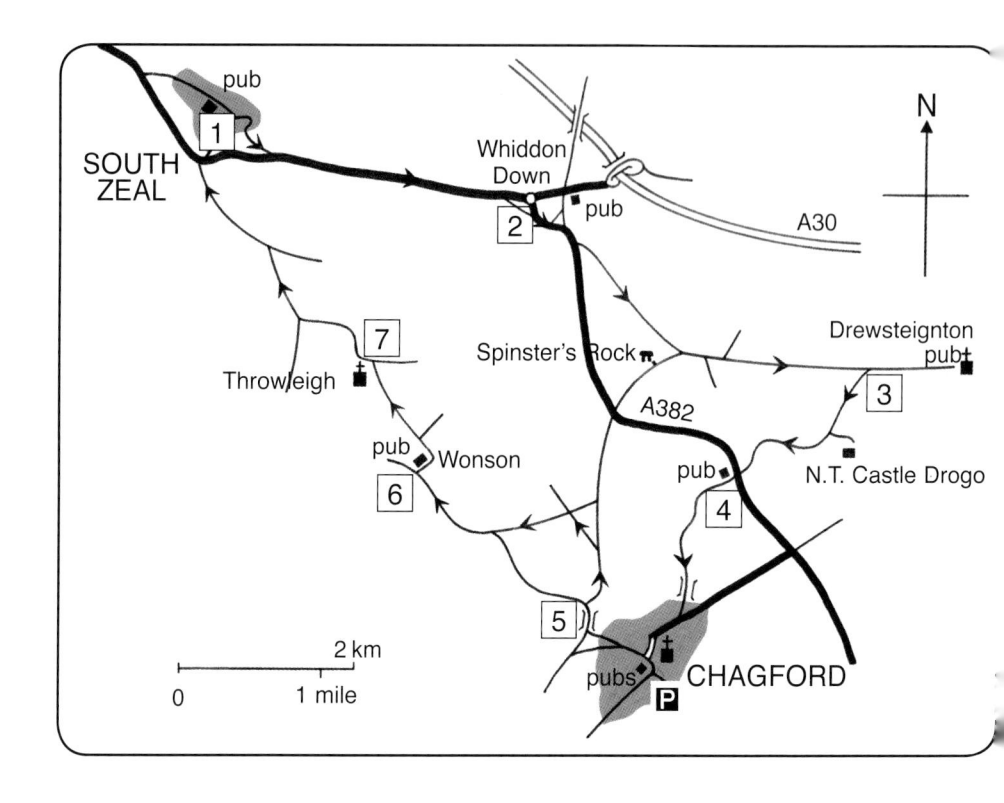

14 South Zeal and Castle Drogo

This enjoyable though demanding ride is mainly by narrow lanes that offer great views of eastern Dartmoor's rugged profile, but involve some steep ascents and descents. It includes England's newest castle and Dartmoor's best preserved prehistoric burial chamber.

Spinster's Rock, a granite dolmen dating from approximately 3500 to 2500 BC, is well worth a detour. The burial mound above it has long gone, but the three huge granite piers and capstone that formed its centre remain. In 1862, they fell down but were re-erected in the same year. According to legend, the monument was built by three spinsters.

Castle Drogo overlooks the Teign Gorge. It was built of local granite, combining an air of medieval grandeur with the comforts of modern life. Sir Edwin Lutyens designed it at the behest of millionaire grocer, Sir Julius Drewe. It took twenty years to build and was completed in 1931.

Chagford is well endowed with stone, cob and thatch buildings, including the Three Crowns Hotel. See page 16 for its stories.

(1) Turn left out of the car park in South Zeal. Turn right and pedal up the main street to the T-junction. Turn left, WHIDDON DOWN EXETER. Cycle on to the roundabout. Take the second exit, MORETONHAMP-STEAD (2).Take the third turning left, DREWSTEIGNTON.

To visit the dolmen, turn first right, SPINSTER'S ROCK. Keep ahead for 400m. Lock your bike by the kissing gate. Return to the Spinster's Rock turning. Turn right, DREWSTEIGNTON FINGLE BRIDGE.

Take the second right, CASTLE DROGO (3). Divert left, CASTLE DROGO. After visiting, return to the lane and turn left. Pedal down to Sandy Park on the A382 (4). Continue ahead SWIMMING POOL, past the pool and on to a T-junction. Turn right CHAGFORD.

At the Market Place, turn right GIDLEIGH THROWLEIGH. Cycle downhill. Fork right GIDLEIGH THROWLEIGH. Descend a steep hill and turn right GIDLEIGH THROWLEIGH. Cross the bridge (5) and continue steeply uphill. Continue ahead at the next turn, THROWLEIGH. Cycle straight on, WONSON THROWLEIGH at White Gate Cross.

Near the crest of the hill, behind an iron gate, is a stone enclosure, 'Chagford Manor Pound', built to contain livestock. Turn left at the next junction, MURCHINGTON GIDLEIGH THROWLEIGH.

Continue ahead, following the WONSON THROWLEIGH signs. The lane leads downhill and over a bridge, then steeply uphill past Providence. Take the next right, WONSON THROWLEIGH (6) past the Northmore Arms and straight on at the next junction.

Arriving in Throwleigh, turn left at the Cross (7) and right in front of the church and church house, SOUTH ZEAL. Continue ahead, SOUTH ZEAL at Clannaborough Cross. Arriving at South Zeal, fork left under the stone road bridge and pedal downhill to the car park.

Start/finish: Free public car park in South Zeal, SX 652935

Distance: 26km (16 miles)

Terrain: Demanding. Several sharp ascents and descents. Country lanes and a section of declassified former main road

Refreshments: Pubs, South Zeal, Whiddon Down, Sandy Park, Chagford and Wonson. Cafés/restaurants, South Zeal, Castle Drogo and Chagford

Public toilets: South Zeal, Chagford

Maps: Landranger 191 or Outdoor Leisure 28

Castle Drogo (National Trust): Open daily, except Tuesdays, in season, plus some winter weekends. Check 01647 433306

Link: Can be linked to Ride 8, Chagford

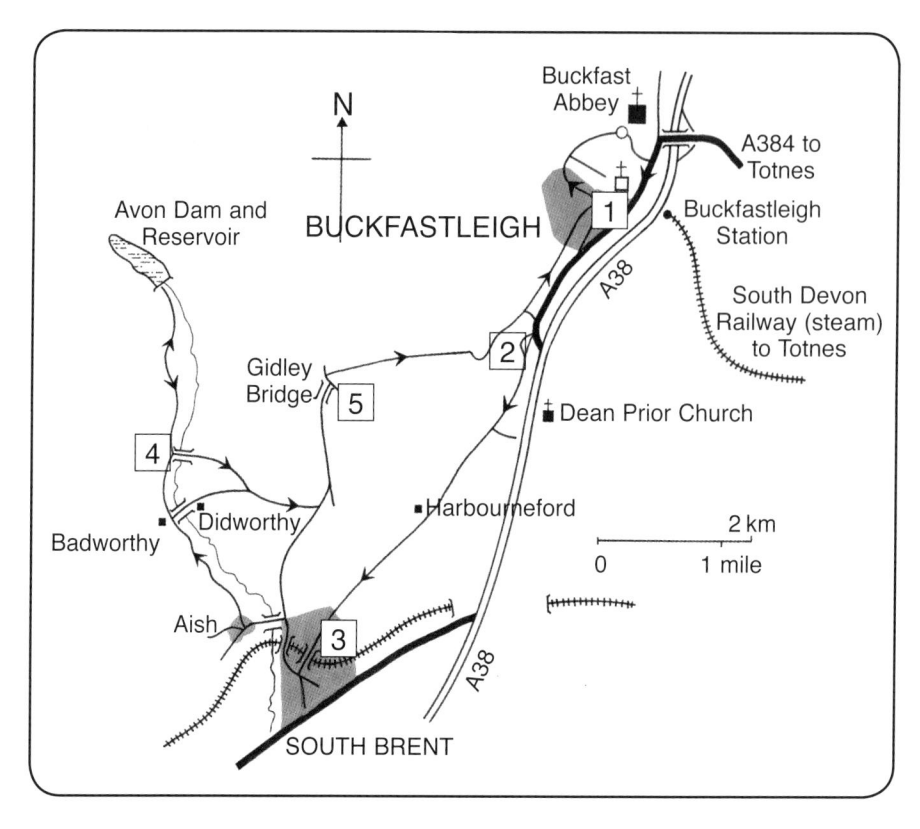

15 Buckfastleigh and Shipley Bridge

Allow plenty of time for this route. It provides a great deal of interest and fine views of southern Dartmoor, but includes several steep hills. There are former mills in Buckfastleigh and at Buckfast Abbey. The Abbey itself is open to visitors and was rebuilt by French monks between 1882 and 1938 in the style of the original medieval abbey.

The skeleton of Holy Trinity church stands on a limestone peak. It was largely destroyed in an arson attack in 1992, but the tower and spire were repaired and the bells rang again in 1996. In the churchyard is the Cabell tomb (1656), source of local legends and inspiration for Arthur Conan Doyle's *Hound of the Baskervilles*.

After a short section of the B3380 the route follows a much hillier and much older route through Harbourneford to South Brent. A 5.6km diversion from Shipley Bridge alongside the boulder-strewn river Avon and its waterfalls leads to the impressive Avon Dam. The return to Buckfastleigh affords superb views of Western Beacon and other tors, plus a long, exciting descent.

(1) Turn right out of the Victoria Woodhouse car park. Follow the road round to the left, ALL ROUTES. Follow the TOWN CENTRE signs right and right again. Turn left into Mardle Way and follow it past the former mills and uphill. Divert right at Round Cross to visit Holy Trinity. Return to Round Cross. Turn right (Higher Mill Lane). Coast downhill to a mini roundabout.

Turn left to visit Buckfast Abbey. Return to the roundabout. Cycle ahead to another mini roundabout. Turn right, LOCAL SERVICES. Follow the B3380 around Buckfastleigh and on to Upper Dean **(2)**. Follow the road right past Dean Forge to a fork. Keep left, SOUTH BRENT. Pedal uphill and continue ahead at Clampitt Cross. The route now joins Cycle Route 2. Follow it through Harbourneford and on to South Brent. Cross the railway bridge **(3)**. Continue to a junction.

Turn right, DIDWORTHY AVON DAM (or divert 50m left to the Pack Horse). Follow the road right past the church and back over the railway. Continue ahead at Oakhill Cross, AISH ZEAL DIDWORTHY. Cross Lydia Bridge and follow the lane steeply uphill through Aish. Keep ahead, DIDWORTHY, at Binnamore Cross.

Divert left at Shipley Bridge **(4)**, PUBLIC BRIDLEPATH BROCKHILL FORD. The tarmac track (a little potted but quite ridable) follows the river Avon to the dam. Please watch for pedestrians and horses. Return to Shipley Bridge **(4)**. Turn left. Pedal on to Gingaford Cross. Cycle ahead, SOUTH BRENT BUCKFASTLEIGH.

At Bloody Pool Cross, turn left, GIDLEY SKERRATON. Turn left at the next T-junction **(5)**, and follow the lane round right, SKERRATON DEANCOMBE. The lane descends steeply – beware loose gravel and slow down when it narrows. Keep ahead at Deancombe Cross. (Do not take the Nurston Addislade turn.) Keep ahead, BUCKFASTLEIGH at Coxhill Cross. Turn left at the sports field (Duckspond Road). Turn right at the next junction and right again. Follow this (Bossell Road) to the start.

Start/finish: Victoria Woodhouse car park, Plymouth Road, Buckfastleigh. (Follow TOWN CENTRE signs from B3380)

Distance: 31.5km (19½ miles)

Terrain: Demanding. Several steep ascents and descents. Mainly quiet country lanes. Short sections of B road, town streets and tarmac track

Refreshments: Pubs, Buckfastleigh and South Brent, café Buckfast Abbey

Public toilets: Buckfastleigh, South Brent, Shipley Bridge

Maps: Landranger 202 or Outdoor Leisure 28

Cycle shops

Please note this list is not an exhaustive guide and details are subject to change. Telephone first to check for cycle hire, repairs and availability of parts.

Ashburton: Bigpeaks Centre, Linhay Business Park, Eastern Road. 01364 654080

Bovey Tracey: Bikus, St John's Lane 01626 833555

Heathfield: Devonbiker, 21 Teignbridge Business Centre, Cavalier Road. 01626 832901

Liverton: The Mountain Bike Centre, Cummings Cross. 01364 654080

Okehampton: Moor Cycles, 6 The Arcade, Fore Street 01837 659677

Okehampton: Okehampton Cycles, Bostock Garden Centre, North Road. 01837 53248

Okehampton: Okehampton Station (cycle hire) 01837 55637

Plymouth: DMT Cycles, Unit 34, City Business Park. 01752 607222

Plymouth: Natural Cycles, 100 Albert Road, Benbow Street 01752 550729

Sourton: Devon Cycle Hire, Sourton Down 01837 861141

South Brent: TC2 Recycles, 9 Station Road 01364 73221

Tavistock: Dartmoor Cycles, 8 Atlas House, West Devon Trading Estate 01822 618178

Tavistock: Tavistock Cycles, 2 Farriers Court, Paddon Row, Brook Street. 01822 617630

Useful addresses

Sustrans: 0845 113 00 65 www.sustrans.org.uk Maps, guides, advice, accessories

CTC Cyclists Touring Club: 01483 417217 www.ctc.org.uk Touring and technical advice, legal aid and insurance

Bike and bus

Two bus services will carry cyclists and their bikes onto Dartmoor:

Dartmoor Easirider: 'ring and ride' Mondays to Saturdays. Normal private hire/taxi rates apply 01803 840 009

Dartmoor Freewheeler: free summer Sunday bus service, offers two routes:

   1. Ashburton-Bovey Tracey-Moretonhampstead-Mardon Down
   2. Plymouth-Yelverton-Princetown

Winston C
his politics a

Contents

1. General Chronological Notes 1
2. Elections and Seats 26
3. Churchill's Government posts 27
4. Churchill's secretaries 27
5. Visits and meetings 28
6. Selected Bibliography 29

Acknowledgements

In producing even a small book such as this one, an Author is indebted to many people. I would like to acknowledge the help and support of my colleagues at Chartwell during the preparation of this work. Particular thanks are due to Carole Kenwright, Tony Mulvany, Neil Walters and Angela Griffin for enabling the project to go ahead and to John Brunsden, John Solway, Neville Snazel and John Whaler for their input to the material. Finally, my thanks go to Margaret, my wife, for her patience; to my colleague and typesetter, Mike Cotterell, for his design skills; and to David Coombs, whose encouragement and kind words are esteemed as much as his incomparable expertise.

Section 1: General Notes

1874
Lord Randolph marries Jennie Jerome, daughter of Leonard Jerome, director of the New York Times.
Winston Churchill is born at Blenheim, November 30; His nurse is Mrs Everest. His grandfather, the 7th Duke of Marlborough, becomes Lord Lieutenant of Ireland under Disraeli

GOVERNMENTS: 74–80 Disraeli. Con. (Maj 50); 80–85 Gladstone. Lib.(Maj 50)

1876–1884
The family moves to Ireland, where they remain until 1879. Churchill attends St George's School, Ascot (82–84) and the Misses Thompsons' School, Brighton (84–88)

GOVERNMENTS: Jun 85–Jan 86 Salisbury. Con. (Not an election. Gladstone. resigned.);
Feb 86–Jul 86 Gladstone. Lib. (Lib 335, Cons 249, Irish 86.)
Jul 86–Aug 92 Salisbury. Con. (Con 311, Lib-Unionists 78, Lib 191, Irish 85)

1885
Lord Randolph is appointed Secretary of State for India.
April 1. Clementine is born.

1886
Lord Randolph is appointed Chancellor and leader of the House of Commons in Salisbury's government. Randolph makes his famous statement 'Ulster will fight and Ulster will be right'. He wants a more liberal budget and Salisbury is against it. He offers to resign, bluffing, but Salisbury accepts. This destroys his political career. Leonard Jerome dies.

1888
Churchill attends Harrow school; he is good at fencing (English Public Schools Champion), swimming, English and rifle shooting. Contrary to popular thought, he passes maths, although the knowledge 'passed away like the phantasmagoria of a fevered dream'. (See *My Early Life*)

GOVERNMENT: Aug 92–Mar 94 Gladstone. Lib.

1893
Churchill enters Sandhurst after three attempts.

GOVERNMENTS: Mar 94–Jun 95 Rosebury. Lib.

1895
He graduates 20th of 130 and is commissioned in the 4th Hussars. He goes on his first reporting trip to Cuba for the Daily Graphic. He is awarded the Spanish OM, 1st class. Churchill is based with the Spanish army who are fighting against the Cubans. Later he writes to his mother saying his sympathies were more with the Cubans.
Lord Randolph dies.

GOVERNMENT: Jun 95–Jul 02 Salisbury. Con.

1896–97
Churchill is posted to India on the northwest frontier under Sir Bindon Blood.

1898
Churchill publishes the *Malakand Field Force* and writes *Savrola,* his only novel. He joins the Nile expeditionary force with Kitchener.
(NOTE: Kitchener was anti-Churchill, thinking him brash. Kitchener was out to avenge Gordon. He also committed war crimes – he desecrated the grave of the Mahdi and removed the body for display.)
Churchill writes *The River War*. He takes part in the Sudan War against the Dervishes. He is seconded to the 21st Lancers and takes part in the British Army's last cavalry charge, at Omdurman.
(NOTE: This was on 02/09/98. Observe the similarity to Theodore Roosevelt, who led the charge at San Juan in the Spanish–American War, July 98.)
Churchill is romantically involved with Pamela Plowden, who later marries Lord Lytton.

1899
Churchill resigns his commission after five years in the army. He stands for the Conservatives at the Oldham by-election. He loses narrowly and goes to South Africa to report on the war for the Morning Post. He takes 60 bottles of alcohol and 12 Rose's Lime Juice. (Claret is two shillings a bottle). He rescues the armoured train and is captured by the Boers. He escapes and hides in a mine (see the film *Young Winston*, which was an accurate record). By the end of 1899 Churchill has earned over £2,000 from journalism, (approximately £100,000 now). This is the highest of any journalist to date. He writes *The River War*.

1900
Churchill returns to South Africa and is commissioned as a Lieutenant in the South African Light Horse (The Cockyolly Birds). He serves for seven months, including action at Spoin Kop. He is rescued by Trooper Roberts from the Boers. He is elected for the Conservatives at Oldham. He spends a long time on his speeches and continues to do so all his life. He prefers speeches to debating.
Savrola is published. He says in *My Early Life*, 1930, that he discouraged his friends from reading it. He also writes *The Life of Lord Randolph*.
He meets Theodore Roosevelt when TR is Governor of New York. There is mutual dislike. TR says later to Alice, his daughter, that it was because Churchill did not stand up when ladies entered the room!
In two years Churchill earns £10,000 from journalism (approximately £500,000 today). The money is invested by Sir Ernest Cassell (the King's banker). He also publishes *London to Ladysmith* and *Ian Hamilton's March*.
The Labour Party is formed.

1900–04
Churchill predicts European wars on a large scale. He disagrees with Joseph Chamberlain and Balfour over Tariffs.
(NOTE: Churchill was in favour of free trade, a Liberal view. The Conservatives were pro-Empire protection. Churchill wanted to reform the Tories and combine with the Liberals to defeat Labour. He saw Labour as the antithesis of his politics.)

GOVERNMENT: July 02–December 05 Balfour. Con.

1904
Churchill leaves the Conservatives and crosses the floor to join the Liberals. He sits next to Lloyd-George, with whom he becomes close. He meets Clementine.

GOVERNMENT: Dec 05–April 08 Campbell–Bannerman. Lib. [Lib 399, Con 156, Lab 29, Irish 83]

1906-07
The Life of Lord Randolph Churchill is published. Churchill receives an £8,000 advance (approximately £400,000 now) from Macmillan.
He is elected at Manchester as a Liberal. Hicks is his opponent and accuses Churchill of saying different things as a Liberal from those he said as a Conservative Churchill replies that he'd had to say silly things as a Conservative and he'd joined the Liberals in order to stop saying silly things. Churchill is appointed to the government as Under-secretary of State for the Colonies.

(NOTE: He turned down the post of Treasury Minister, even though it was a higher-ranking post. This was because Asquith was Chancellor and was in the Commons, but Lord Elgin was Colonial Secretary and was in the Lords, so Churchill was in charge in the Commons.)

He proposes to Pamela Plowden and is rejected. At about this time, Clementine is secretly engaged to Sidney Peel, but she breaks off the engagement. She then becomes engaged to Lionel Earl (aged 42). The engagement is announced on August 15; broken off on October 22.

Edward Marsh is appointed as Churchill's secretary. He will remain for 25 years. They tour East Africa in 1907. Churchill writes *My African Journey*.

GOVERNMENT: April 08–May 15 Asquith. Lib. [Not an election, change of PM]

1908

Asquith becomes PM. Churchill is appointed President of the Board of Trade. This is a Cabinet post and Churchill is only 34. Very few had been appointed to the cabinet so young, viz, Pitt, Palmerston, Peel, Gladstone, Churchill, Harold Wilson and … William Hague. At this time he has to stand for re-election and he is defeated. (The Irish Catholics switch votes because of Churchill's support for the Ulster compromise.) Churchill is immediately selected at Dundee and elected.

(NOTE: Churchill was a social reformer. He agreed in many ways with the Webbs. He was opposed by Scrimgeour, a prohibitionist, who received only 5% of the vote. Scrimgeour kept trying and eventually beat Churchill in 1922.)

Churchill and Clementine marry on September 12. Lord Hugh Cecil is best man. (He was the younger son of Marquis of Salisbury, the former PM.) They live in Bolton St.

(NOTE: Churchill was associated with very few women, Pamela Plowden, Violet Asquith, Muriel Wilson, Ethel Barrymore (he proposed to her, too) and Clementine.)

1909

The Lords reject the budget. This is the event known as 'The Peers vs the People'.
(NOTE: Churchill, the grandson of a peer, was on the side of the people.)

GOVERNMENT: 1910 Jan Asquith. Lib. [Lib 274, Con 272, Lab 40] (82 Irish Nationalists)
GOVERNMENT: 1910 Dec Asquith. Lib. [Lib 272, Con 272, Lab 42] (82 Irish Nationalists)

1910
The Parliament Act curbs the power of the Lords. Churchill is appointed Home Secretary. Churchill is a social reformer. He is anti-socialist, but very much for improving conditions for workers, especially miners. He is considered by the Tories to be a class traitor. He advocates abolition of the Lords and favours unicameralism. The Tonypandy riot takes place; Churchill is accused of using troops, but the troops are sent in by the local police and Churchill in fact intervenes to stop it.
(NOTE: The calumny persisted. As late as 1963 A P Herbert had to write a defence of Churchill in response to an article reiterating the fiction.)
The Sidney St siege occurs, involving Peter the Painter, a Russian anarchist. Churchill is criticised for being there and taking charge. (See his account in *Thoughts and Adventures*.)
Carson becomes leader of the Irish Nationalists.

1911
October: Churchill is appointed First Lord of the Admiralty. Admiral John (Jackie) Fisher is First Sea Lord. Churchill realises the need for naval spending. He predicts that the navy will need to be at full strength by 1914, because Germany will attack Belgium and France and Britain will have to send troops about 40 days later.
(NOTE: Events turn out so, with Britain and France successful at the battle of the Marne, 37 days after war started in 1914.)
Churchill meets Aitkin (later Beaverbrook). Law becomes Tory leader, beating Joseph Chamberlain and Walter Long. (Aitkin was much involved in the choice of Law.)

1912
Churchill supports Liberal policy on Home Rule for Ireland, but agrees with the Ulster Compromise, along with F E Smith (later Lord Birkenhead) and Austen Chamberlain. For this, he is reviled by Tory Unionists as a renegade and by Home Rulers as a defector. Churchill is drawn to Grey, on a common hard line of re-arming against the German threat.
(NOTE: Churchill's belief in the likelihood of war must not be equated with a desire for it. See Jenkins p212.)

1913
Churchill does a lot of work on the fleet. He converts it to oil and increases speeds to 25 knots. The government invests in the Anglo–Persian Oil Co. Churchill ensures the construction of Dreadnoughts and goes for 15" guns, which is a gamble, but it works.

1914
There is nearly civil war over Ulster. The Irish Home Rule Bill is passed. Bonar Law is ready for insurrection, but events are overtaken by the war. On August 2, Churchill authorises the mobilisation of the fleet. On August 4, the war begins. He goes to Antwerp and organises defences that delay the Germans by five days. He offers to resign his government post and take charge of Antwerp. Kitchener offers to appoint Churchill as Lieut-General but nothing comes of it. Antwerp falls and Churchill is criticised. The battles of Mons, the Marne and Ypres take place.
September: The Treaty of London: Britain, France and Russia agree that none of them will allow a separate peace with Germany. November: Russia declares war on Turkey. Enver Pasha is leader of the Young Turks. Mustapha Kemal is the army commander.
Kitchener is appointed Secretary of State for War. Churchill sets up the Royal Naval Air Service.

1915
The Dardanelles campaign begins. The idea comes from Churchill: 'Are there not alternatives to sending our armies to chew barbed wire in Flanders?' It is initially supported by Fisher and the cabinet, but is a failure and it remains to haunt Churchill for any years.
(NOTE: Much has been written about the campaign and about who was to blame. The matter is complex and it is an over-simplification to view it in isolation from the rest of the war. If any one of a number of events had turned out differently, the course of the war could have been significantly changed. The actions of all of the main participants, from Asquith, Churchill and the rest of the cabinet, to Kitchener, de Roebeck, Hamilton and Monro must be examined in order to have a clear view of the reality. See Gallipoli by L Carlyon)
The second battle of Ypres takes place, as do the battles of Loos, Neuve-Chapelle, and the Somme.

GOVERNMENT: 1915 Asquith. Coalition. [Not an election]

The Conservatives enter the coalition on condition that Churchill be sacked. Churchill is appointed Chancellor of the Duchy of Lancaster but resigns and goes to war. He is commissioned as Major in the Grenadier Guards and then as Lieutenant Colonel in the 6th Battalion Royal Scots Fusiliers. He commands this regiment at Ploegsteert (Plug Street, South of Ypres, North-west of Armentiers.) Sir Archibald Sinclair, (later leader of the Liberal party) is his second in command. At a similar (the same?) time, Hitler is with the 16th Bavarian Reserve Infantry Battalion at Fromelles, although according to Alan Bullock, not in the trenches. The verdict on Churchill by A D Gibb, later Regius Professor of Law at Edinburgh

University: *No more popular officer ever commanded…he left behind men who will always be his loyal partisans and admirers…. Beyond question a great man.* He starts painting, encouraged by Goonie (Lady Gwendoline Churchill, Jack's wife) and Sir John and Lady Lavery.

GOVERNMENT: 1916 Lloyd George. Coalition. [Not an election]

1916
Churchill meets Desmond Morton in the trenches. (Morton will figure later in his life.) He returns to parliament as a backbencher, after being encouraged by many, including some Conservatives, who realise his value. There is the famous dinner with Beaverbrook and F E Smith where Churchill learns from Beaverbrook that he is not to be in Lloyd George's government.
(NOTE: Churchill received no congratulations from Parliament on his war service. MPs (frocks) were disdainful of serving officers (brass hats).
The Battle of Jutland takes place. Both sides claim victory. This is the last high seas fleets battle in history. The fleets never see each other.

1917
The Dardanelles report largely exonerates Churchill and he is appointed Minister of Munitions. (Lloyd-George no longer needs to placate the Tories, most of whom still hate Churchill.) He fights and wins the by-election at Dundee, but Scrimgeour's vote goes up to 30%. He equips the US troops and promotes the adoption of tanks. (Later, Churchill is mentioned as one of the prime movers in a Government report.) At a similar time Eisenhower is promoting tanks in the US. Churchill and Clementine move to Lullenden (East Grinstead), for which he pays £6,000 (a lot of money). The Battles of Vimy Ridge and Passchendaele take place, as does the Russian revolution. The Treaty of Brest–Litovsk sees Russia out of the war. Three weeks later the US enters the war.
The Balfour Declaration on the setting up of a Jewish homeland is announced.

GOVERNMENT: 1918 (Dec) Lloyd George. Coalition. (The coupon election.) [Unionists (note, not Conservatives) 382, Lib 163, Lab 57, BUT, 339 of the Unionists and 134 Liberals are Coalition members, so the coalition has majority of 234]

1918
The second battle of the Marne takes place . The War ends on November 11.
He meets Franklyn D Roosevelt on the latter's visit to Europe as Under-Secretary of the Navy in the US. They don't like each other. When they meet again in 1941, FDR remembers the meeting; Churchill says he does not.

1919
Churchill is appointed Secretary of War and Air
(NOTE: Churchill was against punitive reparations for Germany at Versailles. Lloyd-George was also in favour of magnanimity, but said to Churchill on his return: 'I was between Jesus Christ (Wilson) and Joan of Arc (Clemenceau), so I didn't stand a chance. Clemenceau had worked on Wilson, who originally had a more sympathetic view of Germany, because he (Clemenceau) remembered the Franco–Prussian war and was still bitter.)
Churchill is very active in supporting the anti-Bolsheviks in the Russian Civil War. The British Government supports Denniken, Kolchak and Yudonitch.

1920
The Black and Tans are sent to Ireland. The Government of Ireland Act becomes law. The Communist Party of Great Britain is formed and the League of Nations is founded, without the US.

1921
Churchill is appointed Secretary of State at the Colonial Office. He is responsible for the Irish Treaty. Kipling turns against him over this.
(NOTE: Michael Collins said 'Tell Winston we couldn't have done it without him.' Collins also said 'I'm signing my own death warrant' and he was right.)

1922
The Government publishes the White paper on a Jewish homeland in Palestine (based on the Balfour Declaration). A general election is called by Lloyd-George, who wants a mandate. The election is contrived over a Turkish Massacre of Greeks over a dispute in the Dardanelles at Chenak. Churchill threatens Turkey and they back down. Lloyd-George and Churchill are accused of wanting a war.
(NOTE: According to Jock Colville in The Churchillians, Beaverbrook boasted that he forced Lloyd-George into the election by threatening to expose him over selling peerages. This was Beaverbrook being whimsical.)
Churchill is defeated in the General Election by 10,000 votes. He has appendicitis and can't campaign until two days before the election. He says later 'I was without a seat, without a party and without an appendix.' Scrimgeour is finally elected after 14 years of trying.
Churchill starts writing *The World Crisis*, his history of the war. This will net him £20,000. He buys Chartwell for £5,000 and engages Tilden as architect for refurbishment and extension. He spends a further £17,000 over two years.
(NOTE: Churchill was moving away from the Liberals and somewhat towards the Conservatives. There were changes in the nature of the parties, with the Liberals in disarray.)

GOVERNMENT: 1922 (Nov) Bonar Law. Con. [Con 344 Lab 142 Lib 115]
GOVERNMENT: 1923 (May) Baldwin. Con. [Not an election. B-L died]
GOVERNMENT: 1923 (Dec) MacDonald. Lab. (Con 258, Lab 191, Lib 158; minority govt with Libs]

1923
The first two volumes of *The World Crisis* are published. Churchill meets Brendan Bracken.
May: Churchill stands at Leicester as a 'Liberal Free Trader' and loses.
December: Churchill stands in the Abbey Division of Westminster and loses.

1924
Churchill leaves the Liberals and decides to stand as a 'Constitutionalist' at Epping.
The Zinoviev letter is published.

GOVERNMENT: 1924 (Oct) Baldwin. Con. [Con 412, Lab 151, Lib 40. Lib meltdown.]

In the general election, Churchill is elected at Epping as a Constitutionalist. (Still not a Conservative.) He is appointed Chancellor of the Exchequer by Baldwin. He finally returns to the Conservatives. Lenin dies
(NOTE: He said 'To rat is one thing; to rat and re-rat is another thing altogether.' Observe the similarity to Alcibiades, The Duke of Marlborough and Marshall Ney, who each changed sides more than once.)
(NOTE: Baldwin was still anti-free trade and Churchill was still a Liberal free trader.)

1925
Churchill restores the gold standard. (The policy was inherited from Snowdon, the previous Labour Chancellor). J M Keynes opposes this. The country experiences deflation, unemployment and the miners' strike. The Locarno Treaty is a declaration on non-aggression among France, Germany and Belgium, to be guaranteed by Britain and Italy.
(NOTE: Churchill carried out lots of social improvements. He had a paternalistic concern for the under-privileged. He increased pensions – he had been the only one to vote for 7/6d for pensioners during the Asquith government. Later he would support pensions for war widows. Jenkins says he was not a bad Chancellor.)

1926
May: The General Strike takes place, and lasts for only nine days. The British Gazette is published by Churchill. There is controversy about whether it is

inflammatory propaganda or information. From then on Churchill is reviled by the miners. When he dies in 1965, the chant is 'Churchill's dead, ha ha ha.'

(NOTE: Churchill worked to find a solution and was generally sympathetic to the miners' grievances but was against the strike. He said 'I decline to be impartial between the fire brigade and the fire.' He had talks with MacDonald at Chartwell and proposed a solution but was defeated by Baldwin and the mine owners.)

1927-28

The Kellogg-Briande Pact is signed by 65 countries, including the USA and the USSR. The Pact states that 'war is outlawed'.

Volume 3 of *The World Crisis* is published (in two parts.) He takes up bricklaying at Chartwell, and writes to Baldwin: '200 bricks and 2,000 words a day'.

GOVERNMENT: 1929 (May) MacDonald. Lab. [Con 260 Lab 287 Lib 59. Minority Lab with Lib support]

1929

Churchill produces his fifth budget. He is only the fifth Chancellor to do five consecutive budgets.

The last volume of *The World Crisis* is published. Churchill receives an advance of £2,000 (£60,000 now). He starts on his *Life of Marlborough,* for which he receives a £10,000 advance plus £5,000 for the US edition plus £5,000 for the serial rights. (Total £600,000 now.)

At this time, Lord Irwin (later Halifax) was viceroy of India. Irwin is in favour of Dominion Status for India, but Churchill is very much opposed and will remain so.

The government falls (see above). Churchill urges Baldwin to do a deal with the Liberals, but Baldwin won't, so Labour does. Churchill is out of office. This is the start of the Wilderness Years, 10 years of warnings. See *Step by Step*, published in 1939.

He writes to Clementine that if Chamberlain becomes leader of the Conservatives, he will give up politics and take up writing full time.

This is the time of the Wall Street Crash. Churchill loses about £17,000 (£500,000 now). He closes Chartwell and moves into Well Street Cottage to save money. He embarks on many writing projects in parallel to recover his income.

1930

Churchill publishes *My Early Life*, which sells 11,000 in the UK and 6,000 in the US. His total income from writing is £35,000 (approximately £1m now). He recovers his losses and re-opens Chartwell. In all, Churchill writes for *The Morning Post*,

The Telegraph, The Mail, The Daily Mirror, The News of the World and *The Evening Standard*.

(NOTE: Churchill was idiosyncratic regarding the editing of his text. He demanded that it be typeset immediately and would typically go through a dozen revisions. No publisher would do this now, even with electronic typesetting.)

Baldwin makes his famous denunciation of the press barons: 'the prerogative of the harlot – power without responsibility'. Churchill resigns from the Conservative Business Committee (the Shadow Cabinet) over India.

GOVERNMENT: 1931 MacDonald. National Govt. [Not an election. Fear of civil unrest due to the fleet mutiny at Invergordon and a run on the pound]

GOVERNMENT: 1931 (Oct) MacDonald. National Govt. [Con 522 Lab 52 Lib 36. MacDonald remains PM. He is expelled from the Labour party and Lansbury becomes leader]

1931

The is no post for Churchill in MacDonald's government. He continues his *Life of Marlborough*. Churchill has a bad car accident in the US and is incapacitated for some months.

(NOTE: At this time, he started to warn about Germany. He was in favour of the League of Nations and strong re-armament to prevent war. The Times was very pro-appeasement.)

(NOTE: At this time he was very much isolated. The Tories especially considered him a maverick and a guerrilla; Labour saw him as anti-socialist (which he was)).

(NOTE: Churchill makes his famous 'boneless wonder' speech about MacDonald. Notwithstanding this, Churchill remained largely free of malice and rarely carried grudges.)

1932

Thoughts and Adventures is published.

While researching Marlborough, Churchill meets Putzi Hanfstaengle in Munich, who offers to bring Hitler to meet him. Churchill agrees, saying he'd like to ask Hitler why he is persecuting the Jews. Hitler fails to arrive.

He receives a £20,000 advance for a *History of the English Speaking Peoples*, for delivery in 1939. The book is in fact finished on time but is not published until 1957. He is also doing much magazine writing; six articles bring £2,000 (£60,000 now). He produces a series called *Great Stories Re-told* 1932–38, much of it written by Eddie Marsh, who isn't given much of the fee.

(NOTE: Chartwell was used as a base for intelligence gathering during this period.)
(NOTE: By-election candidates were still called National Government candidates.)
(NOTE: Eddie Marsh was an authority on art and a serious connoisseur. He became a trustee of both the National and the Tate.)

The first volume of *Marlborough* is published

1933
Hitler gains power. Franklyn D. Roosevelt is elected President. Churchill begins to work with Desmond Morton, Head of the Home Office Industrial Intelligence Unit

1934
The second volume of *Marlborough* is published

GOVERNMENT: 1935(June) Baldwin. National Govt. [Not an election]
GOVERNMENT: 1935(Nov) Baldwin. National Govt. [Con 429, Lab 154, Lib 21]

1935
There is still no place for Churchill in the government. He has a place on the committee for air defence research. The Hoare–Laval pact recognises Mussolini in Abyssinia. This agreement is viewed as a disaster and ends the credibility of the League of Nations, as well as damaging Hoare's career. The Stresa agreement by Britain, France and Italy for the defence of Alsace against Germany comes to nothing. At the same time, the Anglo–German Naval Treaty allows Germany to build up to 35% of British Naval strength. This treaty, too, is later ignored by Hitler. Churchill begins his association with Ralph Wigram, Head of the Central Department of the Foreign Office

1936
Hitler enters the Rhineland in contravention of the Treaty of Versailles.
The Spanish Civil War begins. This is difficult for Churchill, who sees the Spanish Government as Communist – others call it a popular liberal government – and, while he does not overtly support Franco, he is reluctant to condemn the Fascist uprising.
He makes his famous speech about the Government: 'Decided to be undecided; resolved to be irresolute; adamant for drift; solid for fluidity; all-powerful to be impotent.'
(NOTE: Throughout this period Churchill was strongly opposed to granting independence to India. He predicted the bloodshed that was to occur in 1947 over partition.)
(NOTE: In *Churchill and Appeasement*, R A C Parker says: 'Churchill never calculated.

> *He said what he thought with grandiose rhetorical emphasis and assumed he would be able to convince'*)

Baldwin makes the appalling speech in which he says openly that if he had spoken of re-arming in 1935 it would have lost the Government the election.

Edward VIII abdicates. Churchill and Lloyd-George back the King. This is very unpopular in Parliament. He is shouted down in the House. Harold Nicolson says 'He has undone in five minutes the patient reconstruction work of two years'. Churchill toys with the idea of forming a 'King's Party', (which would, of course, have been a disaster).

Baldwin appoints Sir Thomas Inskip as Defence Minister. Lindemann describes it as 'the most cynical appointment since Caligula made his horse a consul'.
(NOTE: Inskip was very docile and ineffectual and not pro-rearmament.)

GOVERNMENT: 1937 Chamberlain. National Govt. [Not an election]

1937

Churchill becomes further isolated, despite his correct prediction of Germany's actions. Rearmament starts. The Government allocates £400m expenditure.
Great Contemporaries is published. Ralph Wigram dies.
Churchill writes for the News of the World and gets £400 per article. His total income is £15,000 (which would be about £500,000 now). He begins his association with Imry Revesz (later Emery Reves) who becomes his agent for overseas sales of his books and journalism.

1938

Germany enters Austria. The Czechoslovakian Sudetenland is next. Eden resigns over Chamberlain's refusal to accept Roosevelt's proposal for a peace conference. Halifax is appointed Foreign Secretary. Chamberlain visits Hitler three times. On September 15 at the Berghof and September 22 at Godesberg and then a third visit to Munich on September 28 with Deladier and Mussolini. (When this last is announced, there are cheers in the house except for Churchill, Eden (although this is not universally agreed), Amery, Duff Cooper and Harold Nicolson, but Churchill shakes Chamberlain's hand and wishes him well.) Britain and France give up the Sudetenland. Chamberlain comes back with the paper signed by Hitler and proclaims 'Peace in our time' (He later regrets this and retracts it.) Churchill calls the Munich agreement an unmitigated defeat and predicts that Hitler will annex all of Czechoslovakia. He is proved correct. Duff Cooper resigns.
(NOTE: The number of people willing to be seen siding with Churchill at this time were very few: They include Eden, Duff Cooper, Amery, Admiral Keyes, MacMillan, Sandys, Bracken and Boothby.)
(NOTE: The theory that the Munich agreement bought a year's respite for Britain

is confounded in *Inside the Third Reich* by Albert Speer, who says that Germany feared the strength of the Czech army and their defences.)
November 12: Kristallnacht: the Nazis attack Jews and Jewish property in Germany.
The last Volume of *Marlborough* is published.
The Epping Conservatives come close to de-selecting Churchill because of his warnings against Germany. Churchill threatens to stand as an independent. Compromise is reached. Churchill now loses another lot of money on the US stock market. (About £18,000 or £375,000 now.) Chartwell is put up for sale at £20,000. It is advertised with five reception rooms, 19 bedrooms and eight bathrooms.
Churchill is bailed out by Sir Henry Strakosch, who, purely to be of service to him, takes over his financial affairs and restores his fortune. Jenkins says that the procedure would have been questionable under present-day parliamentary rules, but there is no record of Strakosch's ever receiving any benefit. Chartwell is taken off the market. When Strakosch dies, in 1943, he leaves Churchill £20,000 in his will.
Churchill starts work on *The History of the English Speaking Peoples*. He writes half a million words in a year.

1939
Popular opinion is now much in favour of Churchill, but there is still no place for him in the cabinet. Chamberlain is still hoping for peace. Horabin Misquotes Cromwell: 'I beseech you in the bowels of Christ to believe that you may sometimes be a little wrong'. Franco becomes the Spanish Dictator.
August 25: The Molotov–Ribbentrop pact ensures that there will be no war in the East .
September 1: Hitler invades Poland.
September 2: France mobilises. The Commons meets on Saturday. Chamberlain still thinks it possible to have another 'Munich-type meeting'. The House is furious. Amery calls to Greenwood 'Speak for England'. Chamberlain retreats.
September 3: War is declared by Chamberlain. Churchill is appointed First Lord of the Admiralty. Dudley Pound is First Sea Lord. Ismay is appointed CIGS.
Churchill devises the Catherine plan to invade the Baltic. This is not very clever, because the fleet could have been trapped and the plan is rejected.)
(NOTE: The BBC made a radio programme about this in October 2001.)

GOVERNMENT: 1940 (May 10) Churchill (National Govt.) [Not an election]

1940
Mar 20: Deladier resigns. Reynaud becomes PM.
April 9: Germany invades Denmark and Norway

This is the time of the 'Phoney' War.

May 2: The British withdraw from Trondheim. Churchill is prepared to take the blame, but Lloyd-George says he shouldn't act as an air-raid shelter for his colleagues.

(NOTE: Through all this Churchill still worked on the HESP. The publisher was dissatisfied with the ending, thinking it finished too abruptly. Churchill agreed to write some more, but the project was shelved for the duration.)

Amery makes his speech to Chamberlain 'Depart and in the name of God go'.

May 10: Churchill becomes PM. Germany invades Holland and Belgium. Jock Colville becomes Churchill's private secretary (Churchill inherits him from Chamberlain.) Churchill's other private secretaries are Leslie Rowan and John Martin.

(NOTE: The choice for PM was between Churchill and Halifax. The Conservative Party, Downing Street, The Cabinet Office, King George VI and the Royal Family all preferred Halifax. Chamberlain vacillated and Churchill kept silent. Halifax said it was better to have the PM in the Commons, but there is a school of thought that says he (Halifax) thought that Churchill would fail and then he would get the post. See Clarke, The Tories and Rhodes James, Diaries of Henry Chips Channon)

The War Cabinet consists of Churchill, Chamberlain, Halifax, Attlee and Greenwood.

Gamelin becomes Supreme Commander in Europe.

May 13: Churchill makes his first speech in Parliament as PM ('Blood, toil, tears and sweat…') Randolph finally becomes an MP, but the seat is uncontested. This was the only time out of seven attempts that Randolph obtained a seat.

May 18: The defeatist movement in France is led by Helen de Portes (Reynaud's mistress) and Paul Baudoin.

May 19: Gamelin is replaced by Weygand. Deladier becomes Foreign Minister

May 20: Joe Kennedy is telling FDR that Britain is finished and is seeking a negotiated peace. Fortunately, Kennedy is soon replaced by Winant (see below) who is a much more sympathetic person and who gets on well with Churchill.

(NOTE: Winant committed suicide in 1947. There is a photograph of Winant with Churchill in the study doorway at Chartwell.)

May 27–June 3: The Dunkirk evacuation takes place (Operation Dynamo). 224,000 British and 111,000 French are evacuated.

Churchill goes to France to see Weygand and Reynaud. Weygand wants British forces to move south while the French move north to cut off the Germans. Gort refuses on the grounds that it would be a disaster. The French also want Spitfires sent. Churchill is agreeable, but Dowding says no because they are needed for the defence of Britain. (He throws down his pencil and sits back, defying argument.)

May 28: King Leopold in Belgium capitulates.

June 10: Mussolini declares war on Britain and France.
Halifax is in favour of a peace deal with Germany. Chamberlain wavers but comes down against. Attlee and Greenwood are firmly with Churchill.
(NOTE: In The Second World War, Churchill tries to exonerate Halifax and Chamberlain, by being somewhat mendacious on this point and saying that the war cabinet never discussed a peace deal.)
June 11: The French government goes to Tours. Weygand wants an armistice. Churchill goes to see them in Tours. Reynaud, de Gaulle and Mandel are ready to continue. Pétain and Weygand urge surrender. Churchill offers a Union of France and Britain. (How would it have worked?) But the French refuse. Petain describes it as 'fusion with a corpse'. Reynaud resigns. In all, Churchill makes five trips to France to try to persuade the French not to quit.
June 14: Reynaud decides to move the government to Quimper, but is persuaded by de Portes to go to Bordeaux.
June 16: Reynaud resigns.
(NOTE: Churchill authorised funds to promote de Gaulle as leader of the Free French. See later; FDR wanted Giraud in this post. Although de Gaulle infuriated everybody and at times said and did some very bad things, Churchill retained a respect and even liking for him. The problem of de Gaulle and Giraud would later cause friction between Churchill and FDR.)
June 18: Churchill makes his 'Finest hour' speech.
June 20: France falls, Pétain becomes PM of Vichy. Reynaud, and Mandel, the latter being Jewish, are arrested. Mandel will later be murdered by the Nazis.
July 3: Churchill orders the sinking of the French Fleet at Oran, after the French refuse other options. (Admiral Somerville)
July–September: The Battle of Britain takes place
September 1940–May 1941: This is the period of the blitz. At the height of the blitz, there are more than 1000 casualties per night in London
December 15: Halifax becomes Ambassador to the US after the death of Lord Lothian. Eden becomes Foreign Secretary.

1941

Lend–lease is agreed. Hess flies to Britain. The Bismarck is sunk. Crete is evacuated.
July: Hitler attacks Russia (Barbarossa). Auchinlech replaces Wavell in North Africa.
August: Churchill meets FDR at Placentia Bay. This is their first meeting since 1918. The Atlantic Charter is signed.
Harry Hopkins and Averill Harriman arrive in Britain. Both are very supportive. Both become close to Churchill.
(NOTE: Harriman married Pamela, Randolph's former wife, some 40 years later.)

December 7: The Japanese attack Pearl Harbor. The US declares war on Japan. The Prince of Wales and the Repulse are sunk in SE Asia

Hitler and Mussolini declare war on the US. The Grand Alliance (UK, US and USSR) is formed.

Churchill goes to the US for three weeks. Attlee is left in charge. Churchill addresses Congress 'What sort of people do they think we are?'.

December 25: Hong Kong falls. Churchill has a mild heart attack, but Moran, his doctor, doesn't tell him what it was. Churchill faces a vote of confidence. He wins 464–1.

1942

February : Singapore falls. 64,000 troops are surrendered by General Percival.

June: Churchill visits FDR in Washington. Tobruk falls. He comes back to a vote of censure, but survives 475–25 after Wardlaw-Milne suggests the Duke of Gloucester as C-in-C.

(NOTE: The 25 against was the same number as Pitt had in the vote of censure during the Napoleonic War. Churchill will often mention this in later years.)

August: Churchill visits Stalin in Moscow. (In an un-pressurised Liberator bomber, with a modified oxygen mask so he can smoke his cigars.) They discuss the second front but Churchill tells Stalin that it is too soon to invade France and that the N. Africa landings will remove pressure from Russia.

(NOTE: Willie Gallacher, the communist MP, was torn between vilifying Churchill, whom he hated for his class background, or praising him because he was helping Russia.)

(NOTE: Roosevelt and Marshall as well as Stalin were in favour of a second front in France early, but Churchill, the cabinet and the generals were firmly against.)

Alexander replaces Auchinlech as C-in-C Near East Command.

Montgomery assumes command of the 8th Army in North Africa. The Dieppe landing fails.

The Battle of Alamein takes place. The Torch campaign starts in November; led by Eisenhower and Patton. Darlan leaves Vichy and goes to the Allies, but is assassinated. Eisenhower is criticised by FDR and Churchill for accepting Darlan's defection; it is considered fortunate that Darlan is killed before any damage is done to the Alliance.

Churchill makes the 'End of the beginning' speech. The Battle of Stalingrad takes place. Germany takes over Vichy.

(NOTE: The breaking of the Enigma codes was of great importance. The process of cracking the codes was very stop–start. The last codes were cracked at the end of 1942 and after that the U-boats were less effective. In the last week before the codes were broken, the Allies lost 700,000 tons of shipping.)

1943

von Paulus surrenders at Stalingrad.
January: Churchill and FDR meet at Casablanca. FDR announces that the Allies will accept only unconditional surrender from the Axis. He says this without telling Churchill first. Giraud meets de Gaulle.
Churchill goes to Marrakesh with FDR and does his only painting during the war. He gives the painting to FDR. The painting is no longer in the Roosevelt family.
May: Churchill visits FDR in Washington. The *Trident* conference is held (about the atom bomb. Code name: 'Tube Alloys').
July: Mussolini resigns and is incarcerated. 'The Man who Never Was' deceives the Nazis over the Sicily landings. (Operation Husky.)
August: Churchill visits Quebec. He takes Wingate along just to talk to him on the trip.
September: The Armistice with Italy is declared; the Germans rescue Mussolini
November: Churchill and FDR meet in Cairo.
(NOTE: About this time Churchill started talking about a 'United States of Europe')
(NOTE: Churchill was very friendly with Lindemann (later Lord Cherwell) but wasn't close to Tizard. Many considered Tizard a better scientist than Lindemann.)
September: The Salerno Operation (Avalanche) takes place. The Italians surrender. The Germans occupy Rome.
October: An agreement is signed between Eisenhower and Badoglio and Italy joins the Allies. Eden and Cordell-Hull meet Molotov in Moscow. Mountbatten is appointed Supreme Allied Commander, SE Asia.
December: The first Big Three Conference takes place in Teheran – mainly about a second front (see notes above). FDR and Stalin are squeezing Churchill. Stalin was always out to drive a wedge between the western allies.
(NOTE: Churchill had two more heart attacks as well as pneumonia, twice. His health was failing at this time.)

1944

January: The Anzio landings take place (Operation Shingle).
June 6: This is D-Day. 'Operation Overlord'. The Mulberry Harbour was Churchill's idea. Eisenhower is Supreme Commander. Monty is C-in-C in France until Eisenhower arrives there to take over. Tedder is Deputy Supreme Commander. Leigh Mallory is in charge of Air warfare. Generals include: Monty, Patton, Bradley, Simpson, Devers.
3000 are killed on landing. 10,000 had been predicted. 400,000 are landed in 10 days.
June: The V1s start. 1000 homes are destroyed in a month. In all, 6000 are killed by 2500 V1s and 3000 by 1100 V2s. The US and Britain disagree over strategy.

July 20: The von Stauffenberg bomb plot is an attempt to kill Hitler. Rommel is offered suicide.
August: The Allies land in the South of France in Operation Dragoon (formerly Anvil).
September: Churchill and FDR meet in Quebec. Operation Market Garden is the attack on Arnhem (The Bridge too Far). It fails.
October: Churchill goes to see Stalin in Moscow. This is the occasion of the 'Naughty piece of paper', on which Churchill sets out the division of east–west influence he proposes in Europe after the war. Stalin ticks it to show his approval. Churchill suggests they destroy the paper but Stalin tells him to keep it. It still exists.
(NOTE: Stalin kept to this agreement when the communists took over in Greece. He did not intervene.)
December: The Battle of the Bulge in the Ardennes is von Runstead's last effort.
(NOTE: the similarity to Ludendorf's last attempt to break out in WW1.)
The UN Charter is drafted at Dumbarton Oaks.
Churchill visits the Rhine and crosses onto German soil. He is ordered back by US General Simpson because there are snipers still there.

1945

February : The second meeting of The Big Three takes place at Yalta. Churchill wants to deal with Stalin on Europe, particularly Poland; FDR is pre-occupied with Far East. This is the last time Churchill, FDR and Stalin meet. FDR dies on April 12th.
May 8: VE Day

GOVERNMENT: 1945(May) Churchill, Conservative. [Not an election – caretaker government.]

(NOTE: Churchill wanted Eisenhower to push on to Berlin and Prague; indeed, Patton crossed into Czechoslovakia and was making good progress until ordered by Eisenhower to withdraw. The generally accepted view is that Truman and Eisenhower were worried about US casualties. There were 100,000 killed when the Russians took Berlin.)

July: The last Big Three Meeting is held, in Potsdam. Initially the principals are Churchill, Stalin and Truman. The UK election is held during the conference and Attlee becomes PM. Attlee is attending with Churchill in case he gets elected. This happens and Churchill leaves the conference part way through. That is the end of Churchill's participation in the events. (see C L Mee, *Meeting at Potsdam*.)
De Gaulle becomes French President. Tito becomes Yugoslav PM.
July 21 The US conducts Alamagordo A-bomb tests, called Little Boy and Fat Man.

GOVERNMENT: 1945(July) Attlee. Lab. [Lab majority 146]

Churchill is out of office. King George VI offers Churchill the Order of the Garter, but Churchill declines it on the grounds that the country has given him the order of the boot.
Truman decides to use the A-bomb. (See Alperowitz, *The decision to drop the bomb*)
August 6: The first bomb is used at Hiroshima; August 8: Russia declares war on Japan. August 9: The second bomb is used at Nagasaki; August 15: Japan surrenders.

1946
March: Churchill makes the 'Iron Curtain' speech at Fulton Missouri. (He calls the text 'Sinews of Peace') The speech is criticised by, among others, Eleanor Roosevelt. People say he is making noises like he was in the '30s.
Churchill engages Bill Deakin as his main assistant to work on his war memoirs.
September: In a speech in Zurich, Churchill urges the formation of a Council of Europe. Churchill says the first step is a partnership between France and West Germany. (According to Montague Browne, Churchill uses the term, United States of Europe.)
The Bretton Woods conference sets up the World Bank. (John Maynard Keynes and Harry Dexter White.) Deficit financing is introduced. George Bernard Shaw writes approvingly to Churchill: 'You have never been a real Tory.'
At this time, Churchill possesses £120,000 from his writing. He reckons he needs £12,000 a year to live and he resolves to sell Chartwell for approximately £20,000.
October: Lord Camrose and his consortium buy Chartwell for £43,800.
Life offers $1.15m for the serial rights to The Second World War; Houghton pays a $250,000 advance on the US edition of the book. Churchill buys Chartwell Farm for £22,545.

1947
Mary marries Christopher Soames
(NOTE: About this time, Clementine said to Churchill 'You tease me and call me pink'. That is, Clementine remained a Liberal.)
(NOTE: Churchill was always very generous with money. He helped, among others, Moran, Eden, Randolph, Pamela, daughters of his secretaries and many others.)
Churchill buys Bardogs Farm (adjacent to Chartwell Farm) for £8,200.
August 15: India becomes independent.

1948
Churchill begins writing *The Second World War* (six volumes), which will be finished in 1954. Volume 1 is published. It sells 600,000 in the US, 500,000 in Britain.
June: Churchill speaks in favour of support for Israel. The Berlin airlift begins. Churchill attends the Hague Conference on European Unity.

1949
The Tories are worried by Churchill as leader, but he shows no sign of his resigning. Volume 2 is published. The first meeting of the Council of Europe takes place. Churchill urges an invitation for the Germans
May: Churchill buys Colonist II and starts racing. Clementine is bemused; he'd never had any interest in racing since he left India.
August: Churchill has a stroke. This is kept secret.

1950
The general election is won by Labour. Sandys and Soames are elected to Parliament. Randolph is defeated (again). Volume 3 is published.
June: Labour refuse to go to the meeting of European Coal and Steel Pact. The Korean War starts. Randolph goes to Korea as a war correspondent.

GOVERNMENT: 1950 (Feb) Attlee. Lab. [Lab majority down to 6]

1951
September 12: Churchill receives a letter from Attlee: 'My Dear Churchill, I have decided to hold a general election in October. I will announce it tonight after the 9.00 news. Yours sincerely C R Attlee.'
(NOTE: Churchill's manifesto had a profits tax for armaments manufacturers. It was his idea; not really a Conservative view. Eden was hoping he would resign.)
October: The General Election takes place. Churchill becomes PM again. Jock Colville and David Pitblado are appointed as joint PPSs. Randolph is defeated for the sixth and last time. Volume 4 is published.

GOVERNMENT: 1951 (Oct) Churchill. Con. [Majority 26]

1952
January: Churchill visits Washington (He is now 77.) Eden and Dulles are at odds.
February : King George VI dies. Churchill is ill with an arterial spasm (not a stroke).
Labour starts all-night sessions to wear Churchill out. Channon observes young Labour MPs jeering at Churchill about his age. Volume 5 is published.
August: Clarissa (Churchill's niece) marries Eden. (She is Eden's second wife.)

Anthony Montague Browne joins Churchill's secretarial team.
November: Eisenhower is elected President. The first US hydrogen bomb is exploded.

1953
Churchill's thinking is dominated by defence and international considerations.
January: He visits Eisenhower in Washington. He receives an advance of £63,000 for Volume 6, plus $28,000 from Time-Life.
(NOTE: Churchill ordered the de-rationing of sweets and was told that sugar was not available. He insisted and in six months there was a sugar glut.)
March: Stalin dies. Malenkov becomes Soviet leader.
April: Anthony Eden becomes ill. Churchill takes on the role of Foreign Secretary.
May: The coronation of Queen Elizabeth II takes place.
June: Churchill has a severe stroke, which, again, is kept secret. He makes an amazingly swift recovery.
August: The first Russian H-bomb is tested
October: Churchill is awarded the Nobel Prize for Literature. He is disappointed to learn it is for literature. He had hoped to get the Peace Prize. Finally, he is knighted.
December: He goes to Bermuda with Eisenhower and Laniel (the French Premier). They fail to agree on a meeting with Malenkov.

1954
The Geneva accords are agreed. Volume 6 is published
McCarthy criticises Churchill over Formosa (on which he also criticises Eisenhower), saying Churchill is an appeaser.
March: Churchill and Eisenhower are diverging on how to deal with Russia. Eden says of Churchill 'he can't go on'. Churchill makes a speech to cries of 'Resign' and fails to respond as he would have done earlier. (See Channon diaries.)
June: He visits Eisenhower in Washington. Eisenhower now agrees to the idea of a meeting with Malenkov
Churchill reaches his 80th birthday. The Sutherland portrait is presented to him by Parliament. Churchill calls it 'a remarkable example of modern art'.
(NOTE: In Jenkins' book, Churchill, there is a sketch that Sutherland did before the final portrait, which is a much more sympathetic representation. Also, there is another study in the Portrait Gallery, which, again, shows a more human aspect. Clementine later had the painting destroyed.)
Eden is becoming desperate, as Churchill still puts off his resignation.

1955
Calls for Churchill's resignation appear in *The Daily Mirror* and *Punch*.

February: Churchill announces that Britain will make an H-bomb. Malenkov is replaced by Kruschev. Churchill decides to resign in April.

April: He finally resigns during a newspaper strike. Eden becomes PM.

(NOTE: Colville found Churchill sitting with his head in his hands, and he assumed it was because Churchill was depressed by his resignation. When he asked him what the matter was, Churchill said 'I don't think Anthony is up to the job.')

The Queen offers Churchill a Dukedom, only after being assured by Colville that he would decline the honour. (The only dukedom in the last 100+ years was when Gladstone proposed it for the Duke of Westminster in 1874.)

May: Churchill is re-elected at Woodford. He resumes work on *The History of the English Speaking Peoples*.

June: He suffers another arterial spasm. Anthony Montague Browne is seconded to Churchill indefinitely.

GOVERNMENT: 1955 (Apr) Eden. Con. [Not an election]
GOVERNMENT: 1955 (May) Eden. Con. [Majority 82]

1956

Churchill receives the Charlemagne Prize from Adenauer for 'Contribution to European Cooperation'.

February: Emery Reves marries Wendy Russell. Churchill stays with them at La Pausa, as he will do many times from then on. He visits Beaverbrook at La Capponcina. Churchill is looking for a house to buy in the South of France (which he never does). He meets Onassis.

March: Randolph writes an article criticising Eden.

April: Volume 1 of HESP is published. 130,000 copies are printed (eventually becoming over 200,000). Alan Bullock is engaged as Churchill's literary assistant. A L Rowse is also advising. Churchill meets Bulganin and Kruschev with Eden at No 10.

May: Harry Truman visits Chartwell. Churchill's attendance in the House of Commons is becoming rare. His activities in his constituency are reducing.

July: The Suez debacle takes place. (Britain, France and Israel take over the Canal Zone having concocted the scheme secretly from the US, in violation of the tri-partite treaty of 1950 whereby Britain, France and the US would always act together in the Middle East. Eisenhower thought that Churchill might have had a hand in it, (because it had, according to Eisenhower, a 'Victorian feel to it'), but this was not so.) Montague Browne describes the event as the end of Britain as a great power.

Montague Brown negotiates the sale of 'My Early Life' for £100,000. Churchill offers him 25% of the fee, which was very generous. Montague Brown declines.

Later, it is made into the film 'Young Winston'.
November: Volume 2 of HESP is published. Churchill decides to try personally to repair the damage between Britain and the US caused by Suez.
Eden offers Churchill a cabinet post as Minister without Portfolio. Churchill declines the offer.

1957
Eden resigns. Churchill is consulted by the Queen over the appointment of new PM (MacMillan). Reves pays Churchill £20,000 for a 10,000-word epilogue to an abridged edition of the six-volume book that Reves is publishing.
October: Volume 3 of HESP is published. Churchill sells both farms for £37,500.

GOVERNMENT: 1957 MacMillan. Con. [Not an election]

1958
Volume 4 of HESP is published.
June: de Gaulle becomes French PM. Rowse describes Churchill as 'becoming very quiet'.
September: Churchill's and Clementine's golden wedding anniversary is spent at Beaverbrook's villa, La Capponcina. He goes on a cruise with Onassis (first of eight).
December: de Gaulle becomes President. Churchill is appointed Compagnon de la Liberation.

1959
Churchill is elected at Woodford for the last time. He visits Eisenhower in Washington. Around this time is the end of his painting.

GOVERNMENT: 1959 MacMillan. Con. [Majority 101]

1960
Randolph is appointed as Churchill's biographer. Churchill visits de Gaulle. Kennedy is elected US Pfresident. Churchill has a fall and breaks a bone in his back. Many people think he is finished.

1961
Martin Gilbert joins Randolph's writing team. Although Churchill is slowing down, Montague Brown says that there is no evidence of his becoming senile.

1963
Churchill is made an honorary citizen of the US.

1964
Churchill leaves Parliament. He does not stand in the 1964 election

GOVERNMENT: 1964(Oct) Wilson. Lab. [Lab majority 4]

1965
Churchill dies on January 24, age 90.

GOVERNMENT: 1964(Mar) Wilson. Lab. [Lab majority 99]
GOVERNMENT: 1970(Jun) Heath. Con. [Con majority 36]
GOVERNMENT: 1974 (Feb) Wilson. Lab. [Lab minority govt]
GOVERNMENT: 1974 (Oct) Wilson Lab. [Lab majority 29]

1977
Clementine dies on December 12, aged 92.

Section 2 – Elections and Seats

1899	Oldham. Defeated
1900	General Election. Elected at Oldham as Conservative. Crossed to Liberals in 1904
1906	General Election. Elected at Manchester.
1908 (i)	Appointed President of BOT. Had to stand for re-election at Manchester and was defeated. Out of Parliament for four days.
1908 (ii)	Elected at Dundee
1910 (Jan)	General Election. Re-elected at Dundee
1910 (Dec)	General Election. Re-elected at Dundee
1917	Won by-election at Dundee when appointed Minister of Munitions
1918	General Election. Re-elected at Dundee
1922 (Nov)	General Election. Defeated at Dundee (Appendicitis). Out of Parliament.
1922 (Dec)	Stood at Leicester as a 'Liberal Free Trader'. Lost.
1923	Stood at Abbey Division of Westminster as 'Independent Anti-Socialist'. Lost.
1924	General Election. Stood as 'Constitutionalist'. Elected at Epping.
1929	General Election. Re-elected at Epping
1931	General Election. Re-elected at Epping
1935	General Election. Re-elected at Epping
1945	General Election. Re-elected. Constituency changed to Woodford
1950	General Election. Re-elected at Woodford
1951	General Election. Re-elected at Woodford
1955	General Election. Re-elected at Woodford
1959	General Election. Re-elected at Woodford

Section 3 – Government posts

1906	Under secretary of State for the Colonies
1907	President of the Board of Trade
1910	Home Secretary
1911–15	1st Lord of the Admiralty
1915	Chancellor of the Duchy of Lancaster
1917–18	Minister of Munitions
1919–21	Secretary of War and Air
1921–22	Colonial Secretary
1922–24	OUT OF PARLIAMENT
1924–29	Chancellor of the Exchequer
1939–40	1st Lord of the Admiralty
1940–45	Prime Minister and Minister of Defence
1945	Prime Minister and Minister of Defence (Caretaker Govt.)
1945–51	Leader of the Opposition
1951–55	Prime Minister

Section 4 – Churchill's secretaries

Lettice Fisher	Violet Pearman (Mrs P)
Phyliss Forbes	Jane Portal
Chips Gemmell	Doreen Pugh
Elizabeth Gilliatt	Vanda Salmon
Miss Graham	Marjorie Street
Grace Hamblin	Margaret Shearburn* (later Thompson)
Miss Hipwell	Catherine Snelling
Kathleen Hill*	Dorothy Spencer
Marion Holmes* (later Walker Spicer)	Jo Sturdee*
Patrick Kinna*	Miss Taylor
Elizabeth Layton* (later Nel)	Lady Williams
Miss Marston	Gillian Maturin

* wartime secretaries.

Section 5 – Visits and meetings

Visits to US before WW2:
Oct 1895	New York (on way to Cuba). Met Bourke Cochran
Dec 1895	New York (on way from Cuba)
Dec 1900	New York and Canada (lecture tour). Met McKinley and TR
Aug 1929	Three month tour. Canada to W. Coast (painting). SF & NY
Dec 1931	New York (Car accident. He went to Bahamas to recuperate.)

WW2 Visits to US and Canada:
Aug 1941:	Placentia Bay (Atlantic Charter)
Dec 41/Jan 42	Washington DC and Canada ('Chicken' speech to Canadian Parliament). Return through Florida & Bermuda.
Jun 1942	Washington DC and Hyde Park
May 1943	Washington DC
Aug 1943	Quebec, Hyde Park and Washington DC
Sep 1944	Quebec and Hyde Park

WW2 Visits to Russia:
Aug 1942	To see Stalin in Moscow re Second Front (with Harriman)
Oct 1944	To see Stalin in Moscow preparatory to Yalta.

WW2 Meetings with Roosevelt outside the US and of the Big Three:
Jan 1943	Casablanca (W, FDR, de Gaulle and Giraud)
Dec 1943	Cairo (Churchill and FDR) – before and after Teheran
Dec 1943	Teheran Big Three (W, FDR, JS)
Feb 1945	Yalta Big Three (W, FDR, JS)
Jul 1945	Potsdam Big Three (W, HST, JS) (Attlee in attendance) (Churchill left part way through after his General Election defeat.)

Visits to US and Bermuda post WW2: 1946, 1952, 1953, 1954, 1959
Jan 1946	New York, Miami (painting), Cuba, Washington DC, Fulton (Iron Curtain speech)
Jan 1952	New York. Washington, DC. Talks with Truman.
Jan 1953	New York. Talks with Eisenhower. Washington DC. Talks with Truman.
Dec 1953	Bermuda with Eisenhower and Laniel, French Premier. Also to Ottawa
June 1954	Washington DC with Eisenhower.
May 1959	Last visit to US. Washington DC with Eisenhower.

Section 6 – Selected Bibliography

By Winston Churchill:

The World Crisis (six vols)	My Early Life
Thoughts and Adventures	Great Contemporaries
Step by Step	The Second World War (six vols)

War Speeches (Summarised in three vols)

By others

Keith Aldritt	The Greatest of Friends
Gar Alperowicz	The Decision to Drop the Bomb
Geoffrey Best	Churchill, A Study in Greatness
Conrad Black	Roosevelt
E J Bois	Truth on the Tragedy of France
Les Carlyon	Gallipoli
Violet Bonham Carter	Winston Churchill as I Knew Him
John Charmley	Churchill; The End of Glory
Alan Bullock	Hitler: A Study in Tyranny
Randolph Churchill and Martin Gilbert	Winston S. Churchill (eight vols) (abridged in one vol by Gilbert; see below)
Sarah Churchill	A Thread in the Tapestry
Sarah Churchill	Keep on Dancing
Alan Clarke	The Tories
Jock Colville	The Fringes of Power
Jock Colville	The Churchillians
C Eade	Churchill by his Contemporaries
Anthony Eden	Facing the Dictators
Martin Gilbert	Churchill, A Life
Roy Jenkins	Churchill
Ralph Martin	Jennie (Two volumes)
C L Mee	Meeting at Potsdam
Anthony Montague Browne	Long Sunset
Lord Moran	Churchill, The Struggle for Survival
Nigel Nicolson	Diaries of Harold Nicolson (3 vols)
William Manchester	The Last Lion (2 vols)
R A C Parker	Churchill and Appeasement
Robert Rhodes James	The Diaries of Henry 'Chips' Channon
Andrew Roberts	Eminent Churchillians
Celia Sandys	Churchill - wanted dead or alive
William Shirer	The Collapse of the Third Republic
Mary Soames	Clementine Churchill
Albert Speer	Inside the Third Reich
A J P Taylor	English History 1914–45

Notes